Achieving Health Equity

THIRD EDITION

Context, Controversies, and Remedies

Patti R. Rose, MPH, EdD

President and Founder
Rose Consulting, Inc.
Miami, Florida

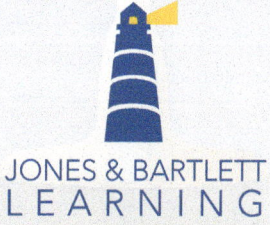

JONES & BARTLETT
LEARNING

World Headquarters
Jones & Bartlett Learning
25 Mall Road
Burlington, MA 01803
978-443-5000
info@jblearning.com
www.jblearning.com

Jones & Bartlett Learning books and products are available through most bookstores and online booksellers. To contact Jones & Bartlett Learning directly, call 800-832-0034, fax 978-443-8000, or visit our website, www.jblearning.com.

Substantial discounts on bulk quantities of Jones & Bartlett Learning publications are available to corporations, professional associations, and other qualified organizations. For details and specific discount information, contact the special sales department at Jones & Bartlett Learning via the above contact information or send an email to specialsales@jblearning.com.

01899-8

Production Credits

Vice President, Innovative Learning and Assessment Solutions: Ada Woo
Senior Director, Content Production and Delivery: Christine Emerton
Director, Product: Melissa Kleeman-Moy
Product Manager: Sophie Fleck Teague
Senior Outsourcing Specialist: Carol Brewer Guerrero
Content Coordinator: Samantha Gillespie
Content Management: S4Carlisle Publishing Services
Manager, Intellectual Properties and Content Production: Kristen Rogers
Content Production Manager: John Fuller
Senior Intellectual Property Specialist: Colleen Lamy
Director, Marketing: Andrea DeFronzo
Senior Product Marketing Manager: Susanne Walker
Director, Product Fulfillment: Aaron McKinzie
Purchasing Manager: Wendy Kilborn
Composition: Exela Technologies
Project Management: Exela Technologies
Cover and Text Design: S4Carlisle Publishing Services
Intellectual Property Specialist: Faith Brosnan
Intellectual Property Specialist: Robin Silverman
Cover Image (Title Page, Section Opener, Chapter Opener): © Jones & Bartlett Learning
Printing and Binding: Lakeside Book Company

Library of Congress Cataloging-in-Publication Data
Library of Congress Cataloging-in-Publication Data unavailable at time of printing
LCCN: 2025005774

6048

Printed in the United States of America
30 29 28 27 26 25   10 9 8 7 6 5 4 3 2 1

Dedication

I lovingly dedicate this book, first and foremost, to my beloved husband, Jeffrey Rose. The depth of your love and commitment to me during the process of my writing this book and all aspects of my life is cherished deeply and I am so grateful that you are also my best friend. Dedication is also extended to our two wonderful adult children, Courtney and Brandon Rose. With these two individuals in my life, I have experienced the true meaning of motherhood, in all of its many facets, and my love for each of you remains boundless. No matter the depth of my experience in doing so, and the consequences, I will always stand up for both of you, knowing the richness of our experience as people of African descent in this nation and the importance of who we are, where we came from, and where we must continue to go. We are the product of our loving ancestors, who gave so much so that we could achieve high levels of education, global travel, the pursuit of our life's work, and continuance of their legacy, entwined with our own goals as Black people. May we continue to move forward, within the context of love and gratitude for each other as a family that God put together, while recognizing that we are blessed by this union.

I also dedicate this work to the specific emerging majority people in the United States who, for generations, have endured a lack of health equity without remedies for this unjust disparity. Efforts must be ongoing towards achieving health equity for all as this accomplishment will be laudable, significant and consequential in a very positive way for the United States and its people. It is a national imperative.

Contents

CHAPTER 7 Health Disparities in Urban Communities as Compared to Suburban Communities: Issues, Concerns, and Remedies. 89

CHAPTER 8 Rural Communities and Health Disparities: Issues, Concerns, and Remedies. 105

CHAPTER 12 Children and Health Disparities: Issues, Concerns, and Remedies 167

CHAPTER 13 Older Adults and Health Disparities: Issues, Concerns, and Remedies 189

Preface

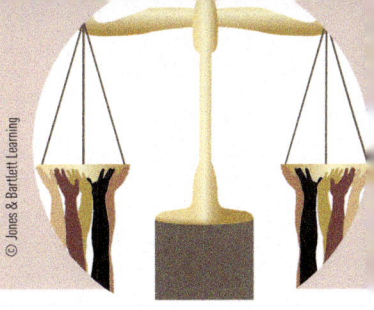

It dawned on me, with great sincerity, after writing the prior edition of this work, that the matters pertaining to health disparities must be resolved. The focus of our attention in public health and health care must be to rectify the problems. The word *solutions* was used in the prior edition of this book. Unfortunately, *solution(s)* is becoming merely a buzzword in these fields, bantered around without tangible action, because little has changed. Moving to the word *remedy* feels more resolute/ actionable. Additionally, the term *diversity, equity, and inclusion (DEI)* took a beating in all sectors of society, including in education and health sectors throughout the United States. Perhaps, one reason, beyond the political motivation of some, is because it is a term that is over-used and has lost its sense of purpose. It was and continues to be a reflection of what should have always been done and must be done, largely remaining unresolved.

In exploring the term *health equity*, there is a similar concern. The matter is not resolved. Who has the capability to resolve the issue of lack of health equity in the United States? The answer includes public health practitioners, state, local, and federal policy makers, and, most importantly, input from people who are experiencing the problems. These are the most important voices, in terms of health equity or the lack thereof. This edition, entitled *Achieving Health Equity: Context, Controversies, and Remedies,* is replete with remedies in nearly every chapter focusing on all types of groups, including children, older adults, emerging majorities, men, women, people in rural and urban communities as compared to suburban communities, etc. This book is a remedy journey, albeit not the destination. It is a walk toward the age-old problems known as health inequity and health disparities, with hopes that readers of this work will consider each remedy and discuss seriously how to implement or use them as starting points. Readers are encouraged to come up with new ideas, with the goal being to fix the problems, not merely lament about them. Research is a necessary means toward understanding the issue, but it is not the destination. In terms of what is discussed in this book, the destination is health equity for all. Until that happens, the question must constantly be, for every problem that pertains to health inequity, "Do we have a remedy for that?" If not, like the water from a broken, fractured pipe flooding everything, the flow of pontification about why it is leaking will continue with no resolution. That is what is happening to the U.S. healthcare system in terms of health equity. It's time to achieve health equity with remedies that work to stop the pain and suffering for emerging majority groups experiencing low economic status and all other people in the same predicament, while others thrive/ fare better, health-wise. The time is now.

What if, instead of focusing on the problems associated with health care, in terms of health disparities, the focus was squarely on remedies? This is a forward thinking text that provides insight regarding the health status gap between emerging majority groups and White people. Throughout, it is replete with remedies, some evidence-based and some based on new, fresh, and existing ideas. It is clear that a paradigm shift is needed to help public health and medical professionals look at the issues associated with the lack of health equity with an eye toward implementation of remedies—fixing problems rather than continuous research, which often explains issues but does not resolve them.

Let's explore the broken pipe analogy a bit further. Imagine there is a leaky, broken pipe in one's home; the plumber arrives, looks at the problem, and then begins research on every aspect of the problem. These are discussed intently with the homeowner and fellow plumbers who are brought into the discussion. The latter concur with him on what went wrong and continue to discuss the problem, but never remedy it. The initial pipe continues to leak, and other pipes in the home begin to leak as well. The problems are exacerbated and never remedied. This is exactly what is happening in health care, particularly in terms of the failure to achieve health equity and this leads to ongoing health disparities.

As a young graduate student at Yale University, pursuing a Master of Public Health degree in the mid-1980s, I stumbled upon a topic that I was unfamiliar with—health disparities in terms of race and ethnicity. I was taking a number of core courses, and within most, there was mention of a gap between the health statuses of Black and White people in the United States. I reflected upon this issue and decided that it would be a key area of interest for me, and indeed, it has been to this day. I took pride in the fact that I was studying in a field—public health—in which I could make a real difference. I would be able to help close the health status gap. Not only did I take courses that emphasized health disparities but I also attended "Closing the Gap" conferences, read books about it, and fiercely debated with classmates, and ultimately colleagues, about the causes.

Some argued that the primary reason for the gap was genetics. I vehemently disagree because I understood then, and understand now, that the illnesses Black people were/are suffering from in the United States were/are not the same as those of Black people in countries in Africa, for the most part. There were some genetic commonalities, such as disposition to sickle cell disease, but that served as a clear indicator that Black people in America were descendants of people in West Africa, primarily as a result of the slave trade. Ultimately, after working in the field of public health for a couple of years, I decided to return to my studies to pursue a Doctorate in Community Health Education at Teachers College, Columbia University. The health disparity still existed without much change, and I continued taking courses and learning more about the proverbial gap and its impact on other emerging majorities beyond Black people. Further, I studied the importance of racial and ethnic diversity in the workforce, in terms of health, as it was touted as one of the many potential solutions to the problem. Many years later, in my role as an academic, I taught about health disparities and diversity, noting that the problems were the same as when I was a young student and that not only was the matter still unresolved but also, in many ways, it was worse.

In the United States, the issues of health disparities and diversity are framed by racial and ethnic considerations. This focus does not preclude the understanding that the term *diversity* is broad, encompassing, beyond race and ethnicity, gender; the lesbian, gay, bisexual, transgender, queer or questioning, and intersex (LGBTQI+) community; people with disabilities; and religious groups. However, this book seeks to identify health disparities along racial and ethnic lines.

Health equity for all in the United States is a lofty goal, particularly given that health disparities are widening. It was felt by some that the Affordable Care Act (ACA), also known as Obamacare, would resolve these issues, leading to greater health equity, but it appears, thus far, that instead, the gap has widened, which is very unfortunate. Nevertheless, it is clear that the ACA is not universal health coverage, as private health corporations remain at the helm of health care in the United States. If we consider the history of the country, perhaps there is some insight, open for debate as to why health equity has not been achieved. However, this cannot be the area of focus. At this point, energy must be focused on how to achieve it. What are the remedies? Once identified, the ensuing steps must be to implement those remedies to see what works and what does not.

In considering Black people and *health inequity*, as one example, we can look at the past to inform the present, in terms of remedies. The year 2019 commemorated the 400th anniversary of the transatlantic slave trade. Some argue that slaves arrived earlier. The timeframe and dates as to when slavery began are important to clarify and remember not only to ensure that no one forgets that this tragedy occurred but also in terms of health disparities. Time should not be spent, however, looking at the dates of origination of slavery, but rather the outcome. Health inequity is pervasive amongst Black people who are experiencing poverty, largely due to social injustice from slavery to the present. Hence, the consideration of universal health coverage is definitely worthy of serious exploration as one approach towards achieving health equity. Universal health coverage and access to care are remedies for the problem, albeit not the sole remedies.

This is a straightforward point regarding universal health coverage and its relationship to lack of equity across the board for Black people and also extends to certain other emerging majority groups. Lower socioeconomic status is at the core of the problem. Whether one agrees with this position or not, what is certain is that in terms of Black, Native American, and the ethnic group of Latino/Hispanic people, health equity in the United States is not the case, relative to White people in the United States. Again, to achieve health equity moving forward, there must be less energy spent discussing the cause, resulting in total emphasis and focus on the remedies. The causes have been studied, researched, argued, and in many instances, established. Therefore, as the *Second Edition* of this work primarily explored causality, as is the case in this text on a more cursory basis, the aim of this *Third Edition* is to highlight and explore remedies.

Additionally, throughout the book, use of the term *minority* is minimized/rarely used in recognition of this term's impending obsolescence. The term is replaced by *emerging majority*, as it is clear that the United States has become more diverse than ever before. *Emerging majority* is used in this book to refer to the various racial groups and the Hispanic/Latino ethnic group. The terms *African American* and *Black* and *Hispanic* and *Latino* are used interchangeably when appropriate.

Additionally, cultural competence is highlighted as one of the many remedies to health disparities, as there is a need within the field of health to value and appreciate the diversity of all people as well as to continue learning about other cultures to ensure optimal provision of services. In this edition, nearly every chapter has lists of remedies, including cultural competency, the importance of education and health literacy and beyond. This edition also includes new chapters and topics, including environmental justice, commercial determinants of health (CDOH), men and health disparities, and artificial intelligence and whether or not it is a remedy for healthcare.

In these chapters, including the new and the revised chapters from the *Second Edition*, the focal point is remedies toward the achievement of health equity. The history of education in the United States is also explored in terms of its relationship to education and health literacy along with remedies specific to the latter. This intersection between education and health in the United States and the parallel injustices within each are enlightening. Understanding these injustices is important as remedies toward health equity are considered.

Many of the remedies explored in this text seem to be based on common sense. For example, let's consider older adults. In the United States, many older adults have aged in prisons while many others are incarcerated as older adults. The consequence is often serious health concerns. A common sense approach to resolving this is to find better approaches to handle older adults, particularly when the crimes they are incarcerated for are not violent. What can be done in lieu of incarceration of older adults? The chapter in this text about older adults explores remedies for this problem. The purpose of the chapter is to interrogate why and how the problems of older adults impact health disparities and to further discuss the need for them to also experience health equity in every aspect of their lives, which must also be the case for people of all ages, throughout their lives.

Furthermore, the title change for this text is about achieving health equity through a forward thinking approach, emphasizing remedies and de-emphasizing the problems, which are understood. The controversies highlighted throughout the text are mainly those associated with topics, such as social injustice, mass incarceration, the new weight loss drugs, artificial intelligence, and more. Rather than simply reiterating and identifying problems related to these controversies, remedies toward health equity remain the focal point. This book is squarely a treatise about remedying health problems, not belaboring them, with the ultimate goal and outcome being the achievement of health equity.

Acknowledgments

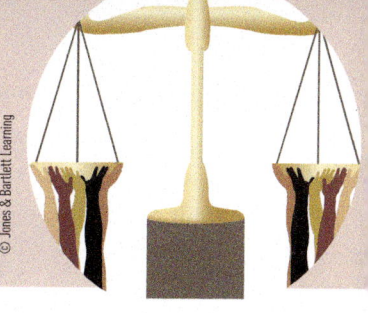

© Jones & Bartlett Learning

Opportunities to express gratitude are often missed as we embark on the complex day-to-day journey of life. Writing a book is an endeavor that involves many in the accomplishment of a goal that is worthy, as a book lasts in perpetuity with the potential to reach the hands of many. In this case, this book may impact lives positively, with hopes that words will turn into deeds toward necessary and positive change. To that end, I do not take lightly this opportunity to express my gratitude to some key, significant people in terms of my writing this *Third Edition*.

I begin by thanking my husband, Jeffrey Rose, for his loving commitment to me and my work, and to his seeing this project through, by my side with never-ending support. He is always the first reader of my books, seeing the words and offering his deft editing for each and every chapter, before I bring them to finalization for manuscript submission. He also assisted by preparing tables of information and the Table of Contents, which was of great help in organizing this work and it was a delight to include his work in this project. I appreciate his attention to detail so much and his love and willingness to share his time from his busy schedule to give me his intelligent, honest feedback and skills, and, most importantly, love and patience.

I also thank my children, Courtney and Brandon Rose. I am profoundly moved by my children and the wonderful adults they are. They both inspire me, just by their existence, and provoke me to think based upon new realities in the midst of social media, their generation, and their personal experiences as intelligent adults navigating this challenging world. Courtney is now a published author of her own book. Watching her do this and providing insight put me in a position to talk to her about my work as a fellow author, which is remarkable. She holds an EdD from Teachers College, Columbia University, one of my alma maters, and she is one of the contributing authors for this text, along with one of her former classmates, Dr. Edmund Adjapong. Their contribution to this work, in the form of a chapter, is as wonderful as their understanding of the history of education, and the intersection between health and educational disparities and the implications regarding health literacy is profound. There are parallels that should not be missed and they clarify this with great skill. I am filled with pride to watch Dr. Courtney Rose walk in my footsteps, as she was 2 years old when I achieved my doctorate at Teachers College. Now, she is a Professor and Director of her program at Florida International University, overseeing the efforts of undergraduate and graduate students (Masters and Doctoral levels).

Brandon is an accomplished young Attorney. Watching him serve as Vice President and General Counsel–U.S. Litigation for a publicly traded international corporation with such skill and adeptness motivates me to move forward with enthusiasm and tremendous energy in all that I do. He is also our family Attorney and a person that I can call upon with 100% trust regarding any matters that require legal attention. As he continues his journey through the legal and professional world in general, I am impressed with how he navigates, figures things out, and remains in the constant quest of determining how he can serve given his legal acumen and other skill sets. His brief, but encouraging words, as I write and share with him how the process is going, are always an inspiration to me, as I am aware of how challenging his day-to-day work is and that so many people depend on him regarding legal matters. Knowing that my book will be in the hands of my husband and children upon completion is a thoroughly rewarding reality. This gives me the energy and enthusiasm to complete the work with pride, knowing that the subject matter—*achieving health equity* in the United States—represents meaningful, important work.

Additionally, I offer gratitude to Dr. Heather Aaron for responding to my interview questions regarding nursing homes with significant expertise for the chapter about older adults and health disparities. She is an important voice in this book and clearly an expert on the subject matter. I also thank Mr. Sunnil Joon for sharing personal insight about his life in the United States as a Trinidadian American immigrant, with parents of Indian descent, but yet he explains that he identifies as a Black person. This is indeed intriguing and compelling and lends insight into how racial classification in the United States confounds individuals in terms of their racial identity in this nation. I also want to thank Dr. Edward Tiozzo, who is of Croatian descent and now an academic in the United States, for sharing his insight regarding men's health.

Other contributing authors that must be acknowledged are Dr. Anthony Munroe, Mr. Clarence Cryer, and Ms. Yolanda Richards. Although their chapters were in the *Second Edition*, with some updates, their laudable work remains in this book because the information is relevant and important to achieving health equity. There is also a new contributing author to this book, Dr. Elizabeth Baquero. She considers me as her mentor, as I have known her since she was a child, through her parents and brother, a close friend of my son. She attended Teachers College, Columbia University, for her doctorate. She wrote, for this text a detailed chapter on the Latino/Hispanic population, which includes important insight, particularly from the interviewee, Dr. Gonzalez, as his insight is thorough and interesting. Ultimately, I offer heartfelt gratitude to all of the contributing authors and interviewees in this book for their time, energy, and knowledge about the subject matter/experiences they share, which truly fortifies this work. I also want to thank John Fuller, Content Production Manager; Indraneil Dey, Project Manager; Will Crain, Copy Editor; and Carol Guerrero, Senior Outsourcing Specialist. Their attention to detail and courteousness throughout the duration of completing this work is greatly appreciated by me.

There is another very important person regarding this work that I want to mention here and that is Sophie Teague, the Product Manager for Public Health at Jones & Bartlett Learning. Our work together now goes back years, as she is the person who approached me about this and prior work, brainstormed with me about the direction the project will take, and who ensured that I was able to move forward with it in terms of the publication process at Jones & Bartlett Learning. I always appreciated her graciousness, thoughtfulness, and confidence in my abilities as an author, and most importantly, her efficiency.

Finally, and above all, I thank God. There is definitely a force in my life that is greater than my mind can imagine, that leads, guides, and protects me and my beloved family. This force inspires my work through an intuitive voice that is forever present. For this blessing, mere words of gratitude are insufficient, but I express them humbly. I always lean on the strength and courage of God, and doing so has never failed me.

About the Author

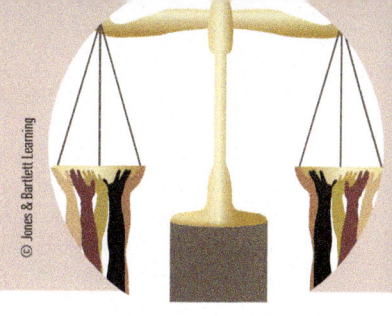

Dr. Patti Rose acquired her Master's degree from Yale University, followed by her Doctorate (EdD) from Teachers College, Columbia University. She has served as a faculty member (from Adjunct Professor to Visiting Professor, to Instructor, to the Associate Professor level) at the University of Miami, Florida, Atlantic University, Florida International University, Springfield College, Worcester State College, Nova Southeastern University, and Barry University. In recent years, courses that she has developed and taught include: Black Women in Medicine and Healing; Psychosocial Health and Healing and Women (online course); Race and Healthcare in America; Culture, Race, and Diversity Issues in the United States; Mass Incarceration and the Impact on the Black Community; and Black Women in Medicine and Healing. In the summer of 2013, she taught Chinese college students as a Visiting Professor at Jiaotong University in Shanghai, China, for 6 weeks, and during the summers of 2014, 2015, and 2016 for 5 weeks in Guangzhou, China, at Jinan University. She also taught at Feng Chia University in Taichung, Taiwan, in 2017, at Jinan University in Shenzhen, China, in 2018, and at Chengdu Polytechnic University in Chengdu, China, in 2019 and 2020. She also served as the Educational Consultant and Liaison for the Essex County College of New Jersey and the JNC International Summer School Program of China Partnership.

Dr. Rose has given keynote addresses, conference presentations, and workshops for many national colleges and universities and other venues, including the Louisiana State University School of Veterinary Medicine; Yale University; Teachers College, Columbia University; LeMoyne College; Ross University; Des Moines University Medical School; Miami Dade College; the American Public Health Association; the National Association of Healthcare Executives; the National Association of Black Veterinarians; and beyond. Her international presentations have included conferences in: Nairobi, Kenya; Barcelona, Spain; Paris, France; Country of Aruba; St. Thomas (U.S. Virgin Islands); and Puerto Rico (a U.S. territory). Her administrative roles include serving as Director and Founder of her own firm, Rose Consulting, her current role, and prior service as President and CEO of Plainfield Health Center in Plainfield, New Jersey and as Vice President of Behavioral Health services at the Jessie Trice Center for Community Health in Miami, Florida, one of the largest community health centers in the nation.

She is the author of several books, including *Cultural Competency for Health Administration and Public Health* (2011), *Cultural Competency for the Health Professions* (2013), and *Health Equity, Diversity, and Inclusion: Context, Controversies and Solutions, Second Edition* (2020), all by the same publisher, Jones & Bartlett Learning. Additionally, she has many published articles, including a piece in the *Harvard Journal of Minority Public Health*, which focused on teenage pregnancy in the Black community. Her work also included serving as administrator and sole writer for her blog, "Natural Is Cool Enough (N.I.C.E.)," that has national and international following, serving as a *Huffington Post* blogger, and being the co-creator and co-host of a podcast, *Ivy Roses*, with her daughter, Dr. Courtney Rose, and the developer of her website, AuthorDrRose.com. She developed a DVD, *Cultural Competency: A Public Health Imperative*, through her consultation for a project directed by the alumni office of the Yale University School of Public Health, where she also received the Public Health Service Award (2004) for her commitment to community health service.

Dr. Rose has language skills in both Spanish and Mandarin, based on her travels and intense study and speaking practice in both languages. Dr. Rose's passion is to travel the globe to understand the world and to share her knowledge of various cultures, history, health education and health promotion, health equity, social injustice (including health disparities), globalism, and diversity through her writing, teaching, and speaking engagements. Her current research is focused on health disparities and health equity, and remedies to achieve the latter, particularly in the United States, from a social justice vantage point, utilizing a cultural lens, and through comparative analysis, from a national and global perspective. Her cultural travel, work, and research have included journeys to Puerto Rico, Mexico, Fiji, Turkey, Africa (South Africa, Kenya, Senegal, Ghana, Morocco, Tanzania, Egypt, Zanzibar, and the Cape Verde Islands), Sri Lanka, Dubai, Australia, New Zealand, Europe (Spain, Italy, Ireland, France, Portugal, Iceland, the United Kingdom, Greece, Croatia, Scotland and the Netherlands), the Caribbean (Jamaica, Tortola, St. Lucia, St. Thomas, Barbados, St. Maarten and St. Bartholomew), Latin and Central America (Cuba, Honduras, Nicaragua, Costa Rica, Panama, the Dominican Republic, and Guatemala), and Asia (Japan, China, Vietnam, Singapore, Bali, South Korea, India, The Maldives, and Thailand).

Her professional affiliations have included the American College of Healthcare Executives, the American Public Health Association, the Black Executive Forum, and the National Association of Health Services Executives. She was appointed by the U.S. Department of Commerce, National Institute of Standards and Technology, to serve in the capacity of Examiner on the 2004 Board of Examiners of the Malcolm Baldrige National Quality Award. She was recently selected as a Yale Alumni Association At-Large-Delegate and served as the President of the South Florida Chapter of the Yale Black Alumni Association and a frequent Yale Alumni Schools Committee college applicant evaluative interviewer. Dr. Rose has been married for 39 years and is the mother of two.

Contributors

Edmund Adjapong, PhD
Associate Professor, Seton Hall University
South Orange, New Jersey

Elizabeth Baquero, EdD, MS
Research Administrator at Weill Cornell Medicine, New York, New York
Adjunct Professor at Florida International University, Miami, Florida

Clarence Cryer, Jr., MPH
Executive Director of Correctional Health Operations, JPS Health Network
Fort Worth, Texas

Annie Daniel, PhD
Founder and CEO, Institute for Healthcare Education Leaders & Profesionals
Baton Rouge, Louisiana

Anthony E. Munroe, MPH, MBA, EdD
President, Borough of Manhattan Community College
New York, New York

Yolanda Richard, MDV
Executive Director, Good Business Colorado
Denver, Colorado

Courtney Elizabeth Rose, MEd, EdD
Assistant Teaching Professor
Program Director, Educational Leadership
Florida International University
Miami, Florida

Reviewers

Mustapha Alhassan, MSW, PhD
BSW Program Director
Associate Professor
Clark Atlanta University
Atlanta, Georgia

Michelle McClave, EdD, MSN, RN
Associate Professor of Nursing
Morehead State University
Morehead, Kentucky

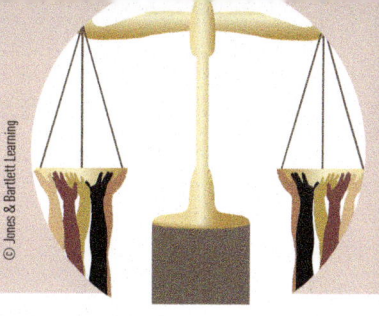

© Jones & Bartlett Learning

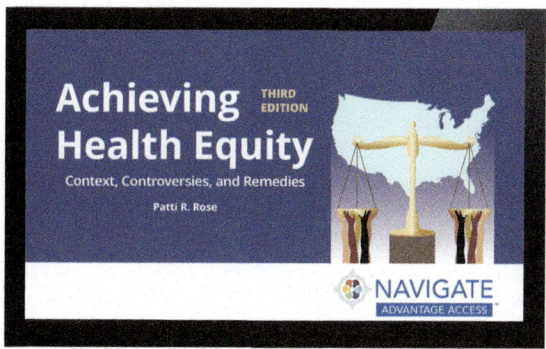

Instructor Resources

Qualified instructors can receive a full suite of instructor resources, including the following:

- Slides in PowerPoint format
- Instructor's Manual
- Test Bank (chapter quizzes, midterm exam, final exam)

Student Resources

Each new purchase of the print textbook or Navigate Advantage course includes an eBook with the following student resources:

- Chapter review slides
- Open educational resources
- Flashcards
- Interactive glossary

We Value Your Feedback

Do you love this text? Spot an error you'd like to report? Follow this QR code to give us your observations and suggestions for improvement.

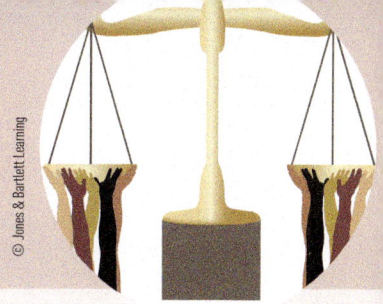

Introduction

Health equity must be achieved in American society. *Achieving Health Equity: Context, Controversies, and Remedies, Third Edition* is intended to address this topic head-on, with an emphasis on how to achieve it. The demographics in the United States are rapidly changing; in the near future, Black, Indigenous, and People of Color (BIPOC) will become the majority group, rather than the minority; their healthcare needs must continue to be met, without the raging disparity that leads to poor health outcomes, human suffering, and a drain on the economy. This text is unique as it is designed not only to speak to individuals in the field of health care, but also to anyone who is concerned about, and committed to, a healthy society for all people. This text also addresses topics, concepts, and issues intended to ensure that those in field of health care understand why the rapid demographic changes currently taking place in the United States add a sense of urgency to the need for remedies for the problems causing a lack of health equity, thereby closing the health status gap. Diversity is essential to this process.

Furthermore, evidence-based research clearly indicates that racial/ethnic diversity in the delivery of health care improves outcomes for emerging majority populations. The discussion of diversity in this text will be contrasted with the concept of cultural competence and will demonstrate that, although distinctly different, the two elements are intrinsically linked in efforts made toward the ultimate goal of closing the health status gap in the United States. In order to truly understand racial and ethnic health disparities and diversity, it is important to gain insight in terms of various groups and to consider how these other groups fare in comparison to the White population from a health vantage point. However, this is not the focal point of this text; it will focus on remedies, rather than problems. Some factors that contribute to health disparities will be explored, along with some indices including infant and maternal mortality, morbidity, longevity, specific diseases, access to health care, and other key concerns. Socioeconomic factors are also explored, as a primary premise of this text is that one of the key remedies toward achieving health equity is to reduce poverty, substantially, in the United States. Because this text aims to provide remedies, interviews with various individuals who lend their insight based on experiential knowledge are included.

Overview of the Chapters

Chapter 2 is an exploration of the notion of health equity. Beyond exploring the meaning of health disparities, another key question involves the true meaning of the term *health equity*. The chapter also provides a thorough explanation of its significance and relevance to health disparities, which will also be defined with a candid exploration of the extent of the healthcare gap and the possibilities that exist toward closing it. Diversity is also explored, focusing on questions, such as "What is diversity, and who defines it?" Various definitions are explored to help with understanding the concept. In addition to the meaning and historical overview, insight will be provided as to the importance of remedies to solve the health disparity problem. Some "models that work" and evidence-based approaches to reducing health disparities will be discussed. Lastly, this chapter also revisits topics thoroughly explored in two earlier books by this author, *Cultural Competency for Health Administration* and *Public Health and Cultural Competency for the Health Professional*, both published by Jones & Bartlett Learning.

Chapter 3 focuses on the Black/African American community, with emphasis on issues pertaining to health equity, including problems and remedies. Initially, it was literally a Black and White issue. That is, it considered the health status of Black people compared to that of White people. This framework has changed as a result of the acknowledgement that there is vast racial and ethnic diversity in the United States, but the largest gap overall is still between Black people and White people; hence these groups are a key focus of this text. Instead of looking at these groups in terms of the problems that exist, exploration is from a remedy-oriented approach to figure out why the health status of White people is so much better than Black people in the United States. What is it about White people's lives that leads to better health outcomes in this nation? By focusing on what is working for this group, remedies can be explored to make sure that whatever is happening to create better health for White people in the United States should be happening to reach the same outcomes with all groups.

Chapters 4, 5, and 6 take the same approach with exploration of the following groups, respectively: people who are Asian American and Pacific Islanders, American Indian and Alaska Natives, and the Hispanic/Latino population. These groups will be categorized, with insight provided regarding the health status of each, as compared to the White population. Remedies will be explored per the disparities that exist.

Chapter 7 focuses on how the health status of populations in urban communities can be improved relative to suburban communities with limited mention of the latter. Understanding the variables unique to the urban setting is useful in exploring remedies toward closing the gap. New topics, which were not covered in the previous edition, are *environmental justice* and *commercial determinants of health*. Definitions and explanations of these terms are provided, followed by recommendations toward remedies.

Chapter 8 explores health disparities in rural communities and the unique issues associated with them that can explain/improve their health status as compared to other populations. The rural community at large warrants specific consideration because the dynamics of the healthcare gap changes in this setting; these communities are sometimes composed primarily, although not exclusively, of White people living at a low socioeconomic level. Through the lens of these communities, further insight is provided as to what factors can be looked upon as remedies rather than problems. In short, what are the models that work in some rural communities?

Chapter 9 explores the link between health and education, including the history of the public school system, the "achievement gap," and the link between educational achievement and health outcomes. Remedies will be explored understanding that education and health go hand in hand. It is a two-prong situation. The goal here is to understand the impact of urban, suburban, and rural education on urban, suburban, and rural health. Improving education for people who are seeking health care is leaning toward a remedy-oriented approach rather than focusing squarely on the problems. Culture, as it relates to teaching and learning, is also reviewed because cultural competence is necessary in a diverse nation that is diverse in terms of education and health. Emphasis will be placed on what must change in the educational system to ensure that health disparities are impacted in a favorable direction. Educational achievement and health outcomes will be considered along with issues pertaining to lack of health literacy and how the educational system can assist with this particular problem.

Chapter 10 explores health equity in terms of remedies among women. Generally, women are the caretakers in families. They bear children, participate in the workforce, and also experience significant health disparities. Socioeconomic status is a major contributing factor to these health disparities. Significant detail is provided to find remedies that are useful to women's health. Essentially, what works, what doesn't, and why?

Chapter 11 provides insight into men's health, including specific issues, concerns, and remedies. The previous edition of this text handled this group in the appendices. This edition goes deeper into the topic by focusing on remedies to ensure dialogue regarding better health for men in this nation. Remedies pertaining to their health, particularly in communities where the health status gap continues to widen, are also discussed.

Chapter 12 considers children as the primary focus. Although children are discussed throughout the text, this chapter takes a serious look at their specific issues, as they are the future of the nation. Consideration is given to remedies for them, in terms of health disparities. Children are key, as they will be the greatest beneficiaries of any successes toward closing the gap.

Chapter 13 covers older adults and health equity. Key health issues impacting older adults are explored with an eye toward remedies. It includes an interview with a healthcare professional who provides cogent insight regarding nursing homes and their relevance to the older population, as well as how they impact the daily living of their patients. In terms of all of the groups mentioned here (women, men, children, older adults, rural and suburban populations, and beyond), Healthy People 2030, which is an initiative that promotes health through the use of objectives, and is the fifth iteration of this process, is considered.

Chapter 14 looks into the future of health care/public health with a focus on artificial intelligence (AI). The question considered is whether AI will be a remedy or a hindrance in terms of problems related to achieving health equity.

Chapter 15 includes case studies pertaining to health disparities and other pertinent issues and considers remedies that will move this nation toward health equity. These case studies offer a look at specific scenarios, which can be explored and discussed to understand how and why remedies must be at the forefront of achieving health equity rather than a focus on problems, as the latter has been the primary approach in healthcare fields. The purpose of these cases is to stimulate discussion about potential remedies, beyond those offered by the author.

Chapter 16 offers a spiritual approach toward remedies, since achieving health equity involves looking beyond typical healthcare and public health approaches. It is not about religion as we typically use the word; rather, it is about self-actualization providing an opportunity to reflect on the key issues of the entire text. This chapter considers the questions "Where do we go from here?" and "How do we actually achieve health equity with a focus on spirituality?"

Features of the Text

Beginning with the next chapter, this text comprises the following elements: learning objectives; a list of key terms; an introduction; remedies; a chapter summary (Wrap-Up); chapter problems; and references. Chapters 6, 7, 9, 12, and 16 are authored by/with this book's contributors. Chapter 15 consists of an introduction, followed by some case studies.

Following the main chapters, appendices are provided to supplement the information discussed throughout the text. These resources include cultural competence assessment surveys, sample components of a diversity plan, a glossary of terms, abbreviations, and more. An index is provided for the reader's convenience.

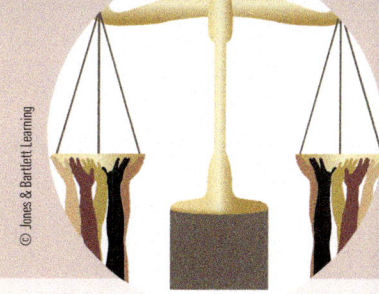

CHAPTER 2

Health Disparities, Diversity, and Health Equity: Meanings and Historical Insights

KEY TERMS

African American/Black
culture
ethnicity
health disparity
health equity

healthcare inequality
mission
race
White

LEARNING OBJECTIVES

After reading this chapter, you should be able to do the following:

1. Understand the role that culture plays in health disparities.
2. List the key factors that influence the health status of various groups.
3. Discuss why the widest health status gap is between Black and White people in the United States.
4. Describe the importance of remedies to solve problems relevant to achieving health equity.

Introduction

Generally, **health disparity** refers to a difference or gap in health status between varying racial and ethnic groups. There are a number of factors to take into consideration when exploring this gap, which will be reviewed in depth throughout this text. These factors include socioeconomic and educational status, race, culture, ethnicity, and other population characteristics. If all of these factors are not taken into consideration when comparing the health status of different groups, then problems may arise in addressing health disparities. For example, it may be erroneously argued that one group is inherently healthier than the other, a type of bias. Or, it may be assumed that one factor is the cause of a disparity, and thus remedies to the problem may be based on a narrow focus. In this text, however, in terms of health disparities, the goal is not to belabor discussion about the problems but rather to explore how to achieve health equity.

Moreover, it helps to consider examples in looking at this flawed approach to understanding the extent of factors that may contribute to health disparities. Specifically, it is generally understood that in the United States, which is the country of emphasis regarding health disparities in this text, the White, currently the majority, population has a higher health status than do members of the African American/ Black population. The goal here is to understand why. What is the reason that White people are healthier than Black people in the United States? There are many reasons, with the first being reliable health care coverage. According to a 2021 Commonwealth Fund report (Radley et al., 2021), cost, affordability, and access to care are all contributing factors as certain groups are impacted by these issues more than others—namely Black, Hispanic/Latino, and Asian and Pacific Islander populations. However, rather than dwelling on what the problems are, as these have been identified in terms of research, books, and beyond over significant periods of time, the question is: What are the remedies for these issues? This same 2021 report from the Commonwealth Fund endeavors to explore remedies from a policy vantage point. The first suggestion is to ensure universal, affordable, and equitable health coverage. This is stated simply but clearly amounts to a difficult process. However, in terms of health care, taking on difficult challenges toward remedies must be at the forefront. The process includes addressing issues with premiums. Premiums, for many, are over the top, and until they are reduced, health care will not be affordable. Another step would be to reduce deductibles. In the past, this was, and now continues to be, an idea for individuals at or below the poverty level. As a brief explanation, a premium is the amount that people pay to their employer or another entity for health care coverage each month and a deductible is the amount people have to pay toward their health insurance, prior to the health insurance payment (*Your Total Costs for Health Care: Premium, Deductible, and Out-of-pocket Costs*, n.d.).

REMEDIES

- Ensure universal, affordable, and equitable health coverage
- Re-evaluate premiums toward affordability for all
- Reduce deductibles

Currently, given inflation and its impact on food, housing costs, and every other aspect of life, deductibles need to be decreased for most people, as many individuals and families are living paycheck to paycheck. Of course, these reductions should not be targeted toward the wealthy, but the rest of society. However, targeted remedies tend to create political divisions that prevent anything from being done. Why not create policies that will assist all levels of society that will inherently include people who are experiencing poverty or struggling financially?

Health Disparities Defined

The concept of *health disparities* has been defined in many different ways. A few formal definitions are presented in **Table 2-1**.

Interest in health disparities has grown over the past 20 years. A primary contributor to this surge is the persistence of health disparities despite improvements in medical care and public health prevention initiatives (Adler & Stewart, 2010). The body of research on health disparities over the past 20–30 years increased rather significantly, and particularly, as national attention was placed on this important issue. Within the past 20 years, one can identify several distinct eras of work on health disparities' association with socioeconomic status. Adler and Stewart (2010) describe the eras as follows: If one considers the eras, the first offers a model to consider the relationship between poverty and health, the second goes further with evidence, in terms of educational, income, and occupational improvements or wealth and how these factors are related to better health outcomes. Socioeconomic status and health are linked in the third era and the fourth considers influences at various levels, while the fifth considers how these factors interact.

Research in health disparities is generally considered to proceed in three generations: (1) research describing relevant disparities; (2) research that addresses the

Table 2-1 Varying Definitions of the Term "Health Disparities" in the United States

Source*	Definition of "Health Disparities"
The Secretary's Advisory Committee on National Health Promotion and Disease Prevention Objectives for 2020 (2008)	A particular type of health difference that is closely linked with social, economic, and/or environmental disadvantage. Health disparities adversely affect groups of people who have systematically experienced greater obstacles to health based on their racial or ethnic group; religion; socioeconomic status; gender; age; mental health; cognitive, sensory, or physical disability; sexual orientation or gender identity; geographic location; or other characteristics historically linked to discrimination or exclusion.
Dehlendorf et al. (2010)	In the United States, discussion of disparities has focused primarily on racial and ethnic disparities. In the international literature, and increasingly in the United States, socioeconomic status and gender disparities, disparities between disabled and non-disabled individuals, and disparities by sexual orientation have also been considered.
Braveman et al. (2011)	Differences in health outcomes and access to health care across different population groups, often driven by social, economic, and environmental disadvantages.

*The full reference for each source is included in the References section at the end of this chapter.

underlying causes of these disparities; and (3) investigations designed to address and resolve these disparities (Dehlendorf et al., 2010). First-generation research studies have provided an abundance of data that significant health disparities exist, including profound differences in life expectancy and cancer-related mortality both by race/ethnicity and by socioeconomic status (Adler & Rehkopf, 2007). Second-generation research studies have provided insight into pathways through which disparities occur, including individual, provider, and healthcare system factors (Kilbourne et al., 2006). Third-generation research studies have been more limited but suggest that targeted interventions do have success at reducing health disparities (Kilbourne et al., 2006).

Table 2-2 highlights select and noteworthy historical U.S. government initiatives over the past 35 years to address health disparities.

Table 2-2 **Select Noteworthy Historical U.S. Government Initiatives to Address Health Disparities**

Date	Initiative
April 1984	The Task Force on Black and Minority Health is established at the U.S. Department of Health and Human Services. This task force is the first coordinated and comprehensive effort facilitated by the department to investigate minority health status in comparison with the majority population.
December 1985	The U.S. Department of Health and Human Services creates the Federal Office of Minority Health. This newly formed office is charged with impacting historical health disparities by developing policy, providing important information that would inform health-related decision making, funding, and providing technical assistance to state minority entities and community-based organizations engaged in improving minority health status.
1986	With significant and increasing gaps in health status among the various racial and ethnic groups, the U.S. Department of Health and Human Services forms the Office of Minority Health. The **mission** of the office is to develop health policies and programs that will eliminate health disparities while protecting and improving the health of racial and ethnic minority groups/populations.
April 1989	National Minority Health month is designated in an effort to bring greater awareness to health disparities, minority health, and racial and ethnic health status differences.
1990	Congress encourages the creation of the Office of Research on Minority Health.
February 1998	President Bill Clinton announces an Initiative to Eliminate Racial and Ethnic Health Disparities.
September 1999	The National Institutes of Health is charged with developing a plan to reduce health disparities.

Date	Initiative
2000	The Minority Health and Health Disparities Research and Education Act is passed. The act leads to the creation of the National Center on Minority Health and Health Disparities at the National Institutes of Health.
March 2002	The Institute of Medicine's impactful, influential report "Unequal Treatment: Confronting Racial and Ethnic Disparities in Health Care" is released.
July 2002	The U.S. Department of Health and Human Services Office of Minority Health holds a National Leadership Summit on eliminating racial and ethnic disparities in health.
2009	The Secretary of the U.S. Department of Health and Human Services releases a report on health disparities and health reform.
April 2011	The U.S. Department of Health and Human Services announces a plan to reduce health disparities. The National Partnership for Action initiates a strategy to expand and strengthen community-led efforts to achieve health equity.

Health Disparities and Emerging Majority Groups

Health disparities remain a central concern in the United States and globally. This difference in health status between emerging majority groups and the White population continues to increase on the whole and has increased over time, adding to the burden of death and illness among emerging majority populations of the country. It is important to look at data to determine what is actually happening in terms of health across racial lines. "All-cause mortality is a primary measure of a population's health" (Benjamins et al., 2021). The definition is nearly self-explanatory: "All-cause mortality means death due to any cause." (Basaraba and Casimiro, 2024).

It is not surprising, given the health inequities, that Black people have higher death rates in the United States than White people. This can be chalked up to social injustice, socioeconomic and educational status, systemic racial inequities, and other factors. Per a cross-sectional study conducted over 10 years by Benjamins et al. (2021), which considered all-cause mortality by city and race, found that the "all-cause mortality rate among Black populations was 24% higher than among White populations nationally (rate ratio, 1.236; 95% CI, 1.233 to 1.238), resulting in 74,402 excess Black deaths annually." According to their research, the overall U.S. all-cause mortality rate is 759 per 100,000. Their study included 26,295,827 death records and they found the following:

> "The all-cause mortality rate among Black US residents was 960 per 100 000 individuals. . . . The all-cause mortality rate among White U.S. residents for the nation was 777 per 100 000 individuals."

Clearly, there is a disparity in which White people are faring better than black people in terms of mortality.

Thus far, the 21st century has been a period of ever-growing globalization resulting in multiculturalism in the United States and elsewhere. The United States is considered a world leader in medical technology. Nevertheless, equity does not exist in the provision of health care because it is not distributed evenly throughout the U.S. population. Beyond the definitions provided in Table 2-1, health disparity is often referred to as **healthcare inequality** or gaps in the quality of health and health care across racial, ethnic, and socioeconomic groups. The Health Resources and Services Administration defines health disparity as "population-specific differences in the presence of disease, health outcomes or access to healthcare" (Carter-Pokras & Baquet, 2002). The focus here is disparities pertaining to the quality of care that different ethnic and racial groups receive. Reasons for disparities in access to health care, specifically, are attributed to many causes, such as low socioeconomic status, lack of insurance coverage, lack of a regular source of care, legal barriers, structural barriers, limits in the healthcare financing system, scarcity of providers, linguistic barriers, lack of health literacy among certain groups and communities, cultural barriers, and lack of diversity in the healthcare workforce. Other factors are education, segregation, and immigration status (Kosoko-Lasaki et. al., 2009).

According to the Centers for Disease Control and Prevention (Office of Health Equity, 2024), "Health equity is the state in which everyone has a fair and just opportunity to attain their highest level of health." There is a long-established understanding that health disparities exist between urban and rural communities. But the geographical aspect of health inequity is complex. As Galvin (2019) pointed out, "Among America's 100 most populous metro areas in 2015, more people lived in poverty in the suburbs than in the major cities nearby." A lack of mass transit and fragmented government resources can exacerbate the issue.

Additionally, immigration is another significant factor pertaining to health disparities, primarily because many immigrant populations do not have access to health care. Although community health centers in the United States are available to serve undocumented people, the problem is that most people, including immigrant and non-immigrant groups, are not aware of these facilities or the fact that people can be seen at these facilities regardless of their ability to pay or their immigration status. Many immigrants, fearing that they will be asked for documentation that could lead to their deportation, seek care only in emergency rooms, or don't seek care at all. A key remedy for this particular concern is making sure that people are aware of community health centers. Marketing of these facilities in all forms of media and direct communication about them would be very helpful and a relatively uncomplicated remedy. Budgets for these centers from the federal government must include significant marketing funds. The health disparities framework in **Table 2-3** provides further insight.

Table 2-3 Health Disparities Framework

Health—Before Care	Access to Care	Health Care Delivery
Income levels, poverty, and other social conditions	Financial resources	Insurance coverage and type
Safety and adequacy of housing	Availability and proximity of providers	Cultural competence levels

Health—Before Care	Access to Care	Health Care Delivery
Employment status and type of employment	Access to transportation	Patient–provider communications
Education levels	Insurance coverage	Provider discrimination or bias
Lifestyle choices—diet, exercise, tobacco, and alcohol use	Regular source of care	Differential propensities for certain diseases by racial/ethnic populations
Environmental conditions—air and water quality, pesticide exposure, green space	Language barriers	Patient preferences and adherence to treatment plans
	Legal barriers (e.g., eligibility restrictions, illegal immigrants)	Diversity of the healthcare workforce
	Prior experience with the healthcare system	Appropriateness of care
	Cultural preferences—care-seeking behaviors	Effectiveness of care
	Health literacy levels	Language barriers
	Diversity of the healthcare workforce	

Courtesy of Health Policy Institute of Chicago (2004, September). Understanding health disparities. Retrieved from http://a5e8c023c8899218225edfa4b02e4d9734e01a28.gripelements.com/pdf/publications/healthdisparities.pdf

REMEDIES

- Make sure that people are aware of community health centers—Federally Qualified Health Centers (FQHC)—that serve people irrespective of their immigration status or ability to pay.
- Budgets for these centers, from the federal government, must include significant marketing funds.
- Health disparity and health equity issues must be addressed at the policy level, not just via discussion and bills that linger in political limbo, but with real action that meets the needs of the people.
- Overall costs need to be reduced to a level that will allow all people to afford health insurance and enable them to access health care services when necessary.
- In order to achieve health equity, the focus must no longer be on repeatedly elucidating the problems but rather on remedies to the problems, including policy, financing, and implementation.

WRAP-UP

As this text moves forward, there will be many more remedies discussed, but the key here is that issues must be addressed at the policy level, not just via discussion and bills that linger in political limbo but with real action that meets the needs of the people. This may be considered pie-in-the-sky idealism, but if as much time was spent discussing and moving toward remedies as is spent on elucidating the problems, we would actually achieve health equity in the United States for all. Racial and ethnic disparities in health care persist despite considerable progress in expanding healthcare services and improving the quality of patient care, although universal health care has not been achieved. As stated by Shi and Singh (2021):

> Future healthcare reform will have to address two broad issues: cost of health insurance for business and individuals and cost of health care services. . . . In essence, overall costs need to be reduced to a level that will allow most people to afford health insurance and enable them to access health care services when necessary.

Although this statement is insightful, it cannot be just *most* people, but must include *all* people. Therefore, universal healthcare is an essential remedy. As for health disparities, many factors contribute to these disparities in complex ways, but the quality of health care can be improved through implementing remedies for all patients/customers with a comprehensive approach that includes ensuring that strategies are implemented to not only reduce healthcare disparities, but also to improve the efficiency and equity of care for all patients (Betancourt et al., 2003). With effective strategies, health equity is achievable. This kind of remedy-oriented focus also includes taking into consideration the improvement of communication and comfort levels between healthcare providers and their patients/customers. Many healthcare organizations are facing dramatic demographic shifts in their customer/patient populations and, therefore, are challenged to provide quality healthcare services to an increasingly diverse patient base. This chapter has discussed complex, sensitive, and challenging issues related to health disparities, emerging majorities, and the health status gap that has historically existed in the United States between different racial groups, with special focus on the substandard health status of Black people (Non-Hispanic/Latino and Hispanic/Latino) with insight regarding contributing factors. Most importantly, this chapter highlights the reality that remedies are the key, so that the problems are not continually identified without resolving them. Hence the summary of remedies delineated in this chapter (and some additional insight) includes:

1. Ensure universal, affordable, and equitable health coverage.
2. Create policies that will assist all levels of society and will inherently include people who are experiencing poverty or struggling financially.
3. Reduce premiums and deductibles.
4. Help Black patients/customers get beyond their feelings of distrust by hiring more healthcare providers of the same race/ethnicity, with whom they may feel more comfortable.

5. Patients/customers should have the opportunity to select which providers they would like to seek care from.
6. Make sure that people are aware of community health centers by marketing these facilities in all forms of media with budgets for these centers, from the federal government that include significant marketing funds.
7. More time, money and energy should be spent on finding remedies for health disparities instead of elucidating the problems (remedy-centered instead of problem-centered).
8. Reduction of healthcare costs.

Chapter Problems

1. List three factors that contribute to health disparities.
2. Explain health disparities in terms of Black people in the United States.
3. What are some possible remedies toward improving access to health care? Explore potential remedies with ideas of your own.
4. What is the difference between a premium and a deductible and what remedy is needed in terms of both of them?

References

Adler, N. E., & Stewart, J. (2010). Health disparities across the lifespan: Meaning, methods, and mechanisms. *Annals of the New York Academy of Sciences, 1186*, 5–23. https://doi.org/10.1111/j.1749-6632.2009.05337.x

Adler, N. E., & Rehkopf, D. H. (2007). U.S. Disparities in Health: Descriptions, Causes, and Mechanisms. *Annual Review of Public Health, 29*(1), 235–252. https://doi.org/10.1146/annurev.publhealth.29.020907.090852

Basaraba, S. (2024, September 18). What does All-Cause Mortality mean? *Verywell Health.* https://www.verywellhealth.com/what-is-all-cause-mortality-2223349

Benjamins, M. R., Silva, A., Saiyed, N. S., & De Maio, F. G. (2021). Comparison of All-Cause mortality rates and inequities between black and white populations across the 30 most populous US cities. *JAMA Network Open, 4*(1), e2032086. https://doi.org/10.1001/jamanetworkopen.2020.32086

Betancourt, J. R., Green, A. R., Carrillo, J. E., & Ananeh-Firemong, O. (2003). Defining cultural competence: A practical framework for addressing racial/ethnic disparities in health and health care. *Public Health Reports, 118*(4), 293–302.

Braveman, P., Egerter, S., & Williams, D. R. (2011). The social determinants of health: Coming of age. *Annual Review of Public Health, 32*, 381–398. https://doi.org/10.1146/annurev-publhealth-031210-101218

Carter-Pokras, O., & Baquet, C. (2002). What is a "health disparity"? *Public Health Reports, 117*(5), 426–434.

Dehlendorf, C., Bryant, A. S., Huddleston, H. G., Jacoby, V. L., & Fujimoto, V. Y. (2010). Health disparities: Definitions and measurements. *American Journal of Obstetrics and Gynecology, 202*(3), 212–213. https://doi.org/10.1016/j.ajog.2009.12.003

Galvin, G. (2019, March 26). The suburban myth of health and wealth. *US News & World Report.* https://www.usnews.com/news/healthiest-communities/articles/2019-03-26/long-island-and-the-suburban-myth-of-health-and-wealth

Kilbourne, A. M., Switzer, G., Hyman, K., Crowley-Matoka, M., & Fine, M. J. (2006). Advancing Health Disparities Research within the Health Care System: A Conceptual framework. *American Journal of Public Health, 96*(12), 2113–2121. https://doi.org/10.2105/ajph.2005.077628

Kosoko-Lasaki, S., Cook, C., & O'Brien, R. (2009). *Cultural proficiency in addressing health disparities.* Jones & Bartlett Learning.

Office of Health Equity. (2024, June 11). What is health equity? Centers for Disease Control and Prevention. https://www.cdc.gov/health-equity/what-is/index.html

Radley, D. C., Baumgartner, J. C., Collins, S. R., Zephyrin, L. C., & Schneider, E. C. (2021, November 18). *Achieving racial and ethnic equity in U.S. health care: A scorecard of state performance* [Report]. The Commonwealth Fund. https://www.commonwealthfund.org /publications/scorecard/2021/nov/achieving-racial-ethnic-equity-us-health-care-state -performance

Secretary's Advisory Committee on Health Promotion and Disease Prevention Objectives for 2020. (2008). *The secretary's advisory committee on national health promotion and disease prevention objectives for 2020 Phase I report recommendations for the framework and format of healthy people 2020.* https://odphp.health.gov/sites/default/files/2021-11/Secretary's%20Advisory %20Committee%20Recommendations%20for%20HP2020%20Framework%20and %20Format.pdf

Shi, L., & Singh, D. A. (2021). *Delivering health care in America: A systems approach.* Jones & Bartlett Learning.

Your total costs for health care: Premium, deductible, and out-of-pocket costs. (n.d.). HealthCare.gov. https://www.healthcare.gov/choose-a-plan/your-total-costs/

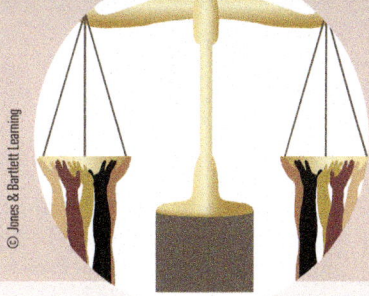
© Jones & Bartlett Learning

The Black/African American Population and Health Disparities: Issues, Concerns, and Remedies

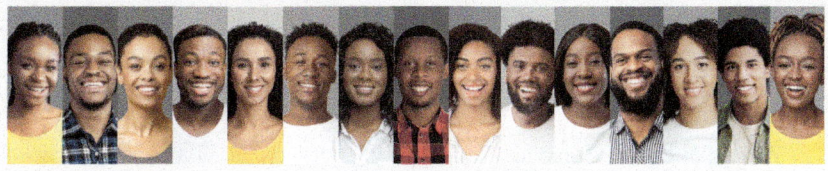
© Prostock-studio/Shutterstock

KEY TERMS

Black/African American
digital divide
FAST
food desert
food injustice
food mirage
health inequality
health literacy

Jim Crow laws
linguistic competence
nationality
people of color
reparation
social injustice
soul food
White hindrance

LEARNING OBJECTIVES

After reading this chapter, you should be able to do the following:

1. Explain why Black/African American people are actually the largest racial emerging majority group, and what factor makes this statement true?
2. Explain the connection between lack of education and health literacy.
3. Discuss social injustice and the role it plays in health disparities.
4. Distinguish between White privilege and White hindrance?
5. List socially unjust factors that impact health status in the United States.

Introduction

Are **Black/African American** people the second largest emerging majority group in America after a long-held position as the largest, and also the largest racial emerging majority group? If we reconsider the status of Black/African American people in terms of which group is the largest emerging majority group, there is a factor that has to be considered, namely Black Hispanic/Latino people. It is appropriate to include Black Hispanic/Latino people in the Black/African American group because, according to the original categorization by race and ethnicity per the Office of Management and Budget (OMB), Hispanic/Latino is not a racial but rather an ethnic group (Office of Management and Budget, n.d.).

Minimum Race and Ethnicity Categories

There have been recent changes to the OMB classifications. According to the revisions to the OMB standards (Office of Management and Budget, 2024), the minimum categories will remain the same, with the addition of two new groups, namely North African and Middle Eastern. The categories that remain unchanged are:

- American Indian or Alaska Native;
- Asian;
- Black or African American;
- Hispanic or Latino;
- Native Hawaiian or Pacific Islander; and
- White.

As part of the revisions, in terms of asking questions used to collect information, the guidance is "Using one combined question for race and ethnicity, and encouraging respondents to select as many options as apply to how they identify." There are also updates to definitions, terminology, etc., and the requirement to ask for more detail beyond race and ethnicity (Office of Management and Budget, 2024). Throughout this text, the terms African American and Black will be used interchangeably to describe people of African descent in the United States.

Although these changes are in effect, it doesn't change the fact that Hispanic/Latino people may be Black, White, or of other racial groups. It gets a bit more complicated when discussing White Hispanic/Latino people because White Non-Hispanic people are not considered an emerging majority group. Therefore, the health experiences of White Hispanic/Latino people may or may not be different than those of the White population for a number of reasons, particularly White privilege (referred to in this text as White hindrance—see explanation later in this chapter). But for Black Hispanic/Latino people, their experience, in terms of health, is very similar to that of Black/African American, Non-Hispanic people, with culture being the salient difference. Essentially, the health status of Black people (both Hispanic/Latino and Non-Hispanic/Latino) in the United States is lower than that of the White population. Changing categorization does not alter the reality for Black people in terms of health disparities whether they are Hispanic/Latino or Non-Hispanic/Latino people.

According to the United States Census Bureau (U.S. Census Bureau Public Information Office, n.d.), "In each of 10 southern states—Texas, Florida, Georgia, North Carolina, Maryland, Louisiana, Virginia, South Carolina, Alabama, and

Mississippi—more than 1 million people reported as Black." Black people have been referred to by many titles in America, including Colored, Negro, Black, Afro-American, African American, and other terms, not mentioned here, that are considered derogatory. These varying terms used to describe people of African descent in America were largely derived within political and historical contexts. Specifically, the term *colored* was used as a result of the following:

> The 1924 law restricting immigration might be the pivotal one here ... [It was] the first ever "comprehensive" immigration restriction law—with a "racial and national hierarchy that favored some immigrants over others." This immigration law treated "race" as obvious and visible as it split the world up into "colored" and "non-colored" races, and into European and non-European (Rubin & Melnick, 2006, p. 8).

The term *Negro* has a different origin. One speculative perspective follows:

> Let us look back into history, then, and strive to discover the origin of this term "Negro." If you look at the unabridged edition of the *Oxford Dictionary*, you will be shown that the origin of the word "Negro," as far as is known in the English language, is in 1555. Nevertheless, that is not the beginning of the term because the English were not the first transgressors in this respect. The English adopted the word from the Spanish. The Spanish may have gotten it from the Portuguese; it isn't yet quite clear (Moore, 1992, p. 35).

By the late 1980s, the term *Afro-American* was largely superseded by *African American*. However, *Afro-American* is still used by the Library of Congress for cataloguing purposes and is also retained in names of organizations or programs, such as Yale University's Afro-American Cultural Center.

Additionally, many still use the term *Black*. According to Spivey (2003), "Ninety Percent of all African Americans have their ancestral roots in the kingdoms of West Africa". Consequently, the term African American is used to make a connection to this ancestral lineage. Some may prefer *Black* as a more unifying term, as they may identify themselves as persons from specific nations, such as Jamaican American and Trinidadian American. In these instances, *African* is not the lead term, although they are also of African descent. Others will solely use the **nationality** of their ancestry (i.e., the nation in which their parents or guardians were born or from which their family descends) to describe themselves, indicating that they are Jamaican or Haitian, for example, and leaving out the term *American* even if they were born in the United States.

A Brief Historical Overview

Sometimes, in order to go forward in terms of potential remedies, it is necessary to go back and look at history to find out what the true genesis of the problem is. As previously discussed, in terms of key health indices, the health status gap between any emerging majority group and the current majority group—White people—is greatest between Black and White people. Because of the significant health disparity between Black and White people, the focus will remain on these two groups throughout this text. Some of the key indices are mortality and morbidity rates and longevity.

In considering longevity, going back to 1850, the average life expectancy of Black people was 21.4 years, in contrast to that of White people, which was 25.5 years (Talamantes et al., n.d.). It was a different time and average lifespans were much shorter than they are today. Nevertheless, the apparent gap was due to heavier labor, inadequate medical care, poorer living standards, and greater environmental exposure for Black people. Additionally, at that time, Black people were enslaved in many parts of the United States, leading to poorer health conditions. Slavery was a complex and brutal system involving many Americans, including White slavers and enslaved Black people. The involvement of medicine in the process is often excluded from historical discussions, but it is very important to the understanding of health disparities. According to Washington (2008), medical science was a key factor in terms of the persistence of enslavement because physicians needed it. It was advantageous to them both economically and for medical research. Physicians were able to advance medically because of slavery by experimenting on the bodies of Black people for their research, sometimes in gruesomely brutal ways.

Life on the plantation was particularly problematic in terms of health care. Enslaved people were fed a suboptimal diet, provided with clothing that did not provide protection from the elements, and were forced to perform labor each day that was long and hard and without the benefit of sufficient rest. When they experienced illness, they often did not receive medication. They became ill largely because of the insufficiency of their work environments. As further stated by Washington (2008), the vulnerability of enslaved Africans was more so than that of White people, primarily because of the poor construction of slave shacks. The enslaved people experienced respiratory infections due to these flimsy shacks, which enabled winter cold and summer heat to enter. Their immune systems were not accustomed to the microbes relevant to pneumonias and tuberculosis.

Moving ahead chronologically, a study in 1997 revealed that White people outlived Black people, living to 77.1 years on average, while Black people lived 71.1 years on average (Talamantes et al., n.d.). This finding leads to an obvious question: Given the ending of slavery in 1865 and a considerable difference in time, why did the gap remain? Simply put, why do White people still live longer than Black people in the United States? In exploring this question further, it is important to note that there was indeed a medical civil rights movement, which allowed for integration of African Americans into healthcare environments, but still the health status gap was not closed.

Medical Exploitation

Specific studies have pointed out that many Black people distrust White people, specifically in relation to health care, as they feel that White institutions are powerful and experiences within them are frustrating (Levy, 1985). This belief creates a scenario of distrust when seeking health care and may impact the relationship between the healthcare provider and the patient/customer. One way that Black patients/customers may get beyond their feelings of distrust is to seek healthcare providers of the same race/ethnicity, with whom they may feel more comfortable (Hopkins Tanne, 2002; Moore et al., 2023). There is often greater understanding between people who share similar cultures, values, and positive and negative experiences (Levy, 1985). Further, a person may seek out providers of the same race/ethnicity if he or she has personally experienced, or knows of, historical instances of maltreatment from one race to another.

Unfortunately, this distrust of the medical establishment by some Black people has been justified. Black people, even after the abolishment of slavery, have still fallen victim to medical exploitation and experimentation (Palmer et al., 2003). Many medical atrocities have been thoroughly documented. A key example is the oft-cited Tuskegee Syphilis Study. Beginning in July 1932, the U.S. Public Health Service enrolled approximately 400 African American men with syphilis in an experiment. The men were told that they were receiving treatment. In reality, they received no treatment for their disease. Instead, they were studied to determine the effects of the untreated disease from the time of diagnosis until their death (Gamble, 1997). Treatment became available during the course of the study, but it was never given to the men (Gamble, 1997). Most of the men were below poverty level, uneducated, and unaware that they had syphilis, and were merely told that they had "bad blood." The men suffered greatly, while their loved ones (who were also unaware that the men were not being treated) watched helplessly. To add to the atrocity, their wives and children were never tested for syphilis. It was not until 1972, 40 years after the study began, that the men who survived were told that they had syphilis and had been subjects in the study. Former President Bill Clinton would later apologize for the Tuskegee Syphilis Study, saying, "Unfortunately, what has happened in the United States cannot be undone." But it should still be discussed. President Clinton's apology was not nearly enough to remedy the atrocity committed against these Black men and their families.

Is it possible to be a unified nation when a significant portion of the people do not have trust and the United States continues to avoid confronting what happened to Black people during slavery and beyond? To discuss the entirety of the history of the atrocities committed against Black people, relative to health disparities and which largely led to the lack of health equity, requires a complete and comprehensive study of historical facts. Suffice it to say that there is shame associated with slavery in the United States and an apology is absolutely necessary as a bare minimum. Many argue that an apology is not enough and what is necessary is **reparations** for all Black people who are descendants of the enslaved people who labored in the United States. This is a contentious, political subject for some, but it is a fact that Japanese American people received reparations and an apology for their internment in the United States during World War II from the administration of President Ronald Reagan (Rosario, 2020). Given the atrocities committed against African American people during slavery, during the Jim Crow laws and beyond, why has this remedy been avoided to try to alleviate some of the pain associated with these events in history? There are explanations to try and explain the logistical differences between the Japanese reparations and offering the same for African American people (Howard-Hassman, n.d.). Howard-Hasmann points out that a number of conditions existed for the Japanese people that may be harder to establish with African American people, in terms of reparations, of which a few are: "the number of victims is relatively small; the victims are easily identifiable; many of the direct victims are still alive; the injustice took place during a relatively short time period; and the amount of reparations asked for is not so large that the public will find it unreasonable." These are some of the reasons Howard-Hasmann posits, which she concludes may make reparations challenging for African American people. Whether one agrees with those potential limitations or not, consideration and implementation of reparations would go a long way in decreasing the socioeconomic gap between Black and White people, which is a key factor in terms of health disparities and lack of health equity between these two groups.

In terms of remedies, arguably, the United States purports to be a nation of brilliant minds, vast capabilities (technologically, militarily, economically, and beyond). If this is the case, why is there a "can't do" attitude/perspective about righting wrongs that occurred involving the descendants of enslaved people in this nation? Some, at governmental levels, want Black people to speak in hushed tones about slavery or, better yet, not mention it at all. The same goes for the issues associated with **Jim Crow Laws** and other atrocities committed in this nation against Black people. According to Pilgrim (2012):

> Jim Crow was the name of the racial caste system which operated primarily, but not exclusively in southern and border states, between 1877 and the mid-1960s. Jim Crow was more than a series of rigid anti-Black laws. It was a way of life.

This involves the banning of books that discuss these topics as well as lambasting or canceling scholars who want to bring these discussions to the forefront. It is an uncanny sense of denial that will never lead to remedies, but rather to more problems. Until this nation addresses the atrocities committed against Black people in the United States and offers an apology and other remedies (e.g., reparations), healing in terms of health disparities and other areas where there is a gap between Black and White people will be difficult to achieve.

In considering the Tuskegee Syphilis Study mentioned earlier, Spencer (2010) offers a poignant response to President Clinton's words: President Clinton offered an apology in 1997, which revealed the pain that individuals believe had ended long ago. However, African American people were impacted gravely. One could examine Tuskegee, as one example of many atrocities, to gain insight as to why there is a lack of trust of the medical establishment, by some African American people, which is contributing, unintentionally, to the continuance of health disparities. This study, and other forms of medical and research mistreatment, has led many Black people to distrust and fear medical care in the United States. Other forms of mistreatment, oppression, and covert and overt racism have led some members of the Black race, and members of other racial groups, to distrust the medical and public health establishments.

REMEDIES

- An official apology from the United States government for slavery.
- Reparations for descendants of enslaved Black people in the United States.
- No hindrance (banning of books, etc.) directed towards people of the United States who want to share the full, true history of the atrocities committed against Black people during slavery, Jim Crow laws and beyond, which directly/indirectly contribute to health disparities and lack of health equity between Black and White people.

Barriers to Seeking Care

Beyond mistrust of the medical establishment, there are other issues, such as lack of cultural competence and a shortage of Black physicians, that impose a barrier for Black people in seeking medical care. The United States has a long history of lack of access to health care for non-White people. This history of unequal access and quality of care created, and continues to foster, an environment of higher morbidity and mortality rates among the various emerging majority groups. This lack of, or insufficient access to, health care in the United States has led to poorer health, **health inequality**, and a widening health status gap between the emerging majority and current majority populations. These trends have raised alarms about the impact of a skewed distribution of societal resources on social and physical well-being. Public health officials have called attention to this problem and pledged to reduce it (Adler & Stewart, 2010).

Myriad Reasons for Health Disparities

It is generally understood that in the United States, which is the country of emphasis regarding health disparities in this text, the White, currently majority, population has a higher health status than do members of the Black/African American population. The goal here is to understand why. Beyond understanding, the next goal is to figure out how to remedy this disparity. What is the reason that White people are healthier than Black people in the United States? There are many reasons, with the first being reliable health care coverage. According to the Kaiser Family Foundation (Ndugga et al., 2024), cost, affordability, and access to care are all contributing factors as certain groups are impacted by these issues more than others—namely, emerging majorities who are Black, Hispanic/Latino, Asian, Native Hawaiian and Pacific Islander, Native American, and American Indian and Alaska Native people. Examples of important health disparities per Heywood (2023) are as follows:

> Despite having lower rates than White people, Black people in the United States are 30% more likely to die from heart disease.
>
> Black adults in the United States are 30% more likely to experience obesity than white adults. This disparity is even greater for children and teens (50%) and women (50%). Obesity is a risk factor for several conditions on this list and can contribute to worse outcomes pertaining to other conditions.

These problems, as examples of many more, persist in the face of research and a constant barrage of information about their existence. Remedies must be sought to resolve them rather than constant long-term discussion about them in various health care fields, including but not limited to public health and medicine.

White Privilege Versus White Hindrance

Beyond the health disparities that exist, there are some factors, outside of the realm of health specifically, that contribute to the problem. One that is quite pervasive is the notion of White privilege. White privilege is a term that is very negative but should be explored briefly. Use of the term *emerging majority* when describing Black people in this nation is critical, as the demographics are rapidly changing to a point where Black and Brown people will be the majority in the United States and are already the majority in some locations (states, cities, etc.). Use of the term *White privilege* should also be reconsidered as "privilege" has a positive connotation. It refers to a right. For example, if you are in a work environment and you meet or exceed a certain standard, you may be given the privilege of having a higher position or promotion or receiving more pay. Privilege actually makes a person proud. There is no way that anyone should be proud of unearned privilege due to their race. Some White people may actually comment about how they benefit from white privilege and how they feel it is not right. Many Black people constantly express concern about the privilege afforded to White people. White skin is not an inherent privilege that anyone should honor above others. In fact, we should re-label the term **White hindrance** rather than white privilege. When people move through life benefitting simply by virtue of the color of their skin, whether they acknowledge it or not, it should be pointed out that this hinders others from achieving what they deserve/earn. Hence, this kind of undeserved benefit must be viewed as an impediment to the progress of others and must be stamped out wherever it is seen.

Specifically, the predominance of White people in academia, healthcare professions, the arts, media, and every walk of life in the United States must end. We see Black people dominating in athletics as athletes, but those at the top, making all of the decisions and earning the most substantial share of the money, are largely White people. All of this is White hindrance because White people are taking most of the premier leadership spots while hindering Black people from achieving the same goals. In terms of health care, acknowledging this hindrance would be tremendous, as it will give the opportunity to ensure more Black educators/practitioners in public health, medicine, and other health professions are represented in their respective fields. Similar actions can be taken to recruit Black students in these fields and beyond. If this society is serious about remedies regarding health disparities, every effort should be made to ensure some level of parity in terms of selection, to eliminate Predominantly White Institutions (PWIs), especially those that have very low numbers of Black people. There are larger issues for some Black applicants of meeting requisite requirements to apply/be accepted to PWIs given that some, resource-wise, may have attended institutions prior to higher education that are not up to standard. Given the socioeconomic status gap between Black and White people, some White communities, when higher socioeconomic status is the case, have many advantages over Black communities where people are experiencing poverty. This speaks to broader educational inequities that must be remedied, to be discussed in a later chapter in this book.

Limited Perspectives

The preceding sections are mere examples of the myriad issues, which exemplify the health disparities that exist between Black and White people in the United States. Factors contributing to poor health outcomes among African American people include discrimination, cultural, linguistic and literacy barriers, and lack of access to health care. Unfortunately, there are also examples of limited perspectives as the rationale for the disparity between Black and White people, specifically the argument that genetics is the key factor. Some may argue that, genetically, there are illnesses that tend to exist within the Black population that contribute to their overall lower health statistics. Race continues to be one of the most politically charged subjects in American life; it involves a sociocultural component that often leads to misleading and inappropriate categorizations (Kittles & Weiss, 2003). According to an Institution of Medicine Committee Report, "genetics cannot provide a single all-purpose human classification scheme that will be adequate for addressing all of the multifaceted dimensions of health differentials" (Hernandez & Blazer, 2006). As stated by Duello et al. (2021):

> . . .the majority of the health disparities experienced by [African American people] are due to social determinants of health, thus, while genetic discoveries and new technologies offer great promise, the public should not be led to believe that genetic solutions to health disparities are imminent given that 34 million Americans have not completed high school, 38.1 million live below the poverty level, 13.55 million are unemployed and 44 million are without health insurance.

The argument of genetics, therefore, has no substantial basis as a valid and sole explanation for health disparities. There are other contributing factors to this gap, to add to those mentioned earlier, such as socioeconomic status, education levels, diet, and health literacy. These factors have a great impact on the gap between the health status of Black people and other emerging majority groups and that of the White population in the United States. Hence, exploring these factors in depth not only leads to a greater understanding, but also creates an opportunity to explore potential remedies. Although the remedies are sometimes complicated, they are not unachievable. The United States leads the world in healthcare spending. However, it is the only industrialized nation that does not ensure that all citizens have health coverage.

REMEDIES

- Universal health care for all, which will increase access to care for Black people in the United States.
- Eliminate White privilege via an acknowledgement that it is actually white hindrance and significantly diversify PWIs to the point that the term PWI (and the reality of it) does not exist anymore in academia, healthcare institutions, and beyond in the United States.
- Recognition that genetics is not an explanation for health disparities in the United States in terms of Black people but rather social determinants as many of the illnesses that exist for Black people in the United States are not prevalent in Africa where Black people in the United States descended from.

Persistence of Health Disparities

A look back over the past 35 years shows acknowledgment, on behalf of the U.S. government, that the worsening health disparity gap between emerging majority and current majority populations warranted attention and resources. Various initiatives were implemented and new federal-level offices were created in an effort to address emerging majority health issues, the tremendous gap in health disparities, and the worsening emerging majority health status. In 1984, the U.S. Department of Health and Human Services released "Health, United States, 1983," a report on the health of the nation. The report documented that although the overall health of the nation showed significant progress, major disparities existed in "the burden of death and illness experienced by Black people and other [emerging majority people in the United States] as compared with the nation's population as a whole" (Gibbons, 2005, p. 2).

In 1985, the release of the "Report of the Secretary's Task Force on Black and Minority Health" significantly raised awareness of the disparate health of the country's minority groups as compared with the White majority population (Gibbons, 2005).

"Unequal Treatment," a 2003 report by the Institute of Medicine (IOM), significantly raised the level of awareness and attention given to emerging majority health and health disparities (Institute of Medicine, 2003). According to the report, in 1999, Congress requested that the IOM: (1) assess the extent of racial and ethnic disparities in health care, assuming that access-related factors, such as insurance status and the ability to pay for care are the same; (2) identify potential sources of these disparities; and (3) suggest intervention strategies (Institute of Medicine, 2003). The study committee reported being struck by what it found (Institute of Medicine, 2003): "Even among the better-controlled studies, the vast majority [of published research] indicated that minorities are less likely than White people to receive needed services, including clinically necessary procedures," even after correcting for access-related factors, such as insurance status. In general, the research showed the following:

- Black/African American and Black Hispanic/Latino people tend to receive a lower quality of health care across a range of disease areas (including cancer, cardiovascular disease, diabetes, mental health, and other chronic and infectious diseases) and clinical services.
- Black/African American people are more likely than White people to receive less desirable services, such as amputation of all or part of a limb.
- Disparities are found even when clinical factors, such as stage of disease presentation, comorbidities, age, and severity of disease, are explored.
- Disparities are found across a range of clinical settings, including public and private hospitals, teaching and nonteaching hospitals, and so on.

Emerging majority people experience many health challenges more frequently and more severely than do Non-Hispanic/Latino White people, and they often receive lower-quality care, which leads to poorer health outcomes. Given the diversity of the U.S. population, comparative effectiveness research should capture the health outcomes of racial and Hispanic groups and investigate whether disparities reflect variations in care or different responses to treatment (Mullins et al., 2010). Racial and ethnic emerging majority patients are less likely to be placed in rehabilitation than are Non-Hispanic/Latino White patients, even after accounting for insurance status, suggesting the existence of systemic inequalities in access. Such inequalities may have a disproportionate impact on long-term functional outcomes of African American and Hispanic traumatic brain injury patients and suggests the need for an in-depth analysis of this disparity at a health policy level (Shafi et al., 2007).

Differences among racial and ethnic groups are pronounced; for example, about twice as many Black and Hispanic/Latino people report being in fair or poor health than do White people (Adler & Stewart, 2010). Differences are even greater by socioeconomic status; almost five times as many adults who are experiencing poverty report fair or poor health compared with those with the highest income (Adler & Stewart, 2010). These findings are consistent with the National Healthcare Quality and Disparities Reports and suggest little progress in eliminating health disparities among emerging majority groups. Additionally, education is significant because there is a correlation between health outcomes and years in school. There is no doubt that education impacts employment, social status, and other factors.

However, in American society, education alone may not be sufficient to explain differences in health outcomes because African American people with high education levels (college) also may have poorer health outcomes when compared to their White counterparts. Differences in health outcomes may have more to do with exposure to positive or negative healthcare practices generationally; for example, African American people are descendants of enslaved people and thus may have inherited the dietary preferences of enslaved people that have been passed on from one generation to the next, including highly seasoned and fried foods and other preparation methods that are less healthy than the foods and preparation methods of other groups. Research was conducted in St. Louis, Missouri, in which the eating habits of the early African Americans were explored. The following was determined:

> During slavery they subsisted on "scraps" from the master's table, second-line (imperfect) crops, and pork. Organ meats, such as brains or liver, fried foods, highly salted vegetables (greens) and unusual animal parts generally discarded by the master were prepared to ingenious fashions to add flavor. Cattle and beef were usually consumed by Whites. Pig snoots, pig feet, brains, chitterlings, and tripe became the cuisine of the African American culture (Kosoko-Lasaki et al., 2009).

Furthermore, African American people, who live largely in poorer socioeconomic conditions, are more apt to be first-generation college students, and may also have issues associated with lack of cultural competence when seeking health care. However, mindfulness regarding the use of the term "first-generation college student" is necessary. It seems that a stigma is placed on students who are referred to in this way, as there are students of all races whose parents or guardians may not have gone to college. This is a term that is often used when referring to emerging majority students, before verifying if this is the case.

Again, the less-than-positive health outcomes for African American people are in part a result of eating patterns and culture; Kosoko-Lasaki et al. (2009) discuss these patterns and their cultural significance:

> A very interesting article from the 2001 *Journal of Archaeology*, entitled "Ham Hocks on Your Cornflakes" examined the role of food in the African American Identity. Excavations in Annapolis, Maryland, and 13 other sites

in the Chesapeake region were explored. Findings were consistent; food remains showed a definite pattern. Pork was much more commonly consumed than beef, and shallow water fish not typically purchased from markets where Whites typically shopped predominated. Apparently, by the late 19th century as Whites turned to beef, Blacks did not … For many people, eating particular foods serves not only as a fulfilling experience, but also a liberating one—an added way of making some kind of declaration. Consumption then is at the same time a form of self-identification and communication. Blacks living under the oppression of slavery, with very few options, gathered at the end of the day for a communal meal with friends and family. They most likely found spiritual strength and regeneration through eating and camaraderie. This experience over generations became a part of the culture.

Soul Food and Diet-Related Diseases

It is important to be aware of those diseases that are food related in exploring **food injustice** issues and how they contribute to health disparities. Included among those diseases are the following (Chowdhury, 2024):

- Hypertension
- Cancer
- Diabetes
- Heart disease
- Obesity

When considering the health status of lower-income communities, it is clear that there is a high prevalence of such diseases. In exploring health disparities per the members of lower-income Black/African American communities, as an example, it is evident that a contributing cause of such diseases is the type of food consumed. For this population, it is necessary to consider foods still eaten today that pertain to slavery and a cultural norm that emerged from it. From a cultural vantage point, eating this type of food, affectionately known as **soul food** or "food for the soul," enables the preservation of a survivalist aspect of a group of people who experienced severe oppression and denigration in a society where they were considered less than human. Soul food was, therefore, more than just food; it was a coping mechanism (Slocum, 2010). Although, for the most part, this food is fatty in content and highly salted, which increases sodium intake and can lead to hypertension and stroke, it continues to be a key aspect of food preparation for many Black/African American people (Airhihenbuwa et al., 1996).

Although most people of African descent in the United States are thought to be from West Africa, you will not find soul food eaten on the continent of Africa. As discussed previously, it was the conditions of slavery in the United States that led to this form of food preparation. Therefore, the role of food in disease processes can be appreciated by comparing the illnesses experienced by African people on the continent of Africa to those experienced by Black/African American people. Indeed, the marked differences found rule out the genetic factor as the cause of many illnesses in Black/African American people. It is clear that the movement of African American people from the continent of Africa, mainly West Africa, to the United States to serve as enslaved people, and the ensuing forms of oppression experienced, including poor-quality food, have contributed gravely to health disparities. Unfortunately, as a consequence of the desire for some Black/African American people to eat soul food, marketing efforts foster this desire, particularly in low-income communities, and fail to promote healthier choices, including organic foods and those that are more healthfully prepared (Airhihenbuwa et al., 1996).

It is unfortunate that the food preparation methods and choices of Black people in the United States, practices that continue for many, evolved from such an awful historical context involving slavery, segregation, and persecution (James, 2004). Why do many Black/African American people continue this eating behavior if it is leading to negative health experiences? This is a complicated question because the problem is multifactorial. Lack of understanding, depending on one's educational level and/or nutritional insight, of the problems associated with eating food that is not prepared with health in mind is the first issue. Additionally, there are factors of socioeconomic status and food deserts and mirages, to be discussed at a later point in this chapter. For those who may want to change, accessibility and affordability of healthy foods is often the problem, depending on socioeconomic status. It is difficult to acquire whole grains, organic fruits, vegetables, and other healthy food items and, therefore, much easier to find, afford, prepare, and then consume foods that have high fat, salt, and sugar content, even if the cost is hypertension and other food-related illnesses (Jetter & Casady, 2006).

Because soul food is very tasty, it connotes a skill set in the kitchen that many Black people have passed on from generation to generation, and enjoying it is often a communal, familial experience. Therefore, some people who appreciate it do not want to let it go. The only way to begin to change/modify this pattern of eating would be to approach it comprehensively, from a multidimensional and multifaceted perspective, taking into consideration the interdependent nature of individual, cultural, and communal factors. Furthermore, the higher prevalence of convenience stores and other entities that mainly provide energy-dense, high-sodium-content and processed foods would need to be eliminated so as to decrease exposure, acquisition, and consumption of unhealthy foods (Smith & Morton, 2009).

Food Injustice

In lower-income communities in the United States, supermarket availability is very limited, and in stores located in these communities, the quality of food is lower than that of food sold in higher-income communities (Bower et al., 2014). Also, in lower-income communities, there are often small grocery shops, known as convenience stores (**Figure 3-1**).

These stores generally have food supplies on their shelves that are high in fat and sugar and are energy dense (Bower et al., 2014). As a result, individuals who live in communities with these types of stores as their predominant source of food acquisition will have diets of lesser quality compared with individuals who live in communities with large supermarkets that offer a great deal of food variety. This disparity/gap in the offering of quality foods has a direct impact on the health status of those who live in communities where this problem prevails (Bower et al., 2014). The old adage, "You are what you eat," therefore, becomes evident.

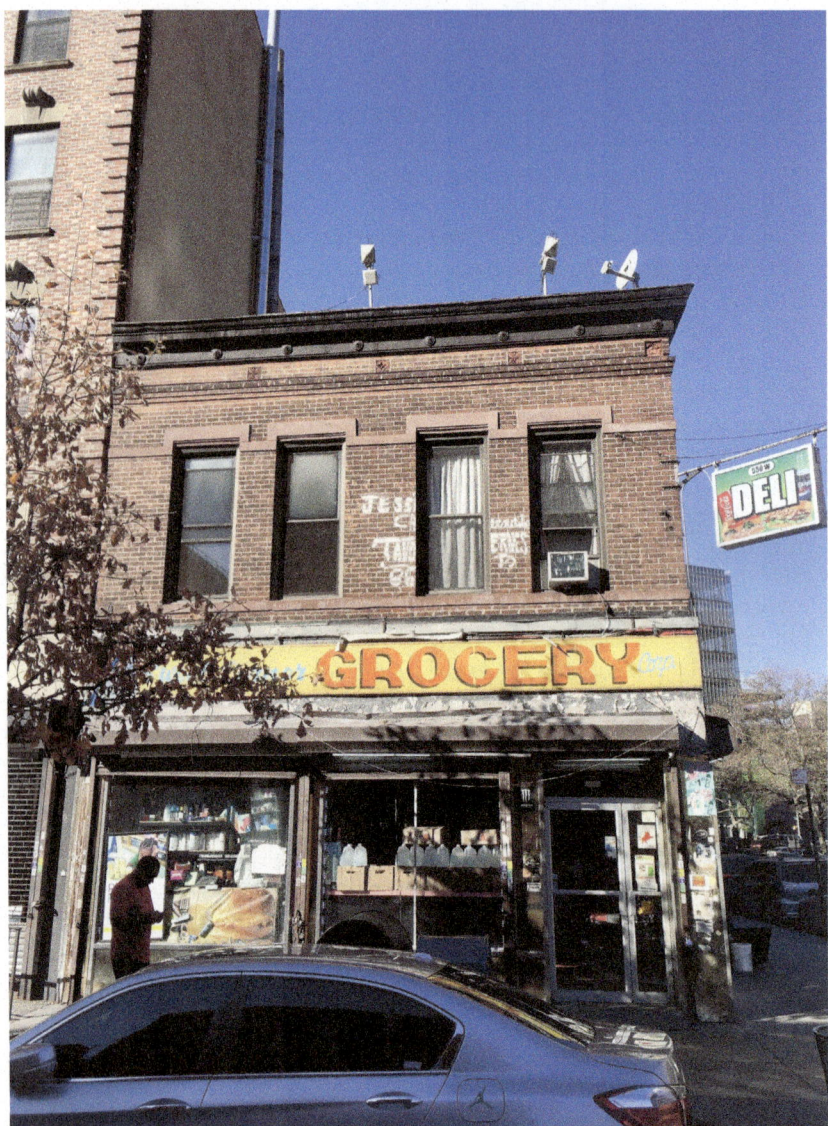

Figure 3-1 Small grocery stores known as convenience stores are found in many communities where people are experiencing low incomes.
© Here Now/Shutterstock

Food Deserts and Food Mirages

Food deserts and **food mirages** are highly problematic and are indicative of an interface between poverty, lack of food access, and poor health outcomes (Breyer & Voss-Andreae, 2013). In the United States, healthy foods are usually acquired through large supermarkets. These types of supermarkets are typically not found in low-income neighborhoods. People living in low-income neighborhoods often have

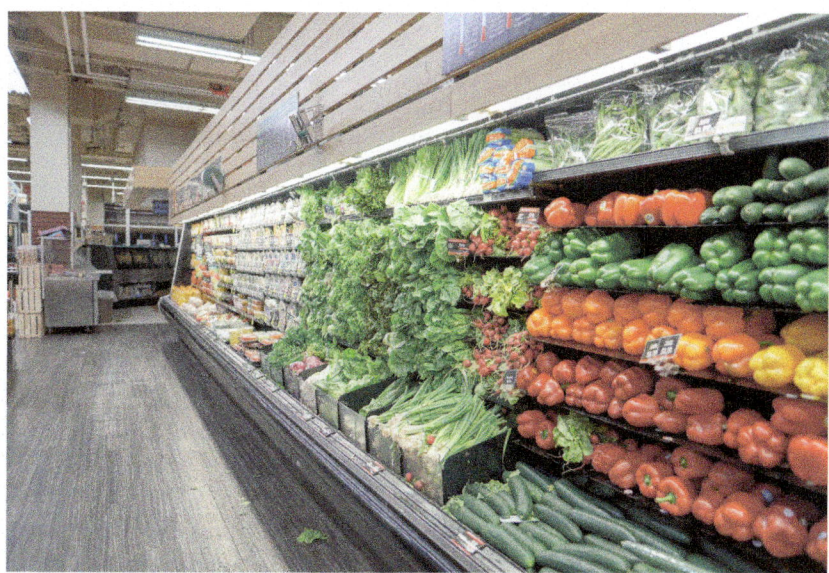

Figure 3-2 Large grocery stores with fresh produce are often not found in communities where people are experiencing low incomes.
© Sorbis/Shutterstock

difficulty accessing the stores because of transportation issues. They are less likely to find stores, such as Whole Foods and other large markets that carry healthy foods, including organic products, without traveling great distances (**Figure 3-2**). These types of markets are generally not in the census blocks of these neighborhoods (Galvez et al., 2008).

Supermarkets are needed in low-income neighborhoods, because without them, community members lack access to healthy foods, including fruits, vegetables, and other essential items that enhance health. In short, this issue of lack of accessibility to healthy foods due to low socioeconomic status is a contributing factor to health disparities (Galvez et al., 2008).

In terms of food mirages, the clarifying fact is the reality that the price of food is skyrocketing, due to inflation in general, in the United States. Consequently, even in low-income neighborhoods where there are actual large grocery stores that include a wide selection of healthy foods, if the individuals who live in the neighborhood cannot afford to shop there, the stores are merely mirages (Breyer & Voss-Andreae, 2013). Specifically, a market may offer a choice between fresh produce and processed food. Individuals will often go into such markets and choose processed foods because they are less expensive. Based on their budgets, choosing the cheaper foods is logical. Budgets and household income are key considerations in food acquisition and quality (Breyer & Voss-Andreae, 2013). It is a complicated situation because if supermarkets are built in low-income neighborhoods, the people cannot afford the food, and food mirages result. Yet, if supermarkets are built outside of poor communities, individuals cannot get to them, and even if they do, they cannot afford the healthy products that are inside of them, which results in food deserts (**Table 3-1**).

Table 3-1 Food Deserts and Mirages

Food Mirages	Food Deserts
Supermarkets build in low-income neighborhoods.	Supermarkets build outside of poor communities.
People cannot afford the food.	Individuals cannot get to them due to lack of transportation and cannot afford the food, were they to reach them, due to limited economic resources.

Foods Available in Communities Having Lower Incomes

Unfortunately, rather than healthy foods with significant variety, in communities where people are experiencing lower incomes, there are many fast-food restaurants (**Figure 3-3**). From a geographic exposure vantage point, in these neighborhoods, which are often predominantly comprised of Black people, eating food from fast-food restaurants is expedient, convenient, and more affordable (**Table 3-2**).

In fact, in many neighborhoods where low incomes are experienced, there are 2.4 fast-food restaurants per square mile compared with 1.5 in predominantly White neighborhoods (Galvez et al., 2008). It would seem that such affordability and accessibility would be positive, but the contrary is true. Obesity is a major problem in communities where people are experiencing low income. There is very likely a relationship between fast food and obesity, making fast food a contributing

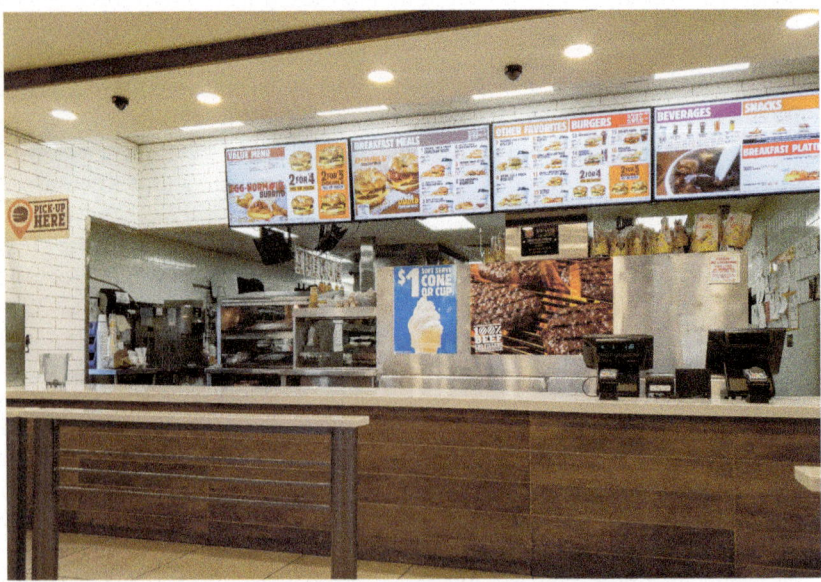

Figure 3-3 Fast food restaurants are pervasive in communities where people are experiencing low incomes.
© Kit Leong/Shutterstock

Table 3-2 **Options in Communities Where People are Experiencing Low Incomes**

Small Community Grocery Stores	Fast-Food Restaurants	Alcohol and Cigarettes
Inventory is convenient but limited.	Food is cheap and easily accessible.	These items are easily accessible in low-income communities.
Prices are higher than in supermarkets.	Individuals with limited income flock to them to feed themselves and their families.	People may turn to alcohol and cigarettes as coping mechanisms.
Access to healthy food choices is limited.	Nutritional value is questionable at best and problematic at worst.	Sellers of these items are available in excess in low-income communities.

factor to the health disparities among these communities and others—namely, between emerging majorities and the White population. Per Jia et al. (2021):

> It is widely accepted that some environmental factors in the neighborhood may interact with personal characteristics to affect individual weight status. Fast-food restaurants (FFRs) are one of such environmental factors, which are defined as food venues primarily engaged in providing food services (except snack and non-alcoholic beverage bars) where patrons generally order or select items and pay before eating.

The nutritional content of foods available in areas where people are experiencing low-incomes is not the only consideration in this discussion. Because the produce and other food items that are accessible are not organic, much of what is available is most likely sprayed heavily with pesticides, and poultry and meat are filled with antibiotics and hormones, etc.

REMEDIES

- The United States government entities that are charged with the quality of health must ensure that Black people receive the same quality of care that is received by their White counterparts in all aspects of health care received.
- Medical professionals, public health and nutrition practitioners, etc. must be taught the history of slavery in the United States and the food culture that emerged for some Black people, known as soul food, so that modification efforts can be suggested with knowledge, insight, respect, and care for Black people.
- The placement of supermarkets in Black communities where people are experiencing low incomes/poverty so that they are able to buy, affordably, fresh produce and foods that are not processed and high in sodium (generally unhealthy).
- Eliminate all food deserts and food mirages in Black communities where people are experiencing lower incomes/poverty.

In specifically looking at food-related illnesses, as mentioned previously, and continuing with the example of Black/African American people, there is a clear indication that hypertension rates are higher in this group compared with any other group, particularly White people (National Center for Health Statistics, 2015). There are other diseases, including cancer and diabetes, that relate to health disparities and food injustice.

Educational Disparities

To fully comprehend health disparities in the United States, another important topic to consider is education. In continuing to explore the two groups for which there is the widest health disparity, one notable fact is that Black/African American people are more likely to attend "high-poverty schools" that are under-resourced than are their White counterparts (American Psychological Association, 2017). Although there are complicated reasons for the educational disparity, one of the primary issues is taxes. A significant portion of local property taxes is used to fund schools. Hence, the amount of money that a school receives is based on the socioeconomic status of the surrounding community. Unfortunately, many Black/African American people experience a lower socioeconomic status, and many do not own property. When they do own property, it often generates less tax revenue due to its comparatively low property value. Consequently, in many largely Black/African American communities, there is less money to fund schools. As stated by Duncan-Andrade and Morrell (2008), "We are not a nation of opportunity for all, but a nation built upon grand narratives of opportunity for all." These issues of educational disparity are relevant to many Black communities in the United States because according to the U.S. Census Bureau, Black people have the highest poverty rate and the lowest median income (DeNavas-Walt et al., 2011).

Because the schools in Black/African American neighborhoods often do not have sufficient resources compared with schools in predominantly White neighborhoods where the tax base is usually higher, Black/African American students largely experience an educational disadvantage, including lack of sufficient textbooks, limited (or altogether absence of) technology, and lack of equipment for labs, physical education, art, music, and other programs. Consequently, their overall curriculum is less rigorous, with lower expectations from the students and teachers as compared to their White counterparts (American Psychological Association, 2017). Unfortunately, the outcome of a lower-quality, less-resourced education is less opportunity to progress by attending college or finding decent work, which often leads to remaining in low socioeconomic status communities, perpetuating the problem from one generation to the next.

Health Literacy

As mentioned, there are serious weaknesses in the U.S. educational system that largely stem from the fact that people of lower socioeconomic status do not have access to the same educational resources as the rest of society. This disparity parallels that of the health status gap in that **people of color** do not fare as well in terms of education or health compared with their White counterparts, as the latter have the power and wealth in society and hence more resources available to them in both education and health.

The definition of **health literacy** is "the ability to obtain, process, and understand basic health information and services needed to make appropriate health decisions" (Institute of Medicine, 2004). Furthermore, according to a report by the Institute of Medicine (2001), patient-centered care is "care that is respectful of and responsive to individual patient preferences, needs, and values."

Furthermore, the problems of poverty and low educational levels lead to diminished health literacy, which impacts the health of individuals. This problem intersects deeply with culture because, often, educational attainment is intertwined with culture and language proficiency, and in the field of health care, there is a lack of awareness of these issues. There must be accountability in the field of health care and assurance that all involved will understand how health literacy and **linguistic competence** impact health to develop creative and innovative approaches to provide patients/customers with health information. Within the context of such innovation, there must be knowledge of the fact that individuals who may be experiencing a lower socioeconomic status, who are predominantly people of color, have less access to the Internet and other forms of technology (**digital divide**). Therefore, innovative approaches must include different mediums for providing health information. Getting around this digital divide may include use of print sources (taking literacy levels into consideration), broadcast media, such as radio and television, and one-on-one discussions with patients.

REMEDIES

- Eliminate the local property tax allocation of resources to public schools process and ensure that funding for all public schools is the same with significant federal contribution.
- Close the digital divide and provide information via other mediums, besides computer related technology, in communities where health information is limited to increase health literacy.
- The government must provide Wi-Fi in every community, especially for those people who are experiencing low incomes and who are experiencing poverty, as well as access to computers and technology training.

Summary of Remedies

Significant detail is provided in this chapter regarding myriad health-related problems impacting Black/African American people. Rather than dwelling on what the problems are, as these have been identified in terms of research, books, and beyond over significant periods of time, the question is: What are the remedies for these issues? The following sections provide an overview of the remedies mentioned for some of the problems/issues listed in this chapter. Perhaps considering some, or all, of these remedies will lead to further consideration and development of new ideas from a forward thinking, positive approach.

Food Injustice Remedies

Ultimately, food injustice is a result of many factors. For example, if one considers the socioeconomic status of Black people compared with White people, the health statuses of the respective groups show some salient differences. Thus, health disparities are not the effect of differences inherent to a particular race, but pertain to outside factors. To resolve the problem, relevant factors must be identified, including the following:

- Politics
- Education
- Culture
- Socioeconomic status

It would seem that community-based models would be most effective, as research has clearly outlined the problems. Changes, such as the development of large supermarkets in communities where there are only convenience stores, will be very helpful in providing an opportunity for healthy eating. Reducing prices in these large supermarkets would be necessary through creative approaches toward providing produce and healthy unprocessed foods. These steps would go a long way toward remedying the problem. Another step would be the elimination of fast-food restaurants and liquor stores appearing pervasively in communities experiencing low incomes.

Self-Help Remedies

Individuals and communities must be provided with health information that will help with the implementation of self-help remedies. For heart disease, it is important to pay attention to one's weight and keep it moderate. Other important steps are to check blood pressure regularly. Inexpensive blood pressure monitors can be purchased/donated via health organizations and the actual entities that make these devices so that individuals can review their blood pressure. This will enable their keeping of their own records to share and discuss with a healthcare provider, if necessary. It also helps if a person knows his or her family health history to identify any potential pre-existing conditions. Providing individuals with insight as to why family health history is important will be very useful for generations of families. In terms of obesity, eating habits matter. In communities where people are experiencing poverty, finding fresh produce and other healthy food items might be difficult. Some communities have established community gardens which can be quite helpful in terms of nutrition, mental health, income, and the sense of companionship in the community (One New Humanity, n.d.).

In terms of diabetes, weight management is also very important, which can be accomplished through a balanced diet and regular exercise. Often, in the White communities, where socioeconomic status is often higher, statistically, many hold gym or country club memberships or live in communities where they can walk or run freely or have space/equipment in their homes to exercise. Black people, who are experiencing lower incomes, need similar opportunities. Blood sugar levels also have to be managed in terms of diabetes. Hypertension also involves a balanced diet so the suggestions provided earlier are also relevant. There is also the additional step of avoiding/managing stress and lowering salt and alcohol intake. Knowing the importance of this health information, along with diet modification, would be very helpful.

As with the case of heart disease, overall, it is helpful to monitor blood pressure as described in this chapter. Some of the same steps can be taken in terms of strokes, with the addition of eliminating smoking, if that is a factor, along with knowing the signs and symptoms associated with stroke known as **FAST**. Per Madell (2018), the acronym FAST stands for:

F for face—a droop or uneven smile on a person's face (warning sign)

A for arms—Arm numbness or weakness (warning sign)

S for speech difficulty—Slurred speech

T for time—time to act fast

Modification of Soul Food Preparation as a Remedy

Based on the history of soul food and its tendency to be simultaneously delicious and unhealthy, depending on how it is prepared, it seems that the best remedy would be modification. For any group of people indulging in these delicacies—particularly the group of focus in this chapter, Black people—the best approach would not be to recommend against eating soul food, but rather to modify the recipes. Soul food, for some, has become a cultural norm and the preparations are quite tasty. Hence, adding a "healthy twist" without compromising the dishes too much and retaining the delicious taste is the way to go. Some approaches to modification, as examples, include:

- Use of organic ingredients
- Cut down salt (e.g., use Himalayan pink salt)
- Hormone and antibiotic free poultry
- Hormone and antibiotic free, grass-fed meat
- No margarine, little butter
- Olive oil instead of saturated fat (e.g., lard)
- Cooking vegetables briefly or steaming them to retain nutrients
- Avoiding the use of excessive sugar and replacing with honey
- Reduction of the consumption of fried food

Although these are mere examples, with explanations by Doctors/Nutritionists as to how and why to modify, important cultural eating norms will be maintained while simultaneously promoting good eating habits.

Unfortunately, most medical school curriculums often do not include nutrition courses. Per David Eisenberg: "Today, most medical schools in the United States teach less than 25 hours of nutrition over four years. The fact that less than 20 percent of medical schools have a single required course in nutrition, it's a scandal. It's outrageous. It's obscene." (Harvard T. H. Chan School of Public Health, 2017) Medical schools that have taken this leap are preparing doctors to take the lead with this remedy, in a positive direction. According to Minor (2019), "Physicians who completed Stanford Medicine's Introduction to Food and Health CME course, for example, reported being far more likely to discuss various aspects of nutrition with their patients. Minor (2019) further states: And a formal study of a patient-facing version of the same course—with more than 200,000 people enrolled to-date—found that it produced positive changes in patients' eating behaviors and meal composition at home. Such courses for patients should be offered in communities where they live, Community Health Centers, at their doctor's offices in waiting rooms, etc. Brochures, Social Media and other mediums should be used to get this information to patients who may/may not have it readily available to them.

Nutritionists are usually seen by referral, based on the identification of the need for one or a request by the patient/customer. Sometimes, due to lack of basic healthcare access, the added request for a nutritionist is not an option. Often times, doctors/nutritionists have no idea about the history of soul food, its indoctrination into the culture of some Black people, and why it has maintained a loving place there. These health professionals may abruptly indicate the removal of such foods from the diet to their patients, which can be interpreted as insulting or impossible for them to fathom. The remedy for the latter is to ensure that nutrition and the history of the foods of various cultures should be added to the curriculum of healthcare practitioners, such as doctors, nurse practitioners, physician assistants, and beyond. Of course, this is not an exhaustive list of healthcare practitioners but mere examples. The same is the case for public health practitioners and health educators. However, it must be acknowledged that although education provides one with more information and insight into what it takes to be healthy, it may not be enough to override social factors and long-term exposure to cultural norms.

The issue of socioeconomic status and other factors are clearly documented but in terms of those individuals who are economically strong and Black, one important step towards remedying this problem is further analysis to understand the essential factors. This research is warranted as a higher income does not necessarily connote health improvement for Black people in the United States. It seems that this is due to factors often beyond the control of Black people, namely social injustice, failed policies, stress, the experience of racism, discrimination and beyond. Understanding the causal factors in depth, and showing causation, rather than correlation, will go a long way in terms of remedying the problem. The healthcare industry is a business in the United States, meaning its objective is not, in and of itself, to meet the nation's health needs, but to maximize profits. Simultaneously, poverty is on the rise leaving many people financially unable to meet their healthcare needs, which disproportionately impacts the Black population. At the federal, state, and local levels, efforts have been less than successful in curbing poverty trends, particularly among individuals of emerging majority groups, especially Black/African American people. There are clear associations between health disparities and **social injustice** in a number of categories based on socioeconomic status, including food quality/availability, education, mass incarceration, and employment. The ultimate remedy is to resolve all of these issues, without further delay as the bulk of the problems have been researched and understood. The goal now must be to fix them in order for Black/African American people to thrive in the United States.

WRAP-UP

Understanding the history of the United States as it pertains to Black/African American people is crucial if remedies are to be implemented to achieve health equity. It is important to understand important factors, such as which foods are eaten by some, why, if any aspect of the preparation is unhealthy, and how the preparation can be modified without disrupting what may have become cultural norms. Every effort must be made to ensure that people who are experiencing poverty in Black communities have opportunities to exercise in safe and aesthetically pleasant places and have access to healthy produce and supermarkets that stock, at affordable prices, products that are conducive to good health. Social injustice plays a critical role in the perpetuation of health disparities in the United States. Issues, such as food injustice, in its various forms, and health illiteracy must be addressed. There is a lack of quality education and health literacy in low socioeconomic status communities, primarily among people of color. Every effort must be made to ensure that the largest racial emerging majority group in the nation has the same opportunity as the White community to thrive in a state of optimal health and well-being without views that are limited in scope (such as blaming genetics) and systemic oppression serving to curtail remedies to fix problems. Emphasis must no longer be placed on the problems but rather the remedies if health equity is to be achieved.

Black people can also be instrumental themselves in looking toward better, healthier outcomes. Of course, in their efforts to do so, society at large, policy makers, healthcare practitioners, public health administrators, and all aspects of society that contribute to health disparities must take into consideration the structural issues that exist in terms of social injustice, including discrimination, lack of access to care, and beyond. These issues must be addressed in order for health equity to be achieved for Black people in the United States. Remedies must be implemented that include but are not limited to the following:

1. Ensure universal, affordable, and equitable health coverage
2. Self-help remedies, including checking blood pressure, weight management, monitoring glucose levels, managing stress, lowering salt intake, etc.
3. An official apology to Black/African American people by the government of the United States for slavery
4. The provision of reparations for descendants of enslaved Black people in the United States
5. Modification of soul food by those Black people who eat it, with an understanding that this should be the recommendation by healthcare providers rather than suggestions to eliminate it completely
6. Nutrition courses as a curriculum requirement for all physicians that covers types of foods eaten within various racial groups, e.g., soul food for some African American people
7. The provision of health literature to individuals in communities with limited access to technology using non-technological forms of information (pamphlets, brochures, etc.) where appropriate, given the digital divide
8. Implementation of processes in the health professions, including medicine and beyond to ensure more Black applicants and graduates leading to better representation in various healthcare fields

Chapter Problems

1. Explain the difference between White privilege and White hindrance.
2. Health disparities, health literacy, and social injustice are all-important issues that people in the field of health care should understand. Why?
3. There are specific differences between food mirages and food deserts. Explain.

4.   List three diet-related diseases that are specifically contributing to health disparities among Black/African American people.

5.   Name one problem and one remedy specifically pertaining to Black people and health equity.

References

Adler, N. E., & Stewart, J. (2010). Health disparities across the lifespan: Meaning, methods, and mechanisms. *Annals of the New York Academy of Sciences, 1186*, 5–23.

Airhihenbuwa, C. O., Kumanyika, S., Agurs, T. D., Lowe, A., Saunders, D., & Morssink, C. B. (1996). Cultural aspects of African American eating patterns. *Ethnicity & Health, 1*(3), 245–260. https://doi.org/10.1080/13557858.1996.9961793

American Psychological Association. (2017). Ethnic and racial minorities and socioeconomic status. https://www.apa.org/pi/ses/resources/publications/minorities

Bower, K. M., Thorpe, R. J., Jr, Rohde, C., & Gaskin, D. (2014). The intersection of neighborhood racial segregation, poverty, and urban communities and their impact on food store availability in the United States. *Preventive Medicine, 58*, 33–39. https://doi.org/10.1016/j.ypmed.201310.010

Breyer, B., & Voss-Andreae, A. (2013). Food mirages: Geographic and economic barriers to healthful food access in Portland, Oregon. *Health & Place*, 131–139. https://doi.org/10.1016/j.healthplace.2013.07.008

Chowdhury, A. (2024, July 5). *The impact of food sufficiency on the health status: The case of households in the North Central Region* [Research Brief]. North Central Regional Center for Rural Development, Purdue University. https://ncrcrd.ag.purdue.edu/2024/07/05/impact-of-food-sufficiency-on-health-status/

DeNavas-Walt, C., Proctor, B., & Smith, J. (2011). Income, poverty and health insurance coverage in the United States: 2010. United States Census Bureau. https://www.census.gov/library/publications/2011/demo/p60-239.html

Duello, T. M., Rivedal, S., Wickland, C., & Weller, A. (2021). Race and genetics versus 'race' in genetics: A systematic review of the use of African ancestry in genetic studies. *Evolution, Medicine, and Public Health, 9*(1), 232–245. https://doi.org/10.1093/emph/eoab018

Duncan-Andrade, J., & Morrell, E. (2008). *The art of critical pedagogy: Possibilities for moving from theory to practice in urban schools.* Peter Lang.

Galvez, M. P., Morland, K., Raines, C., Kobil, J., Siskind, J., Godbold, J., & Brenner, B. (2008). Race and food store availability in an inner-city neighborhood. *Public Health Nutrition, 11*(6), 624–631. https://doi.org/10.1017/S1368980007001097

Gamble, V. (1997). Under the shadow of Tuskegee: African Americans and health care. *American Journal of Public Health, 87*(11), 1173–1778.

Gibbons, M. C. (2005). A historical overview of health disparities and the potential of eHealth solutions. *Journal of Medical Internet Research, 7*(5), e50. https://doi.org/10.2196/jmir.7.5.e50

Harvard T. H. Chan School of Public Health (2017). *Doctors need more nutrition education.* https://www.hsph.harvard.edu/news/hsph-in-the-news/doctors-nutrition-education/

Heywood, A. L. (2023b, February 6). *11 Conditions that disproportionately affect Black people.* Healthline. https://www.healthline.com/health/health-disparities-in-the-black-community

Hernandez, L., & Blazer, D. (Eds.). (2006). *Genes, behavior, and the social environment: Moving beyond the nature/nurture debate.* National Academies Press.

Hopkins Tanne, J. (2002). Patients are more satisfied with care from doctors of same race. *BMJ: British Medical Journal, 325*(7372), 1057.

Howard-Hassman, R. E. (n.d.) *Why Japanese-Americans received reparations and African-Americans are still waiting.* The Conversation. https://theconversation.com/why-japanese-americans-received-reparations-and-african-americans-are-still-waiting-119580

Institute of Medicine. (2001). *Crossing the quality chasm: A new health system for the 21st century: Formulating new rules to redesign and improve care.* National Academies Press. https://nap.nationalacademies.org/catalog/10027/crossing-the-quality-chasm-a-new-health-system-for-the

Institute of Medicine. (2003). *Unequal treatment: Confronting racial and ethnic disparities in health care*. The National Academies Press. https://nap.nationalacademies.org/catalog/12875/unequal-treatment-confronting-racial-and-ethnic-disparities-in-health-care

Institute of Medicine. (2004). *In the nation's compelling interest: Ensuring diversity in the healthcare workforce*. The National Academies Press. https://nap.nationalacademies.org/catalog/10885/in-the-nations-compelling-interest-ensuring-diversity-in-the-health

James, D. (2004). Factors influencing food choices, dietary intake, and nutrition-related attitudes among African Americans: Application of a culturally sensitive model. *Ethnicity & Health, 9*(4), 349–367. https://doi.org/10.1080/1355785042000285375

Jetter, K. M., & Cassady, D. L. (2006). The availability and cost of healthier food alternatives. *American Journal of Preventive Medicine, 30*(1), 38–44. https://doi.org/10.1016/j.amepre.2005.08.039

Jia, P., Luo, M., Li, Y., Zheng, J. S., Xiao, Q., & Luo, J. (2021). Fast-food restaurant, unhealthy eating, and childhood obesity: A systematic review and meta-analysis. Obesity reviews: an official journal of the International Association for the Study of Obesity, 22 Suppl 1(Suppl 1), e12944. https://doi.org/10.1111/obr.12944

Kittles, R. A., & Weiss, K. M. (2003). Race, ancestry, and genes: Implications for defining disease risk. *Annual Review of Genomics and Human Genetics, 4*(1), 33–67.

Kosoko-Lasaki, S., Cook, C., & O'Brien, R. (2009). *Cultural proficiency in addressing health disparities*. Jones & Bartlett Learning.

Levy, D. (1985). White doctors and Black patients: Influence of race on the doctor–patient relationship. *Pediatrics, 75*(4), 639–643.

Madell, R. (2024, April 8). Learn to recognize the signs of a stroke. Healthline. https://www.healthline.com/health/stroke/stroke-warning-signs#takeaway

Minor, L. (2019). *Why Medical Schools Need to Focus More on Nutrition*. Stanford Medicine. https://med.stanford.edu/school/leadership/dean/precision-health-in-the-news/why-medica-schools-need-focus-nutrition.html

Moore, C., Coates, E., Watson, A., de Heer, R., McLeod, A., & Prudhomme, A. (2023). "It's Important to Work with People that Look Like Me": Black Patients' Preferences for Patient-Provider Race Concordance. *Journal of racial and ethnic health disparities, 10*(5), 2552–2564. https://doi.org/10.1007/s40615-022-01435-y

Moore, R. B. (1992). *The name "negro": It's origin and evil use*. Black Classic Press.

Mullins, C. D., Onukwugha, E., Cooke, J. L., Hussain, A., & Baquet, C. R. (2010). The potential impact of comparative effectiveness research on the health of minority populations. *Health Affairs (Project Hope), 29*(11), 2098–2104. https://doi.org/10.1377/hlthaff.2010.0612

National Center for Health Statistics. (2015). *Health, United States, 2015: With special feature on racial and ethnic health disparities*. Centers for Disease Control and Prevention. https://www.cdc.gov/nchs/data/hus/hus15.pdf

Ndugga, N., Hill, L., & Artiga, S. (2024, June 11). Key data on health and health care by race and ethnicity [Report]. Kaiser Family Foundation. https://www.kff.org/key-data-on-health-and-health-care-by-race-and-ethnicity/?entry=executive-summary-introduction

Office of Management and Budget. (n.d.). Office of management and budget (OMB) standards. United States Census Bureau. https://www.census.gov/programs-surveys/metro-micro/about/omb-standards.html

Office of Management and Budget. (2024, March 29). Revisions to OMB's statistical policy directive no. 15: Standards for maintaining, collecting, and presenting federal data on race and ethnicity. Federal Register. https://www.federalregister.gov/documents/2024/03/29/2024-06469/revisions-to-ombs-statistical-policy-directive-no-15-standards-for-maintaining-collecting-and

One New Humanity. (n.d.). The benefits of community gardens. One New Humanity Community Development Corporation. https://www.onenewhumanitycdc.org/blog/the-benefits-of-community-gardens

Palmer, J. R., Wise, L. A., Horton, N. J., Adams-Campbell, L. L., & Rosenberg, L. (2003). Dual effect of parity on breast cancer risk in African-American women. *Journal of the National Cancer Institute, 95*(6), 478–483. https://doi.org/10.1093/jnci/95.6.478

Pilgrim, D. (2012). *What was Jim Crow*. The Jim Crow Museum. https://jimcrowmuseum.ferris.edu/what.htm

Rosario, I. (2020). The unlikely story behind Japanese Americans' campaign for reparations. NPR. https://www.npr.org/sections/codeswitch/2020/03/24/820181127/the-unlikely-story-behind -japanese-americans-campaign-for-reparations

Rubin, R., & Melnick, J. (2006). *Immigration and American popular culture*. New York University Press.

Shafi, S., de la Plata, C. M., Diaz-Arrastia, R., Bransky, A., Frankel, H., Elliott, A., Parks, J., & Gentilello, L. (2007). Ethnic disparities exist in trauma care. *Journal of Trauma Injury, Infection, and Critical Care, 63*(5), 1138–1142. https://doi.org/10.1097/TA.0b013e3181568cd4

Slocum, R. (2010). Race in the study of food. *Progress in Human Geography, 35*(3), 303–327. https:// doi.org/10.1177/0309132510378335

Smith, C., & Morton, L. W. (2009). Rural food deserts: Low-income perspectives on food access in Minnesota and Iowa. *Journal of Nutrition Education and Behavior, 41*(3), 176–187. https://doi .org/10.1016/j.jneb.2008.06.008

Spencer, D. J. (2010). The legacy of Tuskegee: Investigating trust in medical research and health disparities. *Journal of the Student National Medical Association*.

Spivey, D. (2003). *Fire from the soul of the African-American struggle*. Carolina Academic Press.

Talamantes, M., Lindeman, R., & Mouton, C. (n.d.). *Health and health care of Hispanic/Latino American elders*. National Center for Farmworker Health. http://lib.ncfh.org/pdfs/6495.pdf

US Census Bureau Public Information Office. (n.d.). *Majority of African Americans live in 10 states; New York City and Chicago are cities with largest Black populations - Census 2000 - Newsroom - U.S. Census Bureau*. https://www.census.gov/newsroom/releases/archives/census_2000/cb01cn176 .html

Washington, H. (2008). *Medical apartheid: The dark history of medical experimentation on Black Americans from colonial times to the present*. Doubleday Books.

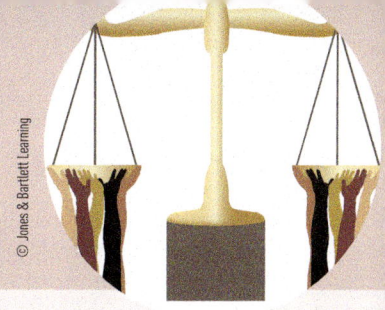
© Jones & Bartlett Learning

CHAPTER 4

The Asian American and Pacific Island Population and Health Disparities: Issues, Concerns, and Remedies

KEY TERMS

Asian American and Pacific Islander
diversity
Filipino American people
Asian Indian American people

Trinidadian people
heterogeneity
mainstream
model minority

LEARNING OBJECTIVES

After reading this chapter, you should be able to do the following:

1.   Explain the heterogeneity pertaining to Asian American and Pacific Islander people.
2.   Discuss health problems that are particularly prevalent in certain Asian American and Pacific Islander groups.
3.   List at least five Asian American groups and their nations of descent.
4.   Explain key health factors and remedies associated with two groups identified as examples in this chapter: Filipino American people, Indian American people, and Trinidadian American people who are also Indian.
5.   Determine if Trinidadian people in Trinidad and Tobago and in the United States are relevant to the discussion of people of Indian descent (Asian), African American/Black people in the United States, or both.

Introduction

Asian American people are generally designated as people in the United States who arrived from Asia, namely from Vietnam, Indonesia, Japan, Korea, China, and other nations. Unlike with the Hispanic ethnic designation, commonality of language is not a factor, as many different languages are spoken among these groups, for the most part. According to Budiman and Ruiz (2021), "A record 22 million Asian American people trace their roots to more than 20 countries in East and Southeast Asia and the Indian subcontinent, each with unique histories, cultures, languages, and other characteristics." They further state that "The U.S. Asian American population is projected to reach 46 million by 2060."

Culturally, there are also significant differences. Some **Asian American and Pacific Islander** people have distinct notoriety in the United States as they have been deemed by many as the "**model minority**," given their tendency to assimilate into the **mainstream**. Nevertheless, all Asian people in America are part of the emerging majority groups. Reeves and Bennet (2003) note the tendency of this emerging majority population to live in metropolitan areas and point out the following:

> Ninety-five percent of all Asians and Pacific Islanders lived in metropolitan areas, a much greater proportion than of non-Hispanic Whites (78 percent). Of the two populations, Asians and Pacific Islanders were twice as likely to live in central cities located in metropolitan areas (41 percent compared with 21 percent). However, among those living in metropolitan areas but not in central cities, Asians and Pacific Islanders were only 3 percentage points below non-Hispanic Whites (54 percent and 57 percent, respectively). (p. 2)

Health Concerns

Due to the vast **heterogeneity** (**diversity**) of the Asian American and Pacific Islander population, it is challenging to try to uniformly categorize their health concerns. Nevertheless, there are some key generalizable issues with the focus being remedies rather than honing in on the problems in depth. According to the Office of Minority Health (Asian American Health, n.d.), "some negative health factors are infrequent medical visits, language and cultural barriers, and lack of health insurance." Asian American and Pacific Islander people are most at risk for the following health conditions: cancer, heart disease, stroke, unintentional injuries (accidents), and diabetes. It appears that the number of Asian American and Pacific Islander people in the United States is growing rapidly as mentioned earlier. Unlike some other emerging majority groups, there is often an assumption that most, if not all, of the Asian American and Pacific Islander population is thriving. This somewhat inaccurate assumption includes health and economic success. This is not always the case. As mentioned earlier, these groups are extremely diverse and in order to understand health problems and remedies, stratification must take place per a number of categories, e.g., nationality of descent, age, socioeconomic status, educational levels, etc. Per Shi and Singh (2017):

> For instance, people of Vietnamese descent are more likely to assess their own health status as fair or poor, compared to people of Korean, Chinese,

Filipino, Asian Indian and Japanese descent. The incidence of overweight and obesity varies greatly, with Filipino adults being 70% more likely to be obese than the rest of the AA/PIs. Nevertheless, 22% of Korean people currently smoke—a rate higher than for Black and Hispanic adults. Compared with White people, Asians of Indian descent are more than twice as likely to have diabetes.

Given the vast heterogeneity of the Asian and Pacific Islander population, and the lack of disaggregation of the groups for the most part, two of the groups, namely people of Filipino descent and Asians of Indian descent, will be explored, as examples, in terms of remedies focusing on obesity, smoking, diabetes, and other issues relevant to these groups. Trinidadian people will also be discussed given the lineage of the people of that nation, as many are Indian people who immigrated to Trinidad and then to the United States, making them of interest here.

Filipino American People

Filipino American people are vibrant and diverse and live throughout the United States. Their occupations are varied ranging from healthcare professionals, including doctors and nurses, builders, architects, engineers, information technology specialists, educators (teachers and professors), retail and hospitality workers, farmers, agricultural workers, and entrepreneurs. In the state of Florida, as an example of one geographic location in the United States where Filipino people live, in the 1960s, according to the website Pinoy OFW (2023), many Filipino nurses and other healthcare professionals came to Florida for opportunities in the state's growing healthcare industry. This trend continued and by the 1980s, Filipino people had become one of the largest Asian-American groups in Florida. Many Filipino people arrived as migrant workers, as was the case for other workers, as the United States has always filled the gaps of its labor shortages with migrants. Filipino people have helped to fill that gap.

Like many other emerging majority groups in the United States who arrived as immigrants, for Filipino people, there are language barriers, feelings of isolation, discrimination and racism, financial concerns, lack of healthcare access, and other issues. Consequently, when we look at their healthcare problems, the correlation begins to surface in terms of their life in the United States and health outcomes.

Obesity

Filipino people experience overweight and obesity disproportionately as compared to other Asian and Pacific Islander groups of people. Per the National Institute of Minority Health and Health Disparities (n.d.), "the longer Filipinos live in the United States, the more likely they are to be obese." The reason for such obesity, upon immigrating to the United States, is not completely clear but it seems that factors contributing to the problem include less physical activity than when they were in their home country and the eating of processed food in the United States.

Per Unicef (2021), "Among Filipino adolescents, overweight has tripled in the last 15 years. There is a higher rate of overweight and obese children in urban areas than in rural areas." The younger population, when living in the United States, may move away from their traditional eating habits, which are healthier, and may move toward more calorie-rich options (National Institute of Minority Health and Health Disparities, n.d.) Healthy food options may also be limited due to difficulties in finding work, for some, and they may send a great deal of their earnings home to the Philippines where their families may be in greater need.

Additionally, per Bhimla et al. (2017):

> According to the National Health Interview Survey (NHIS), Filipino American people face higher rates of hypertension and obesity [as mentioned above] compared with other Asian American subgroups and Non-Hispanic Whites.

They also point out other issues, such as higher rates, compared to other Asian groups, of coronary heart disease. Their leading causes of death are heart diseases, malignant neoplasms, strokes, chronic lower respiratory diseases, influenza, and pneumonia.

Remedies for Filipino American People

It seems that the remedies for the health problems associated with Filipino American people will be complicated but are definitely doable. Most of the issues are seemingly lifestyle-focused, particularly for those who are experiencing low incomes. Hence, approaches involving culturally relevant health education/information is a great start. Since Filipino American people are one of the largest Asian groups in the United States, particularly in Florida. Efforts can be targeted to them, specifically based on a deep understanding of key aspects of their lifestyle. As an example, focusing on language barriers is a good starting point. Harvard University has moved forward with a specific effort to focus on the language barrier issue regarding Filipino American people. Per O'Grady (2024), Harvard offered Filipino languages for the first time in the fall of 2023. She points out that "Filipino, which is based on Tagalog and enriched by other native languages, is the lingua franca on the nation of more than 7,000 islands where more than 100 languages are spoken."

This remedy to the language barrier that Filipino American people experience is very important because it enables the younger generation to speak to the older population in their language and with people at home in the Philippines who may not speak English (although most do). Some Filipino American people speak what they refer to as Taglish, which is a fusion of Tagalog and English (O'Grady, 2024). Of course addressing the language barrier issue is one step of many that needs to be taken, but is a great start that will go a long way in terms of the distribution of health information and enhancing health literacy wherever it falls short within the Filipino American community.

On a broader basis, the biggest mistake that happens with research pertaining to Asian Americans and Pacific Islander people, as is the case with many emerging majority groups, is the aggregation of all into one group with a lack of understanding of the significant differences. Stratification is not just a concept but it is key to understanding how to address the issues and formulate targeted remedies for specific problems in terms of various groups of people. It is necessary to consider nationality, languages spoken, types of food eaten and other cultural norms, socioeconomic status and beyond.

Beyond remedies pertaining to the language barrier issues, other key remedies specific to Filipino American people must include improved diet (less salt and sugar) and understanding of their adaptation of the western, namely American diet, that is often salt-laden, processed food, etc., while encouraging the intake of and making available fruits, vegetables, and non-processed foods. This would be tremendously helpful, especially reducing the intake of salt, to reduce hypertension and other cardiovascular health issues. A reduction of alcoholic beverages, smoking, and foods that are high in sugar (sweets) would also be beneficial along with regular, consistent, daily exercise, as some studies of Filipino American people and their health indicate that these are contributing factors to health issues.

None of these suggestions are meant to imply that remedies to these problems are simple/easy. There are considerations and the need to understand the complexity of the concerns that must be discussed. Given that it is difficult for some Filipino American people to find well-paying jobs in the United States and that many make attempts to acculturate by incorporating the Western diet, focusing on their food customs would be a good place to start from a public health vantage point. In terms of the Filipino American diet, public health, for a considerable period of time, did not disaggregate the Filipino American people from the other Asian American and Pacific Islander people, hence their health issues have not been understood by many, in terms of public health. Therefore, another viable remedy, that must be amongst others, is specific health education programs targeting Filipino American people directly, including stratifying them by where they live, largely, and what they have access to, in terms of health information and healthy lifestyle opportunities in their environments. According to Bhimla et al. (2017) Filipino American people, beyond Florida, live throughout the United States in states that include Pennsylvania, Delaware, California, New York, and New Jersey, where health studies have been conducted about them. It is important not to blame the Filipino people for any health problems that they may have with narrow views that attempt to isolate their health issues to genetics.

The best approach is to dig deep by acquiring information directly from the people in their communities, including their health facilities, gain insight from them as to what they believe are the reasons for any health problems that exist amongst them, and accordingly, provide them with health education/information (after addressing language barriers). Additionally, the exploration of job opportunities for those who are having trouble finding jobs and the identification of exercise facilities that they can use in their communities will be helpful. Filipino American people must be at the forefront of all suggested remedies rather than dictating to them, what needs to be done to ensure that they lead healthy lifestyles.

Efforts must also be made to understand the cultural norms, dietary habits, and health behaviors in the Philippines in terms of the lineage and ancestors of Filipino American people and current Filipino people living in the Philippines. Which Filipino people, living in the Philippines, are healthy overall, what are they doing, and why does it work? Without considering these positive outcomes, it will be impossible to connect with their true heritage/lineage/culture and understand what works for them in terms of their health needs in the United States. Public health practitioners exploring the health of Filipino American people must understand who they are and should not impose American approaches, diets, lifestyles, etc., on them when, inherently, there may be unique cultural experiences and differences that resonate with them more, from generation to generation, no matter where they live in the world. These approaches combined, along with other innovative remedies that need to be explored, will cut down on chronic illnesses and lead to greater quality of life and longevity for Filipino American communities that are experiencing health issues. The answer is not to focus on the problems, but rather the remedies.

REMEDIES

- Distribute culturally relevant health education/information to Filipino American People.
- Focus on language barriers in all efforts with them to ensure that they understand any guidance or information pertaining to their health.
- Consider nationality, languages spoken, types of food eaten and other cultural norms, socioeconomic status, and beyond within the context of developing and implementing health initiatives/programs to help Filipino American people.
- Ensure the availability of fruits, vegetables, and non-processed foods in Filipino American communities, which would be tremendously helpful.
- Encourage Filipino American people to cut down on the intake of salt to reduce hypertension and other cardiovascular health issues.
- Advise Filipino American people about the importance of reducing alcoholic beverages, smoking, and foods that are high in sugar (sweets) along with regular, consistent, daily exercise as some studies of Filipino American people have shown.
- Do not blame the Filipino people for any health problems that they may have with narrow views that attempt to isolate their health issues to genetics.
- Involve them in all efforts toward remedies with their direct input and insight about who they are.
- Explore job opportunities for those in Filipino American communities seeking employment because improving socioeconomic status when/where necessary may help to remedy some health issues.

Asian Indian American People

It is important to make a distinction between people who are labeled as American Indian as compared to Asian Indian American immigrant people. The latter are the subject of this section of this chapter. In the chapter on Indian people, namely Native American people, the term *Indian* is used to describe them. That term is a misnomer and will be clarified in a chapter devoted to them in this text. The names preferred by many Native American people will also be discussed. **Asian Indian American people** are immigrants (unlike Native American people) per the first generation that arrived in the United States. According to Ramakrishna and Weiss (1992):

> Other than occasional immigrants, the first groups of Indians, mainly Sikhs from the Northern Indian state of Punjab, arrived at the turn of the century. Since the 1960s, immigration has increased, primarily through sponsorship.

Ramakrishna and Weiss (1992) also point out that there is limited cohesiveness between Asian Indian people across the United States, with some exceptions, and that most are educated and thrive within professions and businesses that pay well. Details regarding why and how they immigrated to the United States are comprehensive, based on varying reasons, including opportunities for life improvement, in terms of work, sponsorship, professional occupations, arranged marriages, female relatives who arrive from India to care for new Indian parents and their children, etc. These are mere examples, but provide some insight as to the rationale for many Indian people immigrating to the United Sates.

Also, many Indian American people immigrated to the United States from the upper realms of society, largely as engineers. According to Gordon et al. (n.d):

> Recent migration from India to the United States began in 1965, and has mostly included educated Indian citizens from the upper-class. Due to India's University IT system, many citizens have received top-rated engineering educations. However, a previous lack of infrastructure in the country led to few jobs for these students. Frequent power outages, unreliable network concerns and little commerce opportunities drove many qualified engineers to the United States for jobs in computer software development.

Health Issues

There are a number of factors that impact the health of Indian American people from India who immigrated to the United States. This is a very diverse population with various cultures, many languages and religions, so summarizing their health status across the board is challenging. Although Indian people, from India, arrived in the United States as immigrants and there are about 4 million in the United States, unfortunately, data on their health in the United States is limited. The leading causes of death in Asian Indian immigrants are cardiovascular disease (CVD, including strokes and heart disease) and cancers (Gidwani et al., 2021). These authors also state that Indian people who are immigrants have higher rates of diabetes, metabolic syndrome, and CVDs as compared to the United States population overall. The rates vary for men and women.

However, rather than dwell on the extent of these health problems, the question is, what are the remedies? To understand how to resolve health issues among Indian people in the United States, it is important to explore why their health problems exist in the first place. Some of the behaviors that must be considered are diet, particularly the types of food eaten (refined carbohydrates and unhealthy fats), sedentary lifestyles, and smoking.

Remedies for Asian Indian American People

There is a very well-known medical doctor in the United States, Deepak Chopra. He was born in India, where he attended the All India Institute of Medical Sciences. He completed a residency in internal medicine and a fellowship in endocrinology in the United States and ultimately became chief of staff of New England Memorial Hospital in 1980. Although criticized by some in the medical and health professions, he has written many books about medicine and health and shares detailed information about Indian medicine, which goes back thousands of years and is known as Ayurvedic medicine. Without getting into a discourse about the Eastern versus Western controversies associated with this physician, suffice it to say he has brought the discussion of Ayurvedic medicine to the forefront. Chopra, who taught at Boston Regional Center, Boston University, and Harvard University, and opened his own practice in endocrinology after serving at New England Memorial Hospital, states the following in his book *Perfect Health* (Chopra,1991):

> Dating back in India more than 5,000 years, Ayurveda comes from two Sanskrit root words, *ayus*, or "life," and *veda*, meaning "knowledge" or "science." Therefore, Ayurveda is usually translated as "the science of life."

Chopra goes on to discuss further that a modernized version of Ayurveda came to the West in the 1980s and that he was one of the first to offer this "new medicine," training other physicians along with his other training in allopathic (Western) medicine. Although a thorough review and discussion of Ayurvedic medicine will not take place here, suffice it to say, it should be considered as part of the repertoire of remedies for health problems of Indian American people because it is so deeply embedded in their culture.

However, per Ramakishna and Weiss (1992):

> "Allopathic" medicines are now readily accepted for most acute conditions. In fact, allopathy (as mainstream Western medicine is known in India) is the preferred type of care in most places where it is accessible. Resistance to or a reluctance to use Western medicine, however, cannot be ignored. Other systems of medicine are still used in India and are preferred for certain problems, including some forms of mental illness and many chronic illnesses. In such a pluralistic medical system, allopathy (biomedicine) is just one of many kinds of medical care available.

Hence, in exploring remedies for health problems related to people of Indian descent in the United States, it is important to consider both Western (allopathic medicine) and Ayurvedic medicine with equivalent relevance. There are cultural nuances that must be taken into consideration. This involves talking to the people directly to determine what they prioritize and, in some instances, to share information from both vantage points. Often, there is a bias in the United States toward Western medicine without understanding that Ayurvedic medicine, as one example, has been in existence for over 5000 years and that there are many attributes of it that are intrinsic to the culture of Indian American people, whether they immigrated to the United States or were born here. There are numerous remedies that should be considered to deal with health issues associated with Indian American people but all must begin with strong communication, understanding what is important to them, health-wise, and respecting and valuing their culture.

REMEDIES

- Ayurvedic medicine, which is 5000 years old, should be included in the repertoire of healthcare options for Indian American people, along with Western medicine.
- Dialogue and communication with Indian American people must take place to determine their preferences in terms of medical and healthcare choices as their culture must be valued and respected.

West Indian Culture

Comparatively, it is also important to note that there is another group of Indian people in the United States to take into consideration, selected for discussion here. The nation of focus is Trinidad, where the people are Indian, African, and mixed culture (others). This is based on the fact that many African people were brought to the Caribbean Islands, as enslaved people, while those islands also had an indigenous population living there before the Europeans arrived and claimed them, for the primary purpose of acquisition of their natural resources, such as petroleum, gas, etc., specific to Trinidad. Later, other groups were brought to these islands, including Indians from India. This led to mixtures, segregation, and new cultures. There are three distinct groups of islands in the West Indies: the Bahamas, the Lesser Antilles, and the Greater Antilles. There are many of these islands, far too many to discuss here, so, two are selected as examples, namely Trinidad and Tobago, which comprise one country, though it is commonly known as Trinidad.

When individuals immigrate to the United States from Trinidad, often their lineage is clear. They may know that their living parents or recent ancestors are from India or from Africa. However, when they immigrate to the United States from Trinidad, their nationality remains Trinidadian. Based on this phenotype, skin color confounds the situation as many Indians have dark skin, similar to that of Black people in the United States. Based on the racial categorization of the Office of Management and Budget (OMB), which is described in this chapter, it becomes difficult for the children of Trinidadian immigrants to determine how to categorize themselves in the United States. Per the OMB (2024), these are the racial categories:

> The minimum categories for data on race and ethnicity for Federal statistics, program administrative reporting, and civil rights compliance reporting are defined as follows:
>
> *American Indian or Alaska Native.* Individuals with origins in any of the original peoples of North, Central, and South America, including, for example, Navajo Nation, Blackfeet Tribe of the Blackfeet Indian Reservation of Montana, Native Village of Barrow Inupiat Traditional Government, Nome Eskimo Community, Aztec, and Maya.
>
> *Asian.* Individuals with origins in any of the original peoples of Central or East Asia, Southeast Asia, or South Asia, including, for example, Chinese, Asian Indian, Filipino, Vietnamese, Korean, and Japanese.
>
> *Black or African American.* Individuals with origins in any of the Black racial groups of Africa, including, for example, African American, Jamaican, Haitian, Nigerian, Ethiopian, and Somali.
>
> *Hispanic or Latino.* Includes individuals of Mexican, Puerto Rican, Salvadoran, Cuban, Dominican, Guatemalan, and other Central or South American or Spanish culture or origin.
>
> *Middle Eastern or North African.* Individuals with origins in any of the original peoples of the Middle East or North Africa, including, for example, Lebanese, Iranian, Egyptian, Syrian, Iraqi, and Israeli.

Native Hawaiian or Pacific Islander. Individuals with origins in any of the original peoples of Hawaii, Guam, Samoa, or other Pacific Islands, including, for example, Native Hawaiian, Samoan, Chamorro, Tongan, Fijian, and Marshallese.

White. Individuals with origins in any of the original peoples of Europe, including, for example, English, German, Irish, Italian, Polish, and Scottish.

Based on these categorizations, it would seem that a person who immigrated to the United States from Trinidad would be able to identify with one of these categories based on the origin/lineage of their parents, especially if they were not born in Trinidad. In an interview later in this chapter, the complication of this identification process is shared as the person being interviewed was born to parents who are, in fact, from India and moved (immigrated) to Trinidad where their son was born. But their son, the interviewee, who immigrated to the United States with his parents at age 11, identifies as a Black person in the United States. Before considering this interview, see the following information about the West Indies as people from the Caribbean, including Trinidad, often refer to themselves as West Indian.

What are the West Indies? In short, we are again considering a misnomer, based on the fact that Christopher Columbus thought he had arrived in India when he had actually landed in what we now know as the Caribbean. For this reason, Native Americans came to be known as *Indians*. Per Shvili (2021) in the World Atlas:

> The West Indies are a chain of islands located in the Caribbean Sea and the Atlantic Ocean. This chain of islands runs from the north, close to the U.S. state of Florida, all the way south to the northern shores of South America. They were named the Indies by Christopher Columbus, the first European on record to reach the islands. He believed that he had reached India, and thus, called the newly-discovered islands the Indies. Later, when it was discovered that what Columbus discovered was not India, the islands were renamed the West Indies, to distinguish them from the Spice Islands in the Pacific Ocean, otherwise known as the East Indies, which now comprise the territory of Indonesia.

Trinidad has been chosen for this discussion as it is largely comprised of East Indian people. According to the World Factbook, the percentages (2011 estimates) are as follows:

- East Indian, 35.4%
- African descent, 34.2%
- Mixed—other, 15.3%
- Mixed–African/East Indian, 7.7%
- Other, 1.3%
- Unspecified, 6.2%

You will find variations on the data of these groups when conducting research because the Indian and the African peoples are so close in terms of percentages. The populations of African and East Indian people on the islands are clearly the most prevalent, as is the case for **Trinidadian people**, who immigrated to, or who are born in, the United States.

The almost equivalent numbers of East Indian and African people have led to a substantial mixture of East Indian and African people in Trinidad. The following box is an interview with a Trinidadian person who provides some insight as to how this mixture has panned out for him and his family in the United States, as immigrants from Trinidad. Before this interesting discussion, also note the following from the World Factbook (*Trinidad and Tobago - the World Factbook*, n.d.).

First colonized by the Spanish, the islands came under British control in the early 19th century. The islands' sugar industry was hurt by the emancipation of the slaves in 1834. Manpower was replaced with the importation of contract laborers from India between 1845 and 1917, which boosted sugar production as well as the cocoa industry. The discovery of oil on Trinidad in 1910 added another important export. Independence was attained in 1962. The country is one of the most prosperous in the Caribbean thanks largely to petroleum and natural gas production and processing.

Interview with Mr. Sunil Joon

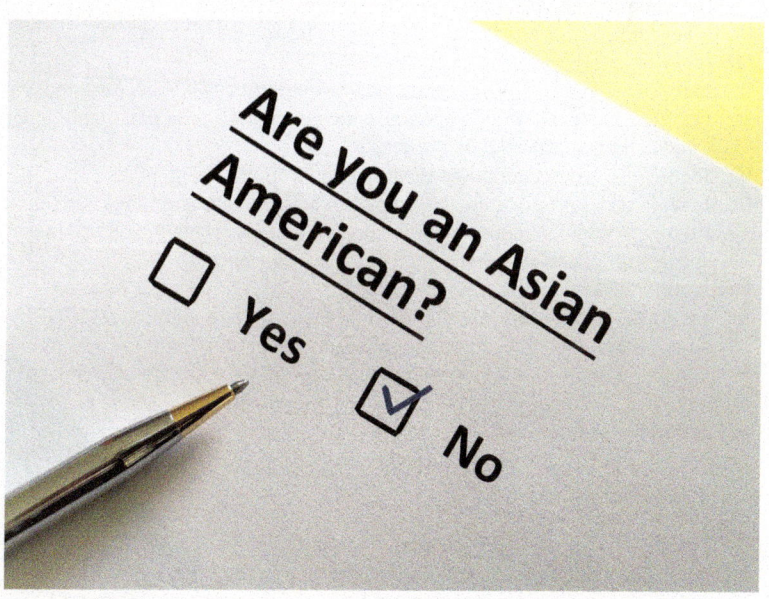

© Yeexin Richelle/Shutterstock

In an effort to highlight a unique aspect of immigration in the United States by some East Indian immigrants and their African counterparts from the same country, this interview with Mr. Sunil Joon will provide some interesting insight. Mr. Joon is a Trinidadian man who lives in the northeast section of the United States with his wife, who is a Black American woman. His parents were East Indian people who immigrated to Trinidad, where Mr. Joon was born. Mr. Joon and his wife have one daughter who is 10 years old. Mr. Joon

(continues)

Interview with Mr. Sunil Joon   *(continued)*

immigrated to the United States from Trinidad in 1981 when he was 11 years old. He is now 52 years old and is an owner-operator of a trucking company. The detail he provides in this interview is based on his opinions, observations, and experiences, and that of his family from his perspective, in Trinidad and the United States. Again, both of his parents were born in India, immigrated to Trinidad and then to the United States. Mr. Joon is affectionately addressed by his nickname "Moody," by his wife and the rest of his family but will be referred to by his formal name, Mr. Joon, for the purpose of this interview. Mr. Joon has a Trinidadian accent so attempts have been made here to retain his speech pattern throughout this interview, whenever possible, based on excerpts from the transcription of an audio recording of the discussion/interview.

Dr. Rose: Tell me a little bit about your background as a Caribbean and Indian person.

Mr. Joon: I was born in Trinidad and Tobago. My father was a bus driver. My mom, she did farming work. We stayed there until I was 11 years old and we came to America. They migrated from India and they went to Trinidad for work. The great-grandparents too. We all came here to the United States from different generations.

Dr. Rose: And so your family's actual origin is from India?

Mr. Joon: Yes.

Dr. Rose: Okay. In terms of your race, what would you say it is because India is the country of your family's lineage, which is their original nationality, before Trinidad, but what would be the race?

Mr. Joon: Well, we call ourselves West Indians from the West Indies.

Dr. Rose: In the United States, there are categories, including Black/African American, White, Asian or Pacific Islander, and American Indian or Alaska Native, etc. Which one would you select to describe you?

Mr. Joon: They also have others.

Dr. Rose: Well, technically, per the Office of Management and Budget (OMB), which determines the racial categories for the nation, there is no "other" category. People can select multiple categories. So what are your selections for you?

Mr. Joon. Well, sometimes I just put West Indian. That is what I usually do.

Dr. Rose: Okay. But you don't categorize yourself in any of the U.S. racial categories?

Mr. Joon: Oh well. I put Black sometimes.

Dr. Rose: OK. But never Asian, which is where Indian falls under?

Mr. Joon: Not really. We don't really consider ourselves Indian.

Dr. Rose: In India, how are you personally viewed there?

Mr. Joon: I've never been there, so I wouldn't know. But, my parents, they've been back there for a visit.

Dr. Rose: I read that most of the Indian people from India came to the United States in the 1960s as professionals because America didn't have enough doctors, engineers, etc. When you look at East Indian vs. West Indian, what are the main differences that exist? Not just looks and so forth, but culturally.

Mr. Joon: Well, we are actually all very similar. Our food is the same type of food, but it is cooked differently.

Dr. Rose: You said the language spoken in Trinidad is English. Why do you think Trinidadian people speak English? In school, everyone learns to speak

English. Is that what you're saying? Are there any other languages spoken in Trinidad and Tobago?

Mr. Joon: No.

Dr. Rose: That's really important because one of the big issues in health care is that people immigrate to the United States and, depending on what country they are from and their primary language, some can't speak English very well or at all, which can lead to problems, essentially language barriers when seeking health care. But with Trinidadian people, everyone speaks English when they come to the United States.

Mr. Joon: Yes.

Dr. Rose: Okay, so before you said there are differences between East Indian and West Indian people, culturally. For example, the food is prepared differently. Can you give me one example of something that is prepared one way by East Indian people and one way by West Indian people.

Mr. Joon: Well, it's how we cook it differently and the seasonings that we use, and the spices they use. Everything we use is different from day one, but it is named the same thing like curry goat, curry chicken, stewed chicken, but we cook differently.

Dr. Rose: So if I had East Indian curry chicken, it would not taste the same as Trinidadian curry chicken?

Mr. Joon: Not at all.

Dr. Rose: And it's because of the seasoning or the way it is prepared?

Mr. Joon: Seasoning and the way it's prepared and the way they cook it.

Dr. Rose: So it's very different. You said that your family went back to India for a visit.

Mr. Joon: Yes.

Dr. Rose: When your family got on the ground in India, did it feel to them like they were at home, finally seeing their true culture?

Mr. Joon: No. They felt like they wanted to come back home. It's not the same.

Dr. Rose: Okay. So it's definitely a different culture. That's really key. Because as I'm comparing the two, Indian people in India and Indian people in Trinidad, I want to make it clear that this is a very different culture, although your family has the same origin, India. Where do you think most Trinidadian people live in the United States?

Mr. Joon: Florida and New York.

Dr. Rose: Why do you think they chose those two places?

Mr. Joon: Well, that's where their family came and whichever family came, they followed them.

Dr. Rose: In terms of East Indian immigrant people, as I said that I read before, the bulk of them came over in the 1960s. They came over because the United States, at that time, didn't have enough of its own professionals, such as doctors, engineers, etc., and the East Indian people were training in those fields, but when they finished their studies, they couldn't get jobs in their country so they came to the United States. Others came over before that to work the railroads and as other types of laborers. So when Trinidadian people come to the United States, what are they doing in terms of work?

Mr. Joon: Construction, real estate, babysitting; they are trying to get their papers; some of them will go to school.

Dr. Rose: Would you say that most Trinidadian people in the United States are at the high, middle, or lower financial level?

(continues)

Interview with Mr. Sunil Joon *(continued)*

Mr. Joon: I think most of them are in the middle income.

Dr. Rose: Okay, this book includes information about the health status of people. We have already talked about the type of food eaten by Trinidadian people, but let's go over that a little bit more. What are the main kinds of foods that are eaten? Is it healthy, not healthy? What do you think?

Mr. Joon: It's not really too healthy. We eat curry duck, stewed chicken, curry goat, a lot of roti, a lot of vegetables, a lot of stuff with oil in it. So a lot of people get cholesterol problems, high levels. We eat like fry bodi [fried string beans]. We eat a lot of fried food. Fried potato (aloo potato), fried tomato, fried cabbage with tomato. . .

Dr. Rose: The cabbage is fried?

Mr. Joon: Yes.

Dr. Rose: Okay. So I'm trying to find out, do Trinidadian people, when they come to the United States, still eat the food of the Trinidadian people who are in Trinidad? It seems that is what you are saying is the case.

Mr. Joon: They still eat the food from back home. We also eat the American food, the junk food. Pizza and all the stuff like that.

Dr. Rose: Is there obesity? Do you think Trinidadian people in the United States are overweight?

Mr. Joon: Yeah. I would say half of them.

Dr. Rose: What about exercise. I know that Trinidad and Tobago are islands, so do people swim a lot? Is exercising a big part of the culture on the islands and what happens when they come to the United States?

Mr. Joon: Well recently, one of the prime ministers of Trinidad, a woman, went and started having exercise machines placed in parks. There was no place to run before, just mostly cricket grounds. So you know, the ladies really had no way to exercise, but now she put exercise machines and tracks so people can walk around a track and run. A lot of people are now exercising in Trinidad.

Dr. Rose: But what about when they come to America? I'm focusing on Trinidadian people in America, primarily. What happens when they come to the United States in terms of exercise?

Mr. Joon: The young ones ... they are in the gym now.

Dr. Rose: Oh, so they are going to the gym. The origin of Yoga is 100% Indian. Do Trinidadian people, particularly the Indian people, practice yoga?

Mr. Joon: You will find not that much. Some people do it but not as much as you think they would.

Dr. Rose: That is so interesting.

Mr. Joon: Trinidadians are into more like partying, hanging out on the beach, cooking. That's their life.

Dr. Rose: Let's talk about Trinidadian children. It seems that when people are healthier, the population, the families and etc. are educated. You said that once some Trinidadian people come here and they get settled, some focus on school.

Mr. Joon: In Trinidad, they are very strict with school. Besides school, they have to do classes after school. They have to do lessons. They are very strict with that ... the parents.

Dr. Rose: What happens when they come to the United States?

Mr. Joon: When they come here, the kids slack off in school. They may cut school or whatever, but they go to school. When you grow up in Trinidad, the parents are very strict about school.

Dr. Rose: So the parents are very strict about education in Trinidad, but when they come here, the children might slack a little bit. So do you think that contributes to health issues? Because the less education you have, perhaps the less you know what to do about your health.

Mr. Joon: Well, I wouldn't say that, because the younger ones, they're more into the American food, those who grew up here. So they eat a lot of junk food and stuff. But yet, they still go to the gym. And they still get an education. In Trinidad you get your full education. It's only a problem with college because those who can't afford it, don't go.

Dr. Rose: Upon arriving in the United States from Trinidad if you get your [immigration] papers and if you get everything settled and you can go to school, namely college, can you get loans and scholarships?

Mr. Joon: You can get scholarships but no loans. Then you might be one person out of 100 people that gets a scholarship.

Dr. Rose: You have a little girl, correct? How old is your little girl?

Mr. Joon: She is 10 years old.

Dr. Rose: What is her life like in terms of Trinidadian and Indian culture, given that her grandparents are from India and then went to Trinidad to live and then came to the United States with you?

Mr. Joon: What she would not be able to get in Trinidad, we make sure she gets that here with education and everything she needs. Plus her mom, who is African American, is very strict with her on school and education. So I'm glad about that. And we really have no problem with her. Everything about her is kind of perfect, so we are kind of lucky right now.

Dr. Rose: Are you raising her as an American? Or are you raising her as a Trinidadian? Or both?

Mr. Joon: I'm raising her as an American.

Dr. Rose: Okay, and can you tell me why you're raising her as American instead of Trinidadian?

Mr. Joon: I try to teach her Trinidadian culture a little bit. But she doesn't really get it too much because she's young. But as she grows up with the food, I make sure that she eats Trinidadian food. My mom gave it to her since she was a baby. She is the only child out of all of our family's kids that eats West Indian food. The rest of them eat American like pizza and other American food.

Dr. Rose: And your wife can cook Trinidadian food, although she is African American?

Mr. Joon: Yes.

Dr. Rose: This seems important to you as part of the maintenance of Trinidadian culture.

Mr. Joon: I make sure she [my daughter] eats Trinidadian food. I want her to grow up at least knowing about what Trinidadian people are eating.

Dr. Rose: Well, that is interesting because in some cultures, for example, the primary language of where the people have immigrated from is not English. So they may emphasize language by telling their children, you have to learn how to speak, let's say Spanish. You have to learn how to speak our language. But since Trinidadian people speak English, you emphasize the culture for your child through the food.

Mr. Joon: Yeah. Plus, she has to learn languages, too. I want her to learn other languages besides English.

(continues)

Interview with Mr. Sunil Joon (continued)

Dr. Rose: Yes, of course, but I'm saying in terms of Trinidad, the way you keep her in touch with the culture is by making sure she understands and eats Trinidadian food. That is so interesting.

Mr. Joon: Also through music. Soca music. Soca is a calypso music. There is a soca fest in Trinidad. My daughter was into it when she was a baby. Soca has something to do with Spanish music. Back in the day, a lot of Spanish people used to come [to Trinidad]. So, it's like the English version now with a lot of drums and steel pans and from there people started singing; now there is the soca fest. It's not just from Latinos but Africans—from when the Africans came to Trinidad. So they mixed everything together. It's like a mixture—the Spanish and the African ... mostly the Africans from the drums.

Dr. Rose: Your wife is African American and your nationality is Trinidadian. Your parents brought you to America from Trinidad, but both of your parents are Indian (from India) and lived in Trinidad when you were born. But, you're also classifying yourself now as Black rather than Indian. When I look around your home, I see many Indian items, in terms of the décor. This is quite complicated.

Mr. Joon: Yes

Dr. Rose: Well you know, interestingly, Indian people are classified here, as I told you at the very beginning, Indian people are in the OMB grouping entitled "Asian." Again, as I mentioned before, in the United States, there is an entity, the Office of Management and Budget, under the President of the United States, that created racial categories, such as Black/African American, White, Asian, etc. East Indian people are classified under the Asian category, no matter their skin color. But, Trinidadian people who identify as Black (those who are of African descent), would fall under Black/African American when they are in the United States. They have separated the two groups, in this country, the Indian and the Black people, by the way they designed the structure, based on country of origin. You can put White if you want, but the question is what nation are you from? If you say Trinidadian, the question is are you Black, or Indian, for the most part. If a person says Black, they will be considered Black per the OMB structure. If they are Indian, then Asian, because it is the origin that meets the OMB structure. So, if a person's parents are Indian, they are considered Indian, which would be Asian in the United States with a Trinidadian nationality (if the person was born in Trinidad). If the person was born in the United States and his/her parents are of Indian descent, technically, they are considered Asian American. Also, what are the major religions in Trinidad?

Mr. Joon: Hindu, Christian, and Muslim.

Dr. Rose: When Trinidian people are living in America what are their major religions?

Mr. Joon: They don't change. Same religions as in Trinidad.

Dr. Rose: So you are practicing Lent right now. That's Catholic.

Mr. Joon: Yeah. Because my mother was a Christian. My father is Hindu and my grandmother is Muslim. We grew up as Hindu. When I was small ... when I was young in Trinidad, I always went to church. I like the church stuff. So when I came here, I was more into the Christian religion.

Dr. Rose: So when there is a marriage ceremony in your family, is it an Indian ceremony or Christian?

Mr. Joon: Well my little sister, she follow Christian. So whatever ceremony it's going to be, it will be Christian. My sisters, they gonna marry in Hindu or they gonna follow what their husbands are.

Dr. Rose: So you don't have brothers?

Mr. Joon: No.

Dr. Rose: Oh okay. So do you have men, besides your father, in your family.

Mr. Joon: Yes, my cousins.

Dr. Rose: Who are Trinidadian?

Mr. Joon: Yes.

Dr. Rose: Those men, how do they get married? Do they have Christian or Hindu ceremonies?

Mr. Joon: Most of them are Hindu. So most of them have a Hindu wedding. But you got some of them who are Christian, like my mother's side. So when they marry, they marry Christian.

Dr. Rose: So the Hindu wedding is like how the ceremonies are in India.

Mr. Joon: Yes. Like in India.

Dr. Rose: Okay. Is there anything else you want to add?

Mr. Joon: No. That's it.

Dr. Rose: Well this has been so interesting. Thank you so much!

Mr. Joon: You are welcome.

It is clear, based on the interview with Sunil Joon, as an anecdotal scenario, that when some people of Indian descent leave their country of origin and immigrate to a place like Trinidad and then the United States, the culture of origin can get removed or changed based on that scenario. Consequently, the health issues associated with the Indian person from Trinidad may be completely different from those of the Indian people in India. Therefore, any remedies to deal with health issues must take cultural and national factors into consideration. There are no broad-based remedies for the Indian population at large, in the United States, as there are many factors that must be considered.

REMEDIES

- The provision of culturally relevant health education/information is imperative.
- Focus on language barriers as a primary focus toward remedies (when languages other than English are spoken).
- In considering remedies for health care issues Asian Indian American people and any group face, there must be strong communication focusing on what is important to the community being served, health-wise, and respecting and valuing their culture.
- In providing health care to Trinidadian American people, it is important to ask them which racial group they consider themselves to be as they may/may not identify with their Indian lineage.

WRAP-UP

The Asian American and Pacific Islander population is very broad, consisting of people from many geographic locations, who speak many languages, eat different foods, and have different cultural norms and beyond. To aggregate them into one group does not lend itself to a situation of determining remedies for health problems without complete stratification by nation, language, culture, age, etc. To do so, even if all are born in the United States, would miss the mark substantially because they cannot be lumped into a category based on the OMB's classification which is:

Asian or Pacific Islander. A person having origins in any of the original peoples of the Far East, Southeast Asia, the Indian subcontinent, or the Pacific Islands. This area includes, for example, China, India, Japan, Korea, the Philippine Islands, and Samoa.

Based on the anecdotal interview with Sunil Joon, outlined earlier in this chapter, there is no place in the OMB categorization for the Indian people in Trinidad who may have origins, in terms of lineage, in India, but who are having an experience in what is labeled a West Indian culture in the United States. Mr. Joon, although of Indian descent, with parents and grandparents from India, who immigrated to Trinidad, and then to the United States, identifies as Black. This is a key factor to consider in caring for a person health-wise as key factors must be considered for those individuals who immigrate to the United States and subsequent generations of their family are born here. There are factors, such as acculturation, or lack thereof, that must be considered, including foods eaten, languages spoken, adaptation to American food, etc., that may impact their health. When these factors are not considered, health problems may be exacerbated. The remedy is in understanding who people really are, how that is handled in their families, their personal existence, and their environment. Appropriate stratification is imperative to understand deeply how health problems have arisen in individuals/groups by talking to them and valuing and understanding to ensure appropriate health remedies.

Chapter Problems

1. What are some of the key health issues for Filipino people?
2. Explain the relevance of Ayurvedic medicine to Indian people.
3. Why is Trinidad relevant to the discussion of Asian Indian people?
4. Discuss some health issues that Asian Indian American people experience.
5. List five remedies for health issues covered in this chapter and identify which groups of Asian people they are relevant to.

References

Asian American Health. (n.d.). Office of Minority Health. https://minorityhealth.hhs.gov/asian-american-health

Bhimla, A., Yap, L., Lee, M., Seals, B., Aczon, H., & Ma, G. X. (2017). Addressing the Health Needs of High-Risk Filipino Americans in the Greater Philadelphia Region. *Journal of community health, 42*(2), 269–277. https://doi.org/10.1007/s10900-016-0252-0

Budiman, A. & Ruiz, N. (2021). Key facts about Asian Americans, a diverse and growing population. Pew Research Center. https://www.pewresearch.org/short-reads/2021/04/29/key-facts-about-asian-americans/

Chopra, D. (1991). *Perfect health: The complete mind/body guide.* Harmony Books.

Gidwani, S., Paul, D., Nalwa, G., Lin, B., Mahadevan, S. V., & Palaniappan, L. (2021). Indian and Asian-Indian immigrant health statistics. In *CARE Data Brief* (Issue No. 1). https://med.stanford.edu/content/dam/sm/care/2021Summerresearchfellowproject/India-Data-Brief.pdf

Gordon, S., Bernadett, M., Evans, D., Shapiro, N.B., & Patel, U. (n.d.). Asian Indian Culture: Influences and implications for health care. The Molina Institute for Cultural Competency. https://www.molinahealthcare.com/providers/mi/medicaid/resource/PDF/resource_MI_AsianIndianCulture-InfluencesAndImplicationsForHealthCare.pdf&ved=2ahUKEwjysL7up_iLAxXK1zgGHQiWIlEQFnoECBYQAQ&usg=AOvVaw0Bzfp2ivNwly-fnNzs_wXw

O'Grady, E. (2024, February 7). Finding community through shared language. *The Harvard Gazette.* https://news.harvard.edu/gazette/story/2024/02/finding-community-through-shared-language/

Pinoy OFW. (2023, January 30). *Filipino community in Florida: What you need to know.* https://www.pinoy-ofw.com/usa/859-florida-filipino-community.html

Ramakrishna, J., & Weiss, M. G. (1992). Health, illness, and immigration. East Indians in the United States. *The Western Journal of Medicine, 157*(3), 265–270. https://pmc.ncbi.nlm.nih.gov/articles/PMC1011274/pdf/westjmed00085-0055.pdf

National Institute of Minority Health and Health Disparities (n.d.) Filipino immigrants are more likely to be obese the longer they live in the United States. https://www.nimhd.nih.gov/news-events/features/community-health/filipino-imigrants-obese.html

Office of Management and Budget. (2024, March 29). Revisions to OMB's statistical policy directive no. 15: Standards for maintaining, collecting, and presenting federal data on race and ethnicity. Federal Register. https://www.federalregister.gov/documents/2024/03/29/2024-06469/revisions-to-ombs-statistical-policy-directive-no-15-standards-for-maintaining-collecting-and

Reeves, T., & Bennett, C. (2003). The Asian and Pacific Islander population in the United States: March 2002 [Current Population Reports, P20-540]. U.S. Census Bureau. https://www.census.gov/content/dam/Census/library/publications/2003/demo/p20-540.pdf

Shi, L. & Singh, D. A. (2017). Delivering health care in America: A systems approach. Jones & Bartlett Learning.

Unicef. (2021, March 4). *Poor diets, failing food systems, and lack of physical activity are causing overweight and obesity in children* [Press release]. https://www.unicef.org/philippines/press-releases/poor-diets-failing-food-systems-and-lack-physical-activity-are-causing-overweight

Shvili, J. (2021, May 23). *West Indies.* WorldAtlas. https://www.worldatlas.com/geography/west-indies.html

Trinidad and Tobago - The World Factbook. (n.d.). https://www.cia.gov/the-world-factbook/countries/trinidad-and-tobago/

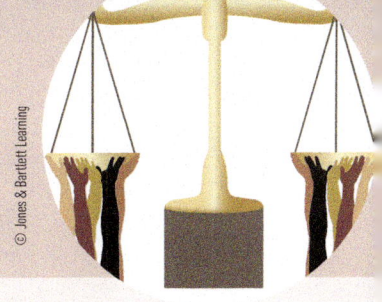

CHAPTER 5

The American Indian (Native American) and Alaska Native Population and Health Disparities: Issues, Concerns, and Remedies

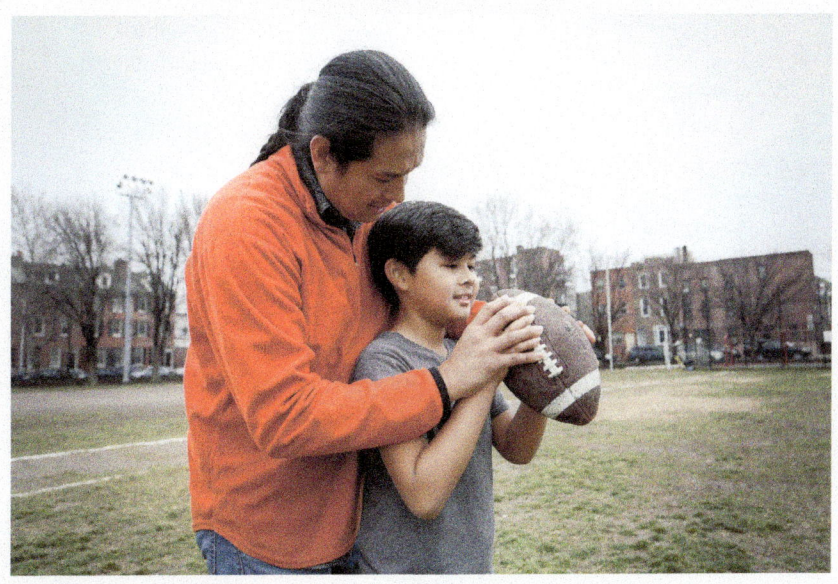

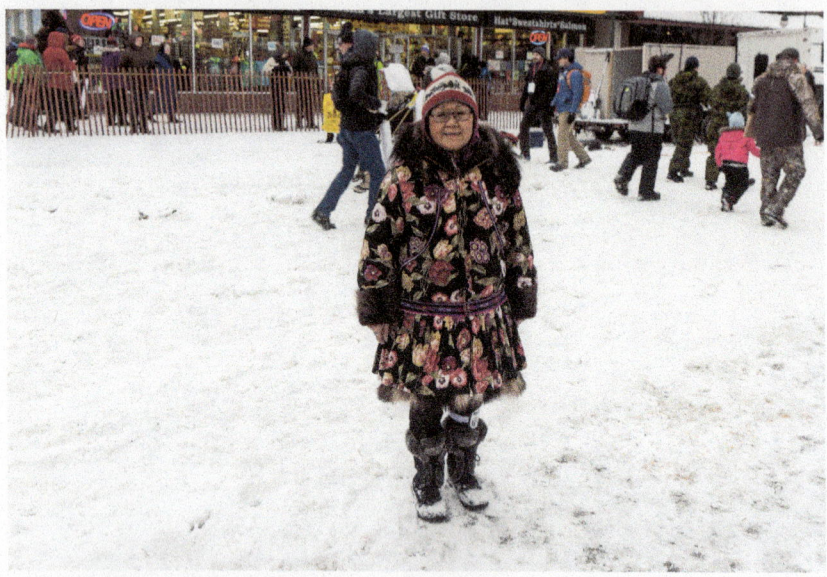

© Steve Jordan/Shutterstock

KEY TERMS

American Indian and Alaska Native
    (AIAN)
chronic disease management program
    (CDMP)
cultural nuances
Office of Management and Budget (OMB)

Bureau of Indian Affairs
Indian Health Care Improvement Act
    (IHCIA)
Indian Health Service (IHS)
Patient Protection and Affordable Care
    Act (PPACA)

LEARNING OBJECTIVES

After reading this chapter, you should be able to do the following:

1. Discuss some of the key health issues among American Indian and Alaska
   Native (AIAN) people.
2. Understand the role of the Indian Health Service.
3. Explain why Native American people are referred to as *Indians* in the United States.
4. Describe some potential remedies to improve the quality of health care among
   AIAN people.

Introduction

The notion of nationality as a key element of understanding culture applies to all of the emerging majority groups. That said, Native American people, who are indigenous to America, have a nationality that is unequivocally American. Other terms have been used to identify them, including *Indian*, but some are considered derogatory. Rubin and Melnick (2006) explain the erroneous nature of the term *Indian* in describing Native Americans:

> Writing in 1941, an Indian immigrant to the United States named Krishnalal Shridharani wrote, with tongue in cheek, about Columbus's "discovery" of America: "We Hindus take a pardonable pride in the fact that had it not been for us 'undiscovered' Indians, America would not have been the same America from 1492 on."

Shridharani is making light of the fact that Native American people were given the title *Indians* because when Christopher Columbus arrived in the Americas during his exploratory voyages, he thought he was in India and incorrectly named the Native people "Indians." Hence, although the **Office of Management and Budget (OMB)** refers to this race as American Indian and Alaska Native people, it is important to note that they were native to American soil before Columbus arrived; therefore, the term *Native American* is somewhat more appropriate. This is not a definitive term, as the terms *indigenous people* and *Indian* are also used by some, as well as "tribal" names. Per Blackhorse (2015):

> This discussion varies in our ever-diverse culture. What I've learned is we can discuss this for hours on end but, when all is said and done, we call ourselves what we want because it is our choice. In fact, choice is something we did not have or were able to practice throughout the annals of U.S. history.

To that end, for the sake of discourse, the term *Native American* is the term used in this text, with the understanding that neither of the terms selected do justice to addressing them accordingly when referring to this specific group within the **American Indian and Alaska Native (AIAN)** racial category, per the OMB. The OMB is an office of the President of the United States that determines racial and ethnic categories for the nation. Thus, the term *American Indian* should be used with understanding that there is controversy associated with it, along with the term *tribe*. As explained by Baker et al. (2021):

> Native nations are independent nations within a nation. The term nation shows respect for sovereignty and the fact that Native nations each have their own systems of government. Globally, we have trivialized the term Tribe (think "bride tribe," "political tribalism," etc.). We don't recommend using Tribe or Tribes to talk about Native nations. Some phrases and even names of Native nations contain the word Tribe or a derivative (Tribal colleges, for example). It's ok to use Tribe in these cases.

As a primary remedy before health issues and other potential remedies are discussed, indigenous people should be asked what they prefer to be called. This will afford dignity as efforts are being made to improve the quality of life for all AIAN people. The history of Native American people in the United States and the atrocities committed against them are complicated and tragic. Once Europeans set foot on American soil, the outcome for Native American people was war, disease, hardship, and suffering. Ultimately, the U.S. government came up with laws particularly related to the provision of health care for Native American and Alaska Native people. Hence, the **Indian Health Service (IHS)** was established in 1955 and was transferred to what was formally known as the Department of Health, Education, and Welfare, which is now the Department of Health and Human Services (Pfefferbaum et al., 1996). The IHS is a federal program that provides comprehensive health services directly to members of federally recognized AIAN groups of people and their descendants. Unfortunately, per Lofthouse (2022), the IHS "has struggled chronically with underfunding and bureaucratic shortcomings."

AIAN people are citizens of the United States. Consequently, they are able to participate in all health programs in the United States, no matter if they are private, public, or state, offered to the general public. In some isolated areas, it is unfortunate, but some Native American people may not have health services available. The IHS provides health care through tribally contracted and operated health programs and services purchased from private providers (Indian Health Service, n.d.-a) and serves approximately 2.56 million AIAN people (Indian Health Service, n.d.-b). The facilities where people are served are either leased or owned by the IHS and exist as either hospitals, school health centers or clinics and, Alaska village clinics. The result of this entity is improvement of the health of AIAN people with shortcomings. Hence, their health status remains problematic.

There is no doubt that as one of the emerging majority populations in the United States, Native American and Alaska Native people should have every opportunity to receive optimal health care to the same degree as their White counterparts and every other race/ethnicity. Although the relationship of this group with the United States has been challenging, the IHS has attempted to be helpful. Per the U.S. Census Bureau, ". . . 2.7 million U.S. residents identified as American Indian and Alaska Native alone. . ." When the U.S. government decided to change its perception from the "termination" of Native American people to "self-determination," as highlighted in the Indian Self-Determination Act of 1975, enabling transfer of programs under the **Bureau of Indian Affairs,** including the IHS, to tribal government (Pfefferbaum et al., 1996), there was the real opportunity to strive toward an improved health status. This is particularly true for Native American women, who, as in many other racial groups, are the primary caretakers of health in their families. As explained by the U.S. Department of the Interior (n.d.):

> At 200 years old, the Bureau of Indian Affairs is the oldest bureau in the Department of the Interior. Our mission is to enhance the quality of life, promote economic opportunities, and to carry out the responsibilities entrusted to us to protect and improve the trust assets of American Indians and Alaska Natives. We accomplish this either directly, through contracts, grants, or compact agreements.

It should be noted that, technically, Native American nations should not be equated with other emerging majorities. The fact is that Native American people,

15 Leading Causes of Death (non-Hispanic AIAN population): 2019

Cause of Death	Percentage
Heart Disease and/or Cancer	36.6
Accidents	10.6
Liver Disease/Cirrhosis	5.2
Lower Respiratory Disease/Diabetes/Stroke	13.7
Suicide	2.9
Kidney Disease/Flu/Pneumonia/Alzheimer's/Septicemia	7.0
Assault	1.4
Other	1.6

Figure 5-1 Mortality profile of Non-Hispanic American Indian or Alaska Native population, 2019.

Data from Arias, E., Xu, J., Curtin, S., Bastian, B., & Tejada-Vera, B. (2021). Mortality profile of the Non-Hispanic American Indian or Alaska native population, 2019. *National Vital Statistics Reports, 70*(12), 1-27. https://stacks.cdc.gov/view/cdc/110370.

by treaty rights, own their own lands and have other rights that are unique to the descendants of the real native people of America. U.S. laws and treaties, officially endorsed by U.S. presidents and Congress, confirm that status (Gover, 2014). No other emerging majority group within the United States is in a similar legal position. Native people view themselves as separate nations within a nation (Baker et al., 2021).

Despite steps in the right direction, such as the establishment of the IHS, Native American and Alaska Native people suffer great health disparities, including alcoholism, obesity, diabetes, and heart disease. Per Arias et al. (2021), in 2019, the 15 leading causes of death for the non-Hispanic AIAN population accounted for 79% of all deaths occurring to this population (**Figure 5-1**).

Cultural Nuances

There are **cultural nuances** relative to the various AIAN groups that often involve the need for healthcare providers to understand their traditional beliefs, which are not monolithic in terms of all AIAN people. Most AIAN people live in rural and urban areas outside of reservations or off-reservation trust lands and many are experiencing unemployment and poverty as well as significant health disparities (Jim et al., 2012; Urban Indian Health Commission, 2007). Although the IHS helps to cross that barrier, to further resolve some of the health issues relevant to Native Americans people, additional key steps must be taken. The delineation of health problems regarding AIAN people is mentioned earlier and is accessible and available via basic research from the IHS, DHHS, and beyond, but the question is what are the remedies to resolve these issues?

REMEDIES

There have been specific initiatives, beyond the IHS, to try to improve the health status of AIAN people, in terms of health disparities. For example, the **Indian Health Care Improvement Act (IHCIA)** of 1976, amended in 1980, created a 7-year approach to resolving some of the issues, with attempts to eliminate health disparities relative to this group of people. Per the IHS, this document is the cornerstone legal authority for the provision of health care to AIAN people (Indian Health Service, n.d.-a) The act was made permanent when President Barrack Obama signed the bill on March 23, 2010, as part of the **Patient Protection and Affordable Care Act (PPACA)**, which was a program under the Obama Administration to assist with affordable access to care for the general population (Indian Health Service, n.d.-b).

It seems that although the IHS and the IHCIA are laudable approaches to assist the AIAN populations in terms of their health, there is a need to consider heavily proven, evidence-based resources to continue/enhance these efforts. In order to do so, some additional factors have to be taken into consideration. All approaches involving remedies for particular groups must be culturally competent. Cultural competence, to be discussed in depth in another chapter in this book, involves ensuring that the cultures and languages of the people to be served are taken into consideration at the forefront of any efforts to address their health needs. Beyond those who are offering the services, the community itself must be involved at every step, with their input being at the center, valued, respected, and appreciated.

Additional Remedies:

- To enhance the efforts of the IHS and the IHCIA, consider heavily proven, evidence-based resources and apply them widely toward the AIAN populations.
- Ensure that all approaches toward improving the health status of AIAN groups are culturally competent.
- The AIAN communities must be involved at every step, with their input being at the center, valued, respected, and appreciated.
- Stratification is imperative based on understanding the history of the group receiving services, age, and other factors.

Evidence-Based Practices

Per Lorig (2022), there are three evidence-based practices to be considered, which are geared toward older people, as one group example. She discussed several evidence-based programs that are worthy of consideration for older AIAN people and may serve as a basis for development of approaches for other age groups. Two are highlighted in this text. The first is the **chronic disease management program (CDMP)**, which is:

> . . . an educational workshop geared toward engaging people who are living with variety of chronic health conditions. Overall, the CDSMP [Chronic Disease Self-Management Program] aims to build participants' confidence in managing their own health and staying engaged in their

own lives. In offering CDSMP within tribal communities, program leaders have used several important strategies to promote cultural competence and appropriateness among Native elders.

The second is Wisdom Warriors, which:

> . . . was developed by tribal specialists and federal leaders at the Northwest Regional Council in Northwest Washington state. Wisdom Warriors is a program that relies on traditional tribal foods, cultural activities, and deep-rooted traditions to help tribal elders improve their health by better managing chronic illnesses . . . The program demonstrates several important strategies that other programs can incorporate to be culturally relevant while adhering to program integrity.

These are examples of effective, evidence-based, culturally competent, nation-centered programs. The bottom line is that any remedy related to helping AIAN people with their health concerns must be culturally competent, involve them at every level and, stratified based on understanding the history of the group receiving services, age, and other factors. There is no "cookie cutter" solution related to AIAN people. Working toward resolving their health problems cannot be accomplished by considering them as a monolithic group. The diversity involved is significant and a key aspect of understanding what their health needs are. Furthermore, other remedies suggested by Lofthouse (2022) are the increase of funding to the IHS by Congress, policy changes and instrumental reforms (both long- and short-term) focused on improving the health of AIAN people, and the removal of barriers to economic growth and the reduction of poverty. In short, he recommends as one example:

> Simplifying the processes and regulations for using, selling, or leasing trust land would reduce the transaction costs facing individual tribal members and tribal governments. Removing or reducing other forms of red tape would more easily allow both individual entrepreneurs and tribal businesses to have more opportunities for economic success. Without continuing the reforms that lower transaction costs, Native Americans are likely to remain impoverished and suffer from higher rates of health problems.

REMEDIES

- Ask Indigenous people what they prefer to be called and then use that terminology, rather than what OMB requires.
- Improve the capabilities of the IHS by the provision of significant additional funding from the U.S. government.
- Ensure that culturally competent approaches are at the forefront of any and all efforts to improve the health status of AIAN people.
- The community itself, namely AIAN people, must be involved at every step, with their input being at the center, valued, respected, and appreciated. The

(continues)

REMEDIES *(continued)*

"White savior" approach should not be considered or implemented at any level, including when government funding is sought and provided.

- Evidence-based approaches should be considered in all efforts to improve the health of AIAN people toward eliminating disparities and achieving health equity.
- Any efforts related to helping AIAN people with their health concerns, in addition to being culturally competent, must involve them at every level, as leaders, and be stratified based on understanding the history of the group receiving services, along with age and other factors.
- There must be changes (both long- and short-term) that, in addition to being focused on improving the health of AIAN people, are also focused on the removal of barriers to economic growth and the reduction of poverty.

WRAP-UP

Since it is a fact that the experience of poverty is a significant determinant in terms of health problems, great emphasis on eliminating this particular issue for AIAN people would be a key remedy, albeit not the only one. AIAN people have contributed greatly to the United States, specifically because they were the caretakers of the land before Europeans ever set foot on it. This contribution was not considered as attempts were made to eliminate/annihilate them from the face of the Earth. Even after centuries of attempts to annihilate them, many AIAN people remain in the United States today. However, many among them are in a state of struggle in terms of their health. They deserve the respect and dignity that is afforded to those who usurped the land from them, namely White people, and who placed them in suboptimal living situations that contribute to poor health outcomes.

The goal should be to no longer simply discuss, delineate, and highlight their health problems but rather to focus on immediate remedies with the AIAN people involved at the forefront in every step of the process. Involvement is not enough; they need to be the leaders of all initiatives pertaining to them. They know better what is necessary for their people to experience the optimal quality of life that they deserve as they were living and thriving before White people entered and tried to destroy them. How long will their health problems be discussed in the United States without the primary goal being, with fierce determination and monetary provisions, to resolve the problem? In short, achieving health equity must be the primary goal of all health entities that serve them, with AIAN leading the process.

Chapter Problems

1. What are some of the main health issues that impact AIAN people?
2. Name two evidence-based programs indicated for elderly AIAN people.
3. What is the relevance of cultural competency in terms of remedies for AIAN health issues?

4. Explain why using the term *tribes* may be a problem when discussing Native American people.
5. Discuss how poverty may impact the health of Native American people.

References

Arias, E., Xu, J., Curtin, S., Bastian, B., & Tejada-Vera, B. (2021). Mortality Profile of the Non-Hispanic American Indian or Alaska Native Population, 2019. National vital statistics reports: from the Centers for Disease Control and Prevention, National Center for Health Statistics, National Vital Statistics System, 70(12), 1–27.

Baker, T., Elk, W. L., Pollard, B., & Bird, M. Y. (2021). *How to talk about Native Nations; A guide.* Native Governance Center. https://nativegov.org/news/how-to-talk-about-native-nations-a -guide/

Blackhorse, A. (2015, May 22). Do you prefer 'Native American' or 'American Indian'? 6 prominent voices respond. *ICT News.* https://ictnews.org/archive/blackhorse-do-you-prefer-native -american-or-american-indian-6-prominent-voices-respond

Gover, K. (2014). Nation to nation: Treaties between the United States and American Indian nations. *American Indian, 15*(2). https://www.americanindianmagazine.org/story/nation-nation -treaties-between-united-states-and-american-indian-nations#:~:text=Happily%2C%20the %20story%20does%20not,the%20rights%20enshrined%20in%20treaties

Indian Health Service. (n.d.-a). About IHS. U.S. Department of Health and Human Services. https:// www.ihs.gov/aboutihs/

Indian Health Service. (n.d.-b). Disparities. U.S. Department of Health and Human Services. https://www.ihs.gov/newsroom/factsheets/disparities/

Jim, N., Martel, R., Yellow Horse Brave Heart, M., Menino, B., Hein, D., Goze, M., & Sommer-Pedebone, D. (2012, September 27). *Expert Panel on homelessness among American Indians, Alaska Natives, and Native Hawaiians* [Report]. Substance Abuse and Mental Health Services Administration. https://www.usich.gov/sites/default/files/document/Expert_Panel_on _Homelessness_among_American_Indians%252C_Alaska_Natives%252C_and_Native _Hawaiians.pdf

Lofthouse, J. (2022). Reducing Poverty to Improve Native American Health Outcomes. Health Care Policy Briefs. Mercatus Center, George Mason University. https://www.mercatus.org/research /policy-briefs/reducing-poverty-improve-native-american-health-outcomes

Lorig, K. (2022, August 4). *How can proven evidence-based resources better reach Native elders?* National Council On Aging. https://www.ncoa.org/article/how-can-proven-evidence-based -resources-better-reach-native-elders

Pfefferbaum, B., Strickland, R. J., Rhoades, E. R., & Pfefferbaum, R. L. (1996). Learning how to Heal: An analysis of the history, policy, and framework of Indian health care. *American Indian Law Review, 20*(2), 365, 376–377.

Rubin, R., & Melnick, J. (2006). *Immigration and American popular culture: An introduction.* New York University Press.

Urban Indian Health Commission. (2007). *Invisible tribes: Urban Indians and their health in a changing world* [Report]. U.S. Census Bureau. https://www2.census.gov/cac/nac/meetings/2015-10-13 /invisible-tribes.pdf

U.S. Department of the Interior. (n.d.). *Bureau of Indian Affairs | Indian Affairs.* https://www.bia.gov/bia

The Hispanic/Latino Population and Health Disparities: Issues, Concerns, and Remedies

Elizabeth Baquero, EdD, MS

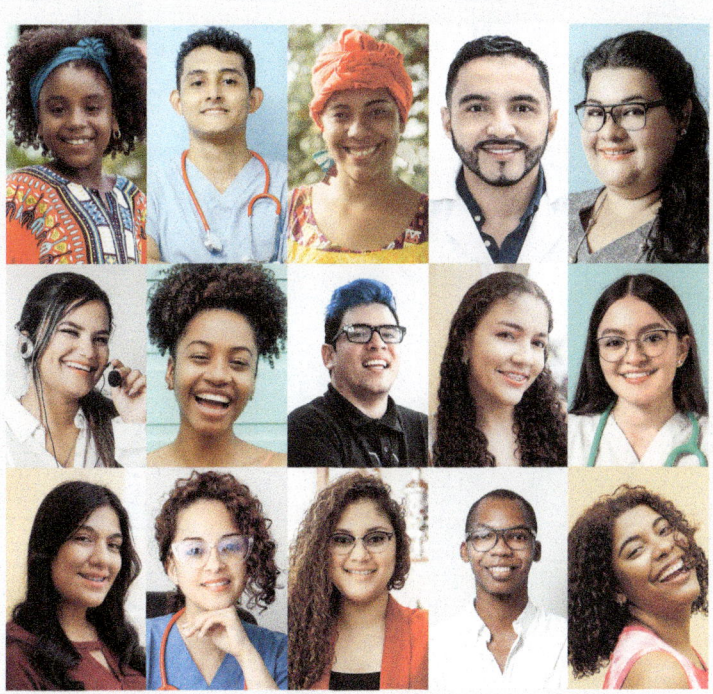

KEY TERMS

cultural competence
Federally Qualified Health Center
    (FQHC)
food insecurity
health literacy
Hispanic

Hispanic health paradox
Latina birth outcomes paradox
Reserve Capacity Model (RCM)
social determinants of health
    (SDOH)

LEARNING OBJECTIVES

After reading this chapter, you should be able to do the following:

1. Explain the difference between the terms Hispanic and Latino.
2. List the leading health challenges experienced by Hispanic/Latino people.
3. Explain how socioeconomic status impacts the health of Hispanic/Latino people.
4. Discuss at least three remedies for improving the health of Hispanic/Latino people.

Introduction

According to the United States Census Bureau, there are over 65 million Hispanic/Latino people in the United States and there are 10 states where they are primarily located (**Figure 6-1**) (U.S. Census Bureau, 2024). Language/cultural

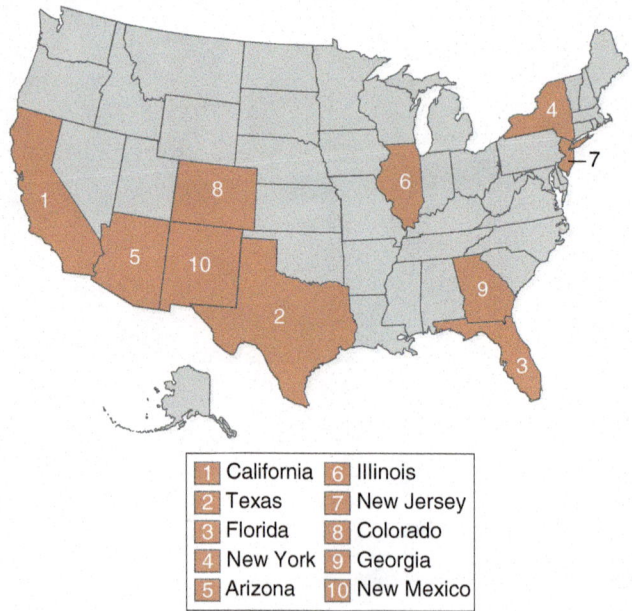

1	California	6	Illinois
2	Texas	7	New Jersey
3	Florida	8	Colorado
4	New York	9	Georgia
5	Arizona	10	New Mexico

Figure 6-1 Top 10 states with the largest percentage of Hispanic/Latino people.

Modified from U.S. Department of Health and Human Services (USDHHS), Office of Minority Health (OMH) (2024). Hispanic/Latino Health. Retrieved from https://minorityhealth
.hhs.gov/hispaniclatino-health

barriers, lack of access to preventive care, and lack of insurance significantly impact the health of Hispanic/Latino people in the United States. This chapter will explore the context, controversies, and remedies relevant to achieving health equity amongst them.

Health Concerns

A major health concern for the Hispanic/Latino population is obesity, which is a significant risk factor for a variety of health conditions, including diabetes and cardiovascular disease (CVD) (Escarce et al., 2006). Hispanic/Latino people have a higher rate of diabetes and obesity compared to non-Hispanic White people (Escarce et al., 2006; Office of Minority Health, n.d.), and nearly half of Hispanic/Latino men and women aged 20 and older are obese (44.8% and 46.8%, respectively). As of 2024, the leading cause of death among the **Hispanic** population is heart disease (a range of conditions that affect the heart, also known as CVD), cancer (abnormal cell growth), and accidents (unintentional injuries) (Centers for Disease Control and Prevention, 2024a).

Hispanic/Latino people are also disproportionately impacted by conditions influenced by structural and social factors known as the **Social Determinants of Health (SDOH)** (Velasco-Mondragon et al., 2016) (**Figure 6-2**). The SDOH are categorized as economic stability, education access and quality, healthcare access and quality, neighborhood and built environment, and social and community context.

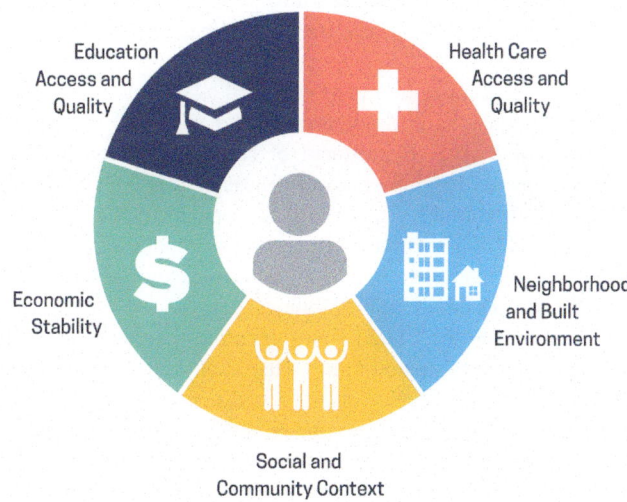

Figure 6-2 Social determinants of health.

Healthcare Access and Quality

Hispanic/Latino people have the highest rates of uninsured individuals of any racial or ethnic group in the United States (Office of Minority Health, n.d.). Over a quarter (28%) of Hispanic adults ages 18–64 years do not have health insurance (Centers for Disease Control and Prevention, 2024a) as compared to the White non-Hispanic population at 7.5% (Centers for Disease Control and Prevention, 2024b). This is problematic as health insurance enhances access to preventive and primary care services while lowering out-of-pocket medical expenses. Central and South American people are more than three times as likely, and Mexican people are six times as likely, to be uninsured as compared to non-Hispanic people. Additionally, a larger percentage of Hispanic people born outside the United States, particularly recent immigrants, lack insurance compared to United States-born Latino people (Greer et al., 2017).

Lack of health insurance is a key predictor of access to health care and the quality of health care received (Buchanan & Smokowski, 2009). For example, lack of insurance can also lead to barriers to preventive screening. Hispanic/Latino people have lower screening rates for some cancers compared to other racial/ethnic groups, and due to the high rates of cancer in this population, screenings also need to be prioritized and more accessible (Velasco-Mondragon et al., 2016).

Education Access and Quality

According to the Centers for Disease Control and Prevention (CDC) (Beckles & Truman, 2011), education is strongly associated with life expectancy and morbidity. For example, lower levels of education are associated with a greater risk of CVD. Higher education levels are associated with a greater likelihood of employment, and a higher degree is typically associated with higher-paying jobs (U.S. Bureau of Labor Statistics, 2021).

Hispanic/Latino people are not as educated as their White counterparts, with 71.8% having a high school diploma compared to 94.6% among non-Hispanic/Latino White people (U.S. Department of Health and Human Services, 2024). Hispanic/Latino people also have a lower college graduation rate than their African American and White counterparts (Arbona & Nora, 2007). These researchers found that more than half of Hispanic/Latino students initially enrolled in community colleges but did not complete bachelor's degrees at four-year institutions due to financial restraints and family responsibilities.

This contributes to the United States unemployment rate being higher among Hispanic/Latino people compared to non-Hispanic/Latino people (10.4% compared to 7.5%, respectively) (U.S. Bureau of Labor Statistics, 2021). Hispanic/Latino people account for 18% of the total employment in the United States, and most Hispanic/Latino people in the labor force are Mexican people (60%). If one is not employed, having health insurance can be more challenging and expensive because, in the United States, health care is accessed mainly through employer-sponsored plans. Although there are Hispanic/Latino people who are doctors, lawyers, politicians, and all types of other professions, they are overrepresented in occupational categories, such as painters (51%), maids and housekeepers (46%), and construction laborers (46%). Valenzuela (2003) reviewed the research on "day labor," which can mean employment distinguished by hazards in or undesirability of the work, the absence of fringe benefits, and other typical workplace benefits. In the United States, day laborers are mainly unauthorized Hispanic immigrants concentrated in metropolitan areas.

Health Literacy

According to the Institute of Medicine Committee on Health Literacy (2004), **health literacy** is how individuals obtain, process, and understand basic health information and services needed to make health decisions. Health literacy is generally low, with 36% of United States adults having basic or below-basic health literacy levels (Kutner et al., 2006). However, Hispanic/Latino adults had lower average health literacy than adults in any other racial/ethnic group.

A central focus of Healthy People 2030 (2024) is health literacy with an emphasis on the fact that most individuals want to be involved in health decisions and how shared decision-making, where patients and healthcare providers collaborate, can enhance patient satisfaction and improve health outcomes. Training providers to build collaborative relationships and use decision aids can facilitate this process.

Low health literacy means people cannot follow healthcare recommendations for diagnostic tests or medications, identify signs and symptoms that prompt seeking care and early detection, and understand what insurance will or will not cover (Kutner et al., 2006). To exacerbate the situation, visit lengths in the exam room with a healthcare provider are short, typically 20 minutes on average, resulting in fewer health issues being addressed and a reduced depth of understanding (Linzer et al., 2015; Shaw et al., 2014).

Economic Stability

Socioeconomic status (SES) is a construct of multiple factors, such as income, education, and employment status. Lower SES is associated with a higher risk of CVD, which is a leading cause of death among Hispanic/Latino people (Beckles & Truman, 2011). Additionally, per the CDC (Beckles & Truman, 2011), individuals with lower incomes face disadvantages, such as inadequate education, poor working conditions, housing insecurity, and living in unsafe neighborhoods. Individuals with lower incomes are more likely to face negative psychosocial factors (occupational stress, social support or isolation, sleep quality, and mental health) that can provoke a physiological stress response, such as increased cortisol and higher blood pressure, which also contributes to the risk of CVD. For Hispanic/Latino people, SES is a particularly important factor since they have the highest poverty rate in the country at 17% (Shrider et al., 2021). Furthermore, Hispanic/Latino women are the lowest-paid individuals across job industries and the gap is closing at a slower rate compared to women in other groups (American Association of University Women, 2025).

Pay inequity requires structural remedies that policymakers must lead. The American Association of University Women recommends the following remedies to close the wage gap:

1. Congress should pass a law prohibiting employers from using salary history to set pay and requiring employers to provide equal pay for jobs of equivalent value.
2. Congress should invest in affordable childcare and create a national paid family and medical leave insurance program for all workers.
3. As states wait for congressional action, they should reform their pay equity laws.

4. Employers should conduct pay audits, have better salary transparency, and prohibit retaliation against employees for discussing or inquiring about their wages.

5. Individuals should educate themselves about pay inequities and how to negotiate their finances in their workplace.

Importantly, in exploring SES in terms of Hispanic/Latino people, it is imperative to consider remedies. Gallo and Matthews (2003) introduced the **Reserve Capacity Model (RCM)**, which provides a framework for exploring the connections between poverty, low SES, and health outcomes. Types of reserves include interpersonal resources, such as social support and social integration or intrapersonal resources, such as self-efficacy, sense of perceived control, optimism, and hopefulness. The RCM suggests that low SES environments are stressful and reduce individuals' reserve capacity to manage stress, thereby increasing vulnerability to negative emotions. These negative emotions can negatively impact physical health by promoting unhealthy behaviors, causing heightened chronic physiological responses. They also found that greater reserve capacity is associated with improved health outcomes and may lower mortality risk, particularly for those with low SES.

Gallo et al. (2009) released a culturally expanded version of the RCM to analyze disparities among Hispanic/Latino people by integrating specific cultural stressors and reserves that could exacerbate or buffer the association between SES and health (Bennett, 2017; Gallo et al., 2009). For example, priorities for Hispanic/Latino people, such as familism (a tendency to put family above an individual's personal interests) and prosocial/nonconfrontational interactions, may help combat the association between low SES and poor health. Their research also indicates that low SES can lead to greater exposure to "risky family" environments, such as parental conflict, neglect, and insufficient nurturing. These conditions can hinder the development of essential social-emotional coping skills needed for healthy psychological and social functioning. More longitudinal studies among Hispanic youth are needed, as SES persists from childhood into adulthood and across generations.

REMEDIES

Remedies Relevant to SES

Available research indicates that remedies, such as interventions to reduce stress and increase resilient psychosocial resources could effectively reduce health disparities related to SES. Prioritizing family and community-building initiatives that enhance social capital may cultivate a sense of control and social connectedness among Hispanic/Latino people who are experiencing a lower SES. Employers should offer flexible work hours or allow more control over shifts, effectively building resources. Healthcare workers should consider family important to the Hispanic/Latino community and create welcoming spaces and communication with the family in mind. Considering that psychosocial risk trajectories often begin early in life, school-based programs should develop protective resources and focus on prevention efforts for families who are tackling economic hurdles. Further understanding and leveraging some Hispanic/Latino cultural reserves and assets, such as social support, familism, and religiosity, may promote more resilience in the face of challenges.

Gallo et al. (2012) measured demographic factors, psychosocial resources (personal and social), and risk (negative emotions and cognitions) variables among 304 middle-aged Mexican-American women. They found that low SES was associated with higher waist circumference and fasting glucose via lower psychosocial resources and higher psychosocial risk. This path was significant in the overall sample and the more acculturated subsample.

Additional studies are needed to examine the psychosocial pathways proposed in the RCM, particularly for objective physical health outcomes and using prospective designs (Gallo et al., 2009).

Neighborhood and Built Environment

Hispanic/Latino people are predominantly located in urban areas where there is often high stress, pollutants, and segregation. Malambo et al. (2016) systematically reviewed the literature to identify built environment attributes associated with CVD. Among the 18 studies, neighborhood environmental attributes were significantly associated with CVD risk and outcomes. Residential density, safety from traffic, recreation facilities, street connectivity, and a high walkable environment were associated with physical activity. A low-walkable environment, fast-food restaurants, and supermarket/grocery stores were associated with high blood pressure, diabetes mellitus, and metabolic syndrome. High-density traffic, road proximity, and fast-food restaurants were associated with CVD outcomes. Fields et al. (2013) studied Hispanic people to understand better how the built environment impacts their health behaviors. They found an association between meeting physical activity recommendations and the presence of sidewalks and safe parks. Residential density and shops nearby were related to active commuting. Sedentary behavior was negatively associated with having a bus stop, bike facilities, a secure park, things to look at, and seeing people active.

These findings, which are consistent with other studies among Hispanic/Latino people (Bayly et al., 2022; Carlson et al., 2022), underscore the significant role of the neighborhood in influencing health behaviors. They also point to a promising avenue for future research and neighborhood change efforts. By targeting built environment variables, we can potentially improve health outcomes among Hispanic/Latino people, offering hope for the future of public health in urban areas.

Additionally, economic segregation, in which wealthier people reside in affluent neighborhoods while people experiencing low incomes live in areas with fewer resources, is another key factor. Neighborhoods where people are experiencing low incomes are less likely to have access to high-quality health care (Beckles & Truman, 2011). Another consequence of poverty and economic segregation is housing insecurity, which can be described as the burden of high housing costs in relation to income, inadequate housing quality, unstable living arrangements, overcrowding, and residing in unsafe neighborhoods. Neighborhoods where people are experiencing poverty and low incomes are often food deserts, which leads to food insecurity.

Food insecurity refers to the inability to access adequate food due to limited economic resources, and the prevalence of food insecurity is high among segments of the Hispanic/Latino population (Varela et al., 2023). For example, people who do not have access to stores with healthy and affordable food cannot prepare nutritious meals for their families, which leads to a higher risk of heart disease, diabetes, and obesity (U.S. Department of Health and Human Services, 2024).

However, providing healthier options is not enough. The built environment needs to be improved to foster transportation to the stores and safe places to exercise. More programs like SNAP (Supplemental Nutrition Assistance Program) are critical in alleviating food insecurity.

Life Expectancy

Overall, Americans are expected to live longer in the coming decades. In 2060, foreign-born men and women are projected to live longer than their native-born peers, regardless of race or Hispanic/Latino origin (Medina et al., 2020) (**Figure 6-3**). Native-born is anyone who is a United States citizen at birth, including people born in the United States, Puerto Rico, a United States Island Area, the United States Virgin Islands, or born abroad to a United States citizen parent. Despite Hispanic/Latino people having a lower socioeconomic status than their non-Hispanic counterparts, Hispanic/Latino people have lower mortality rates and longer life expectancies, also known as the **Hispanic health paradox** (Medina et al., 2020; Morales et al., 2002).

It is essential to recognize that vital statistics data may underreport mortality rates for Hispanics/Latino people due to the under-identification of Hispanic/Latino ethnicity on death certificates. This leads to an uncomprehensive understanding of why Hispanics/Latino people in the United States have longer lifespans and research on this subject is limited. Some suggest that social and cultural effects and the

Projections of Life Expectancy at Birth by Sex, Race, Hispanic Origin, and Nativity: 2017 and 2060

Year	Group 1: Non-Hispanic White alone, non-Hispanic Asian alone, and non-Hispanic Native Hawaiian or Other Pacific Islander alone			Group 2: Non-Hispanic Black or African American alone and non-Hispanic American Indian or Alaska Native alone			Group 3: Hispanic or Latino alone (of any race)		
	Total	Males	Females	Total	Males	Females	Total	Males	Females
Native-born									
2017	79.6	77.3	81.9	75.1	72.1	78.0	80.8	78.2	83.3
2060	85.5	83.9	87.2	84.3	82.4	86.2	86.0	84.3	87.8
Foreign-born									
2017	83.7	81.6	85.5	83.0	80.6	84.8	83.5	81.2	85.5
2060	86.9	85.4	88.5	86.8	85.1	88.4	86.9	85.2	88.5

Figure 6-3 Population estimates and projections per the U.S. Department of Commerce.

migration effect might be starting points for understanding this phenomenon (Medina et al., 2020). Hispanics/Latino people have strong communities and are more likely to live in multigenerational households, which can have positive benefits; however, infectious diseases can spread more quickly. The salmon bias hypothesis (a.k.a. the unhealthy out-migrant hypothesis) suggests that healthier Hispanics/Latino people migrate to the United States, leaving their less healthy counterparts in their home country. It also indicates that foreign-born immigrants who become sick are more likely to report to their home country before dying (Turra & Elo, 2008). However, the paradox does not affect all Hispanic/Latino subgroups or health conditions equally. For example, Mexican, Central American, and South American populations typically exhibit a greater mortality advantage than Puerto Ricans or Cubans (Escarce et al., 2006).

Another phenomenon is known as the **Latina birth outcomes paradox**. Hispanic women in the United States have higher birth rates compared to other racial/ethnic groups, but this varies within subgroups (Velasco-Mondragon et al., 2016). For decades, research has indicated that despite having low SES, Hispanic women in the United States have favorable pregnancy outcomes compared to other racial/ethnic groups (Fuentes-Afflick & Lurie, 1997; Velasco-Mondragon et al., 2016). Studies have found that protective factors, such as cultural support for maternity and various maternal-based traditions, may exist (Velasco-Mondragon et al., 2016). However, a recent review synthesis suggests that due to a lack of standardization in documentation, the status of pregnancy outcomes among Hispanic women is not conclusive and may be diminishing (Richardson et al., 2020).

The longer Hispanic immigrants are in the United States, the more likely they are to acculturate, which involves adapting to the customs and norms of the host culture. Acculturation is a complex process and can impact health and well-being. For example, length of residence is directly associated with increased body mass index (BMI) and obesity among Hispanics/Latino people (Bates et al., 2007; Gonzalez et al., 2023; Gordon-Larsen et al., 2003; Kaplan et al., 2004). Gonzalez et al. (2023) found that the generational composition of social networks alters the association between the generational status and weight of adolescents, and therefore, social factors within those networks may contribute to those associations.

These paradoxes also suggest that there might be a migrant health selectivity, where healthy people migrate into the country and unhealthy people migrate out (Crimmins et al., 2007).

Immigration

The U.S. Department of Homeland Security estimated that there are around 11 million undocumented immigrants in the United States (Baker & Warren, 2024). There is speculation regarding this number, but nevertheless, the key is that the number is significant. Hispanic/Latino immigrants share some characteristics, such as younger average age, a higher proportion of married households, and lower educational attainment than the United States population (Alarcón et al., 2016). Given that Mexican people are the largest subgroup within the Hispanic/Latino community, they are the largest national group of legal and unauthorized immigrants (Hoefer et al., 2012; Tienda & Sanchez, 2013; Baker & Warren, 2024). Individuals and families may seek to immigrate for reasons, including, but not limited to, economic disparities, civil unrest, political instability, and family reunification. Conditions before, during, and after migration can affect the health of migrant populations, considering the different stages of immigration, from pre-immigration to the immigration journey to post-immigration.

While immigrating, there is a high risk for stress and trauma, which can increase the risk of depressive symptoms and anxiety (Mikolajczyk, 2007). There has been evidence to show that, once immigrants are in the United States, stress from acculturation influences family and friend relationships, which in turn affects adolescent mental health problems and substance use (Buchanan & Smokowski, 2009; Cavazos-Rehg et al., 2007). These health issues are disproportionately affecting the undocumented and uninsured in the United States. Cavazos-Rehg et al. (2007) found that being undocumented can generate stress and fear in seeking and possibly being denied health services. Many families include both documented and undocumented members, resulting in complex family dynamics that influence healthcare-seeking behavior.

Cultural and Linguistic Competency

Most Hispanic/Latino people (71.1%) speak a language other than English at home, and over a quarter (28.4%) are not fluent in English (Office of Minority Health, 2024). Only 7% of all physicians and surgeons are Hispanic/Latino in the United States (Funk & Lopez, 2022). About 8 in 10 (81%) of Spanish-language-dominant individuals prefer to have a Spanish-speaking healthcare provider (Funk & Lopez, 2022). Furthermore, in a study about the language barriers in urban Hispanic/Latino people, David & Rhee (1998) found that the lack of explanation of the side effects of medication correlates negatively with compliance with medication, and the language barrier correlated negatively with patient satisfaction.

While training enough Spanish-speaking physicians will take time, a remedy for this concern is cultural competency training, which can enhance providers' knowledge, skills, and attitudes related to cultural competency, leading to improved access to and utilization of healthcare services (Williams et al., 2019). One specific remedy for this concern is evidence-based frameworks, such as the Inventory for Assessing the Process of Cultural Competence Among Healthcare Professionals (IAPCC). Another tool is the Cultural Competence Assessment Tool for Health Professionals (see Appendix V). These assessment mechanisms should be utilized to evaluate **cultural competence** training programs/healthcare professionals to address the issue of exploring the skill sets and attitudes regarding the provision of culturally competent care (Campinha-Bacote, 1999). Both cultural competence and patient-centeredness are remedies to improve the quality of health care for individual patients, communities, and populations (Saha et al., 2008).

Since Hispanic/Latino people in the United States originate from diverse countries and cultures, to improve their health it is essential to tailor programs to their unique qualities and preferences. Accessing appropriate healthcare depends on having the skills to read and complete medical and insurance forms, communicate effectively with healthcare providers, and understand basic instructions and medical advice. Therefore, another essential remedy is that healthcare institutions need interpreters, translators, and bilingual healthcare providers on-site to assist with patient care. There is a need for better patient education materials delivered not simply in Spanish but in a culturally appropriate way, keeping in mind that some in the community have low health literacy.

Camacho-Rivera et al. (2020) conducted a study to examine trust in cancer information from various media sources among U.S. Hispanic/Latino adults as it is one of the leading causes of death in this population. They found that Cuban and Puerto Rican people were twice as likely to rely on cancer information from print media compared to Mexican-American people. Hispanic/Latino people aged 75 and older were nearly three times more likely to trust cancer information from religious organizations than those aged 18–34. Additionally, Hispanic/Latino women were 59% more likely than men to trust cancer information found online. Therefore, trust in cancer information sources among Hispanic/Latino people varies significantly by nationality and other sociodemographic factors, which has important implications for how cancer information is shared. Research indicates that race-concordant pairings often result in higher patient trust and a greater likelihood of adhering to care plans than race-discordant pairings (Williams et al., 2010). Cultural and language barriers, short visit times, and low overall literacy rates can worsen the challenges of effective communication between patients and the healthcare system (Vernon et al., 2007).

Health Coaching and Peer Coaching

Another remedy, which is in the research phase, is health coaching. Several studies have investigated the effects of health coaching on health issues and different types of coaches, such as Nutritionists, Medical Assistants, and peers. Fortmann et al. (2024) conducted a randomized controlled trial (RCT) of 600 adults with type 2 diabetes. They found that blood sugar level significantly improved in the intervention group who received medical assistant health coaching. Kivelä et al. (2014) systematically reviewed health coaching effects on chronic disease management among adults. They found that health coaching positively affects chronically ill patients' lives by motivating lifestyle changes, improving physical and mental health status, and managing chronic diseases.

Other studies have analyzed the effects of peer coaching, which utilizes people from the communities who either have the same health challenge, have overcome the health challenge, or are caretakers of someone with the disease. These peer coaches meet with the study participants and help set and achieve health goals, often using modalities, such as motivational interviewing (Safford et al., 2015; Safford et al., 2023; Safford et al., 2024). Moreover, health coaching is an effective, evidence-based approach to patient education and care among high-risk populations. It can inspire and harness a patient's readiness to change their lifestyle while supporting self-care at home (Kivelä et al., 2014; Olsen & Nesbitt, 2010); hence, it is indeed a remedy.

The Community Preventive Services Task Force (2009) suggests using technology-supported multicomponent coaching or counseling interventions to influence weight-related behavior or outcomes. Technology-supported counseling may offer increased access for people living in remote areas, people with difficulty traveling, or with unconventional work hours. It also allows anonymity and can be available 24 hours a day.

Insight from a Hispanic/Latino Physician Scientist

In an interview with Christopher Gonzalez, MD, MS, he offered insight into achieving health equity among the Hispanic/Latino population. Dr. Gonzalez is a Clinician-Researcher dedicated to addressing health inequities affecting diverse Hispanic/Latino populations across the United States. He received his MD from the Vagelos College of Physicians and Surgeons, Columbia University, and completed his Internal Medicine training at New York-Presbyterian/Columbia University Medical Center. He was the inaugural Health Equity Research Fellow of the HRSA Diversity Center of Excellence at Weill Cornell Medicine, where he is currently an Assistant Professor of Medicine. He has received funding from the National Heart, Lung, and Blood Institute and the National Institute of Diabetes and Digestive and Kidney Diseases, and is a scholar of the Robert Wood Johnson Foundation's Harold Amos Medical Faculty Development Program. He develops and evaluates interventions that leverage social and cultural factors to reduce cardiometabolic inequities and optimize care for historically marginalized, predominantly Hispanic communities.

Interview with Dr. Christopher Gonzalez

Dr. Baquero: Based on your clinical experience and health equity research, what do you perceive as some of the main challenges faced by Hispanic/Latino people in the United States?

Dr. Gonzalez: Approximately 65 million people in the United States, nearly a fifth of the total population, identify as Hispanic/Latino. This is an enormous population with unique characteristics and diverse needs which, from my experience as a Physician and Health Services Researcher, I believe our current healthcare system is not prepared to manage. First, this incredibly heterogeneous population is constantly evolving, making it challenging to measure the health inequities it faces. We tend to overlook that the terms "Hispanic" and "Latino" are themselves relatively novel, and that they were mainly developed for political reasons, with plenty of debate over whom the terms included and excluded. From its inception, the term was criticized because it seemed to obscure the population heterogeneity it intended to identify. Since then, the terminology has evolved, with similarly controversial terms newly emerging. For example, the use of the term Latinx has been widely debated. Some argue that it is gender inclusive, with an etymology incorporating indigenous origins, while yet others argue that it excludes the population it is meant to represent and anglicizes an inherently gendered language. And that's just the terminology; the population itself also continues to evolve. Recent global and international policies have changed immigration patterns, and therefore, has changed the national identities represented by Hispanic/Latino people in the United States (often referred to as "Hispanic origin"). Because health outcomes vary by Hispanic origin, these evolving migration patterns have important implications for the health of the aggregate Hispanic/Latino population. Furthermore, even at the individual-level, this population is substantially evolving. Over a third of the Hispanic/Latino population in the United States is less than 18 years old. Unlike the adult population, much of the Hispanic/Latino child population is born in the United States, which is, for Hispanic/Latino people, a predictor of numerous (often unfavorable) health outcomes. This young population with unique social determinants and new needs is naturally growing into adults, for which care and resources are much more limited. These examples illustrate the heterogeneity of this population, its evolving nature, and the challenges of measuring its health outcomes. Second, despite the population's heterogeneity, there are important social determinants of health, including those at the policy level, that disproportionately impact the health outcomes of Hispanic/Latino people in the United States. At the most basic level, limited access to health care continues to be a primary challenge for many Hispanic/Latino people, manifesting most clearly as a lack of health insurance, but also as a lack of access to care that is concordant with the linguistic, cultural, and/or literacy needs of the population. Poverty and limited educational attainment, associated with unfavorable health outcomes across all groups, are disproportionately more prevalent among Hispanic/Latino people. A lack of healthy food options, overcrowded households, air pollution, and several other unfavorable neighborhood-level social determinants of health, are all more common in predominantly Hispanic/Latino communities. At the policy level, immigration policies often exacerbate xenophobia, acculturative stress, and fears of utilizing healthcare services or engaging in clinical research. Cumulatively, and at times cyclically, these factors contribute to health inequities, including disparities in obesity, diabetes, cardiovascular disease, cancer, pulmonary disease, and mental health. Unfortunately, our healthcare system, infamously disconnected from many public health initiatives, has just recently started aiming to measure social determinants or consider intervening upon them. But reasonably, studying these factors and their intersectionality can be challenging. Third, despite the unfavorable social determinants of health mentioned, it is critical that we acknowledge that the Hispanic/Latino population, in aggregate, has several favorable health outcomes compared to other racial and ethnic groups, including mortality (termed the Hispanic paradox). Several cultural and social factors, including social cohesion, are thought to contribute to resiliency that may be protective to health, but the mechanisms underlying these observations remain under investigation. This investigation requires interdisciplinary study that incorporates diverse expertise, including but not limited to expertise in sociology, epidemiology, medicine, public health, implementation science, and health policy.

Dr. Baquero: How does your work aim to address some of the health disparities observed among Hispanic/Latino people in the United States?

Dr. Gonzalez: My primary goal is to contribute to the optimization of care provided to Hispanic/Latino people in the United States, primarily by addressing some of the challenges I've mentioned thus far. On the one hand, I am a bilingual primary care Physician practicing at a **federally qualified health center (FQHC)**, which is a health center or clinic that serves medically underserved areas and populations serving a predominantly Hispanic/Latino community. As such, I am one member of an increasingly diverse healthcare workforce that aims to address the lack of access to linguistically concordant primary care observed among populations that are underinsured or uninsured and that are historically marginalized and underserved. On the other hand, I am a Social Epidemiologist, health services researcher, and implementation scientist whose work is informed by real-world clinical experience. My research aims to address or leverage

(continues)

some of the social determinants of health predominant among Hispanic/
Latino people in the United States. This includes better characterizing the
heterogeneity of the Hispanic/Latino population, particularly in relation
to how they prefer to receive health information, which can inform how
population-targeted public health awareness campaigns are tailored or
delivered. It also includes identifying the social mechanisms underlying
acculturated health behaviors, including the processes that facilitate or
hinder the adoption of obesity-promoting behaviors; this allows us to pinpoint
particularly vulnerable subpopulations that may benefit from targeted social
interventions. At present, my research primarily focuses on issues more
proximal to the clinical encounter and, more specifically, on the provision of
care within FQHCs, which serve a large proportion of Hispanic/Latino people
in the United States. My ongoing research explores how unique factors of
these health centers, including their reach, their social capital, and their
cultural humility, can be leveraged to provide patient-centered linguistically
and culturally responsive care to address disparities in diabetes.

Dr. Baquero: Beyond your specific research, what other steps do you feel are
needed to improve the health outcomes of Hispanic/Latino people in the
United States?

Dr. Gonzalez: Much of my work is inspired and informed by often under-
acknowledged leaders in health equity, many of whom are from groups
historically underrepresented in medicine. Addressing complex issues
requires a diverse workforce willing to take innovative approaches; our
current healthcare workforce, and the leaders within it, do not represent the
diversity of our population. Hispanic/Latino-identifying individuals remain
acutely underrepresented in medicine and in science. There is a need to
invest in rigorous programming that consistently supports the educational
advancement of predominantly Hispanic/Latino communities, and that
does so from a very early age. In addition to diversifying the workforce, this
would address several financial and educational disparities prevalent among
Hispanic/Latino people in the United States. From a research perspective,
there remains a need to go beyond simply measuring social determinants,
health disparities, and the heterogeneity of the Hispanic/Latino population.
Instead, we must develop and evaluate interventions that (1) address health
inequities using innovative multi-disciplinary methods and (2) pragmatically
provide person-centered care. Even beyond that, we need to understand how
these interventions can be rapidly implemented in real-world settings that
effectively reach the populations of interest as those issues emerge. Most
importantly, however, research is just the first step: effective interventions
need to be supported and incentivized at the policy level so that that they
can be implemented. Numerous interventions have proven to be effective,
but they remain underutilized because there is no funding to support their
infrastructure. As an example, peer and community health worker-led
interventions have continually shown overwhelming promise across a
number of health outcomes, particularly among historically marginalized
communities, yet they are generally not reimbursed by insurers nor are they
sustainably and sufficiently funded through public health initiatives. In sum,
improving the health outcomes of Hispanic/Latino persons in the United
States requires far-reaching, interdisciplinary, and pragmatic person-
centered interventions that are sustainably supported by equitable policies.

WRAP-UP

The majority of Hispanic/Latino people in the United States are young. Key factors influencing the health outcomes of some members of this group include low education rates, high poverty rates, and language and cultural barriers. Many Hispanic/Latino adults are less likely to have health insurance, health literacy, access to quality care, and receive preventive healthcare. These determinants lead to a higher risk of heart disease, cancer, and injury. However, Hispanic/Latino immigrants have longer life expectancies, possibly due to their resilience, social ties, and migrant bias. More research and insight is needed regarding this paradoxical reality. Remedies should be community- and family-centered and tailored to specific Hispanic/Latino nationalities and cultures. Health education materials that are cultural and linguistically competent must be available and designed with health literacy in mind. Furthermore, healthcare institutions need to offer trained interpreters and translators to assist with patient care and more flexible hours given the demands of working several jobs, which is the case for some Hispanic/Latino people who are experiencing a low socioeconomic status. Policymakers should focus on a health equity agenda to ensure that Hispanic/Latino people achieve the health equity they deserve.

Chapter Problems

1. What is a Federally Qualified Health Center (FQHC)?
2. List three leading causes of death for Hispanic/Latino people in the United States
3. What are the categories of the social determinants of health (SDOH) per Healthy People 2030?
4. What is the relationship between the Reserve Capacity Model and stress?

References

American Association of University Women. (2025). The simple truth about the gender pay gap. 2020 update. Retrieved July 7, 2024 from https://www.aauw.org/resources/research/simple-truth/

Alarcón, R. D., Parekh, A., Wainberg, M. L., Duarte, C. S., Araya, R., & Oquendo, M. A. (2016). Hispanic immigrants in the USA: social and mental health perspectives. *The Lancet Psychiatry, 3*(9), 860–870. https://doi.org/10.1016/s2215-0366(16)30101-8

Arbona, C., & Nora, A. (2007). The Influence of Academic and Environmental Factors on Hispanic College Degree Attainment. *Review of Higher Education, 30*(3), 247–269. https://doi.org/10.1353/rhe.2007.0001

Baker, B., & Warren, R. (2024, April). Estimates of the unauthorized immigrant population residing in the United States: January 2018–January 2022. Office of Homeland Security Statistics, U.S. Department of Homeland Security. https://ohss.dhs.gov/sites/default/files/2024-06/2024_0418_ohss_estimates-of-the-unauthorized-immigrant-population-residing-in-the-united-states-january-2018%25E2%2580%2593january-2022.pdf

Bates, L. M., Acevedo-Garcia, D., Alegría, M., & Krieger, N. (2007). Immigration and generational trends in body mass index and obesity in the United States: Results of the National Latino and Asian American Survey, 2002–2003. *American Journal of Public Health, 98*(1), 70–77. https://doi.org/10.2105/ajph.2006.102814

Bayly, J. E., Panigrahi, A., Rodriquez, E. J., Gallo, L. C., Perreira, K. M., Talavera, G. A., Estrella, M. L., Daviglus, M. L., Castaneda, S. F., Bainter, S. A., Chambers, E. C., Savin, K. L., Loop, M., &

Pérez-Stable, E. J. (2022). Perceived neighborhood factors, health behaviors, and related outcomes in the Hispanic Community Health Study/Study of Latinos. *Preventive Medicine, 164,* 107267. https://doi.org/10.1016/j.ypmed.2022.107267

Beckles, G. L., & Truman, B. I. (2011, January 11). Education and Income — United States, 2005 and 2009-. *Morbidity and Mortality Weekly Report, 60*(1), 13–17. https://www.cdc.gov/mmwr /preview/mmwrhtml/su6001a3.htm

Bennett, K. (2017). Reserve Capacity Model. In V. Zeigler-Hill & T. K. Shackelford (Eds.), *Encyclopedia of Personality and Individual Differences* (pp. 1-3). Springer International Publishing. https://doi.org/10.1007/978-3-319-28099-8_1154-1

Buchanan, R. L., & Smokowski, P. R. (2009). Pathways from acculturation stress to substance use among latino adolescents. *Substance Use & Misuse, 44*(5), 740–762. https://doi.org/10 .1080/10826080802544216

Camacho-Rivera, M., Gonzalez, C. J., Morency, J. A., Blake, K. D., & Calixte, R. (2020). Heterogeneity in Trust of Cancer Information among Hispanic Adults in the United States: An Analysis of the Health Information National Trends Survey. *Cancer Epidemiology Biomarkers & Prevention, 29*(7), 1348–1356. https://doi.org/10.1158/1055-9965.epi-19-1375

Campinha-Bacote, J. (1999). A Model and Instrument for Addressing Cultural Competence in Health Care. *Journal of Nursing Education, 38*(5), 203–207. https://doi.org/doi:10.3928/0148 -4834-19990501-06

Carlson, J. A., Sallis, J. F., Jankowska, M. M., Allison, M. A., Sotres-Alvarez, D., Roesch, S. C., Steel, C., Savin, K. L., Talavera, G. A., Castañeda, S. F., Llabre, M. M., Penedo, F. J., Kaplan, R., Mossavar-Rahmani, Y., Daviglus, M., Perreira, K. M., & Gallo, L. C. (2022). Neighborhood built environments and Hispanic/Latino adults' physical activity in the U.S.: The Hispanic community health study/study of Latinos community and surrounding areas study. *Preventive Medicine, 160,* 107073. https://doi.org/10.1016/j.ypmed.2022.107073

Cavazos-Rehg, P. A., Zayas, L. H., & Spitznagel, E. L. (2007). Legal status, emotional well-being and subjective health status of Latino immigrants. *Journal of the National Medical Association, 99*(10), 1126–1131.

Centers for Disease Control and Prevention. (2024a). Health of Hispanic or Latino Population. *National Center for Health Statistics.* Retrieved July 7, 2024 from https://www.cdc.gov/nchs /fastats/hispanic-health.htm

Centers for Disease Control and Prevention. (2024b). Health of White non-Hispanic Population. *National Center for Health Statistics.* Retrieved July 7, 2024 from https://www.cdc.gov/nchs /fastats/white-health.htm

Crimmins, E. M., Kim, J. K., Alley, D. E., Karlamangla, A., & Seeman, T. (2007). Hispanic paradox in biological risk profiles. *American Journal of Public Health, 97*(7), 1305–1310. https://doi.org /10.2105/ajph.2006.091892

David, R. A., & Rhee, M. (1998). The impact of language as a barrier to effective health care in an underserved urban Hispanic community. *The Mount Sinai journal of medicine, New York, 65*(5-6), 393–397.

Escarce, J. J., Morales, L. S., & Rumbaut, R. G. (2006). The health status and health behaviors of Hispanics. In M. Tienda, & F. Mitchell (Eds.), *Hispanics and the future of America* (Chapter 9). National Academic Press. https://www.ncbi.nlm.nih.gov/books/NBK19899/

Fields, R., Kaczynski, A. T., Bopp, M., & Fallon, E. (2013). Built environment associations with health behaviors among Hispanics. *Journal of Physical Activity and Health, 10*(3), 335–342. https://doi.org/10.1123/jpah.10.3.335

Fortmann, A. L., Soriano, E. C., Gallo, L. C., Clark, T. L., Spierling Bagsic, S. R., Sandoval, H., Jones, J. A., Roesch, S., Gilmer, T., Schultz, J., Bodenheimer, T., & Philis-Tsimikas, A. (2024). Medical Assistant Health Coaching for Type 2 Diabetes in Primary Care: Results From a Pragmatic Cluster Randomized Controlled Trial. *Diabetes Care, 47*(7), 1171–1180. https://doi .org/10.2337/dc23-2487

Fuentes-Afflick, E., & Lurie, P. (1997). Low birth weight and Latino ethnicity. Examining the epidemiologic paradox. *Archives of Pediatrics and Adolescent Medicine, 151*(7), 665–674. https:// doi.org/10.1001/archpedi.1997.02170440027005

Funk, C., & Lopez, M. H. (2022, June 14). *Hispanic Americans' experiences with health care.* Pew Research Center. https://www.pewresearch.org/science/2022/06/14/hispanic-americans-experiences-with -health-care/

Gallo, L. C., Fortmann, A. L., Roesch, S. C., Barrett-Connor, E., Elder, J. P., de los Monteros, K. E., Shivpuri, S., Mills, P. J., Talavera, G. A., & Matthews, K. A. (2012). Socioeconomic status, psychosocial resources and risk, and cardiometabolic risk in Mexican-American women. *Health Psychology, 31*(3), 334–342. https://doi.org/10.1037/a0025689

Gallo, L. C., & Matthews, K. A. (2003). Understanding the association between socioeconomic status and physical health: Do negative emotions play a role? *Psychological Bulletin, 129*(1), 10–51. https://doi.org/10.1037/0033-2909.129.1.10

Gallo, L. C., Penedo, F. J., De Los Monteros, K. E., & Arguelles, W. (2009). Resiliency in the face of disadvantage: Do Hispanic cultural characteristics protect health outcomes? *Journal of Personality, 77*(6), 1707–1746. https://doi.org/10.1111/j.1467-6494.2009.00598.x

Gonzalez, C. J., Copeland, M., Shapiro, M. F., & Moody, J. (2023). Associations of peer generational status on adolescent weight across Hispanic immigrant generations: A social network analysis. *Social Science & Medicine, 323*, 115831. https://doi.org/10.1016/j.socscimed.2023.115831

Gordon-Larsen, P., Harris, K. M., Ward, D. S., & Popkin, B. M. (2003). Acculturation and overweight-related behaviors among Hispanic immigrants to the US: the National Longitudinal Study of Adolescent Health. *Social Science & Medicine, 57*(11), 2023–2034. https://doi.org /https://doi.org/10.1016/S0277-9536(03)00072-8

Greer, S., Naidoo, M., Hinterland, K., Archer, A., Lundy De La Cruz, N., Crossa, A., Gould, L. H. (2017). *Health of Latinos in New York City.* New York City Department of Health and Mental Hygiene. https://www.nyc.gov/assets/doh/downloads/pdf/episrv/2017-latino-health.pdf

Healthy People 2030. (2024). *Health communication and health information technology workgroup.* Office of Disease Prevention and Health Promotion. https://health.gov/healthypeople/about /workgroups/health-communication-and-health-information-technology-workgroup

Hoefer, M., Rytina, N., and Baker, B. C. (2012). *Estimates of the Unauthorized Immigrant Population Residing in the United States: January 2011.* Office of Immigration Statistics, Policy Directorate, United States Department of Homeland Security. https://2008election.procon.org/sourcefiles /Estimates_of_the_Unauthorized_Immigrant_Population_Residing_in_the_United_States _January_2011.pdf

Kaplan, M. S., Huguet, N., Newsom, J. T., & McFarland, B. H. (2004). The association between length of residence and obesity among Hispanic immigrants. *American Journal of Preventive Medicine, 27*(4), 323–326. https://doi.org/https://doi.org/10.1016/j.amepre.2004.07.005

Kivelä, K., Elo, S., Kyngäs, H., & Kääriäinen, M. (2014). The effects of health coaching on adult patients with chronic diseases: A systematic review. *Patient Education and Counseling, 97*(2), 147–157. https://doi.org/https://doi.org/10.1016/j.pec.2014.07.026

Kutner, M., Greenberg, E., Jin, Y., Paulsen, C., & White, S. (2006). *The health literacy of America's adults: Results from the 2003 National Assessment of Adult Literacy.* U.S. Department of Education. https://nces.ed.gov/pubs2006/2006483.pdf

Linzer, M., Bitton, A., Tu, S., Plews-Ogan, M., Horowitz, K. R., & Schwartz, M. D. (2015). The end of the 15–20 minute primary care visit. *Journal of General Internal Medicine, 30*(11), 1584–1586. https://doi.org/10.1007/s11606-015-3341-3

Malambo, P., Kengne, A. P., De Villiers, A., Lambert, E. V., & Puoane, T. (2016). Built environment, selected risk factors and major cardiovascular disease outcomes: A systematic review. *PLoS One, 11*(11), e0166846. https://doi.org/10.1371/journal.pone.0166846

Medina, L., Sabo, S., & Vespa, J. (2020). *Living Longer: Historical and Projected Life Expectancy in the United States, 1960 to 2060.* United States Census Bureau. https://www.census.gov/content/dam /Census/library/publications/2020/demo/p25-1145.pdf

Mikolajczyk, R. T., Bredehorst, M., Khelaifat, N., Maier, C., & Maxwell, A. E. (2007). Correlates of depressive symptoms among Latino and Non-Latino White adolescents: Findings from the 2003 California Health Interview Survey. *BMC Public Health, 7*(1). https://doi.org/10.1186/1471-2458-7-21

Morales, L. S., Lara, M., Kington, R. S., Valdez, R. O., & Escarce, J. J. (2002). Socioeconomic, cultural, and behavioral factors affecting Hispanic health outcomes. *Journal of health care for the poor and underserved, 13*(4), 477–503. https://doi.org/10.1177/104920802237532

Office of Minority Health. (n.d.). *Hispanic/Latino Health.* U.S. Department of Health and Human Services. https://minorityhealth.hhs.gov/hispaniclatino-health

Olsen, J. M., & Nesbitt, B. J. (2010). Health coaching to improve healthy lifestyle behaviors: An integrative review. *American Journal of Health Promotion, 25*(1), e1–e12. https://doi.org/10.4278 /ajhp.090313-LIT-101

Richardson, D. M., Andrea, S. B., Ziring, A., Robinson, C., & Messer, L. C. (2020). Pregnancy outcomes and documentation status among Latina women: A systematic review. *Health Equity, 4*(1), 158–182. https://doi.org/10.1089/heq.2019.0126

Safford, M. M., Andreae, S., Cherrington, A. L., Martin, M. Y., Halanych, J., Lewis, M., Patel, A., Johnson, E., Clark, D., Gamboa, C., & Richman, J. S. (2015). Peer coaches to improve diabetes outcomes in Rural Alabama: a cluster randomized trial. *The Annals of Family Medicine, 13*(Suppl_1), S18–S26. https://doi.org/10.1370/afm.1798

Safford, M. M., Cummings, D. M., Halladay, J., Shikany, J. M., Richman, J., Oparil, S., Hollenberg, J., Adams, A., Anabtawi, M., Andreae, L., Baquero, E., Bryan, J., Clark, D., Johnson, E., Richman, E., Soroka, O., Tillman, J., & Cherrington, A. L. (2023). The design and rationale of a multicenter real-world trial: The Southeastern Collaboration to Improve Blood Pressure Control in the US Black Belt – Addressing the Triple Threat. *Contemporary Clinical Trials, 129,* 107183. https://doi.org/10.1016/j.cct.2023.107183

Safford, M. M., Cummings, D. M., Halladay, J. R., Shikany, J. M., Richman, J., Oparil, S., Hollenberg, J., Adams, A., Anabtawi, M., Andreae, L., Baquero, E., Bryan, J., Sanders-Clark, D., Johnson, E., Richman, E., Soroka, O., Tillman, J., & Cherrington, A. L. (2024). Practice facilitation and peer coaching for uncontrolled hypertension among Black individuals. *JAMA Internal Medicine, 184*(5), 538. https://doi.org/10.1001/jamainternmed.2024.0047

Saha, S., Beach, M. C., & Cooper, L. A. (2008). Patient centeredness, cultural competence and healthcare quality. *Journal of the National Medical Association, 100*(11), 1275–1285. https://doi.org/10.1016/s0027-9684(15)31505-4

Shaw, M. K., Davis, S. A., Fleischer, A. B., & Feldman, S. R. (2014). The duration of office visits in the United States, 1993 to 2010. *The American Journal of Managed Care, 20*(10), 820–826.

Shrider, E. A., Kollar, M., Chen, F., & Semega, J. (2021, September 14). *Income and Poverty in the United States: 2020.* United States Census Bureau. https://www.census.gov/library/publications/2021/demo/p60-273.html

Tienda, M., & Sánchez, S. M. (2013). Latin American immigration to the United States. *Daedalus, 142*(3), 48–64. https://doi.org/10.1162/daed_a_00218

Turra, C. M., & Elo, I. T. (2008). The impact of salmon bias on the Hispanic mortality advantage: New evidence from social security data. *Population Research and Policy Review, 27*(5), 515–530. https://doi.org/10.1007/s11113-008-9087-4

U.S. Bureau of Labor Statistics. (2021). Labor force characteristics by race and ethnicity, 2020. https://www.bls.gov/opub/reports/race-and-ethnicity/2020/home.htm

U.S. Census Bureau. (2024, September 16). *Hispanic Heritage Month: 2024.* https://www.census.gov/newsroom/facts-for-features/2024/hispanic-heritage-month.html

U.S. Department of Health and Human Services. (2024). Social Determinants of Health. Retrieved July 7, 2024 from https://health.gov/healthypeople/priority-areas/social-determinants-health

Valenzuela, A. (2003). Day labor work. *Annual Review of Sociology, 29*(1), 307–333. https://doi.org/10.1146/annurev.soc.29.010202.100044

Varela, E. G., McVay, M. A., Shelnutt, K. P., & Mobley, A. R. (2023). The determinants of food insecurity among Hispanic/Latinx Households with young children: A narrative review. *Advances in Nutrition, 14*(1), 190–210. https://doi.org/10.1016/j.advnut.2022.12.001

Velasco-Mondragon, E., Jimenez, A., Palladino-Davis, A. G., Davis, D., & Escamilla-Cejudo, J. A. (2016). Hispanic health in the USA: a scoping review of the literature. *Public Health Reviews, 37*(1), 31. https://doi.org/10.1186/s40985-016-0043-2

Vernon, J. A., Trujillo, A., Rosenbaum, S., & DeBuono, B. (2007). Low health literacy: Implications for national health policy. Department of Health Policy, School of Public Health and Health Services, The George Washington University. https://hsrc.himmelfarb.gwu.edu/cgi/viewcontent.cgi?article=1173&context=sphhs_policy_facpubs

Williams, D. R., Lawrence, J. A., & Davis, B. A. (2019). Racism and health: Evidence and needed research. *Annual Review of Public Health, 40*(1), 105–125. https://doi.org/10.1146/annurev-publhealth-040218-043750

Williams, D. R., Mohammed, S. A., Leavell, J., & Collins, C. (2010). Race, socioeconomic status, and health: complexities, ongoing challenges, and research opportunities. *Annals of the New York Academy of Sciences, 1186,* 69–101. https://doi.org/10.1111/j.1749-6632.2009.05339.x

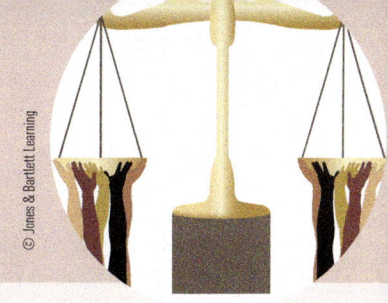
© Jones & Bartlett Learning

Health Disparities in Urban Communities as Compared to Suburban Communities: Issues, Concerns, and Remedies

Anthony E. Munroe, MBA, MPH, EdD and **Patti R. Rose**, MPH, EdD

KEY TERMS

commercial determinants of health (CDOH)

environmental justice

health disparity

Ozempic

population health

poverty

semaglutide

social determinants of health (SDOH)

suburban communities

urban communities

Wegovy

LEARNING OBJECTIVES

After reading this chapter you should be able to:

1. Define "health disparity."
2. Explain how social determinants of health are mostly responsible for health inequities.
3. Discuss environmental justice and its impact on communities.
4. List key concerns related to commercial determinants of health.
5. Describe potential remedies that may be useful to resolve health issues in urban communities.

Introduction

In March 1966, during the Medical Committee for Human Rights meeting at the University of Chicago, Dr. Martin Luther King, Jr., who at that time was the head of the Southern Christian Leadership Conference, spoke about the disparities in health care among Black people. Currently, there are still significant health disparities in communities of color, especially urban communities of African American and Hispanic people.

As we examine health disparities, particularly in urban communities, it is important to recognize the social, political, and economic implications. Such disparities, particularly among urban communities of color, give us some insight into the "social justice platform into health care and access to quality healthcare services" (Braveman, 2006). In this chapter, details will be provided about health disparities, socioeconomic status, social determinants of health, environmental justice, commercial determinants of health (CDOH), **poverty**, access to quality healthcare services, and the types of providers who typically serve emerging majority **urban communities**. These are all major factors and issues worth reviewing to better understand the complex nature of health disparities in urban communities.

Health Disparities: Issues, Concerns, and Remedies

In the United States, health disparities are well documented among various groups, as defined by race/ethnicity, type of community (e.g., rural, urban), gender, environment, economic status, and other group dynamics. Groups not identified as the White majority tend to have poorer health, higher mortality and morbidity rates, and less access to quality healthcare services. **Health disparity** can fundamentally refer to the differences in health status across various populations, as influenced by numerous factors. Some of the factors are behavioral—for instance, whether one uses tobacco products, overconsumes alcohol, does not or cannot exercise, or has limited access to healthy food options.

The term health disparities appears to represent a concept that can be intuitively understood, yet there is much controversy about its exact meaning (Dehlendorf et al., 2010). A central aspect of the most accepted definitions is that not all differences in health status between groups are considered to be disparities; rather, only differences that systematically and negatively impact less advantaged groups are classified as disparities (Braveman, 2006). The Kaiser Family Foundation (Ndugga et al., 2012) offers the following definitions:

> "Health disparity," generally refers to a higher burden of illness, injury, disability, or mortality experienced by one population group relative to another group. A "healthcare disparity" typically refers to differences between groups in health coverage, access to care, and quality of care. While disparities are commonly viewed through the lens of race and ethnicity, they occur across many dimensions, including socioeconomic status, age, location, gender, disability status, and sexual orientation.

The most concise and accessible definition of health disparities/inequalities/ equity was articulated by Margaret Whitehead in the early 1990s as differences in health that "are not only unnecessary and avoidable but, in addition, are considered unfair and unjust" (Braveman, 2006).

In a 2012 report titled "Disparities in Health and Health Care," the Kaiser Family Foundation offers historical insight into the issue of health disparities in the United States (Ndugga et al., 2012):

> Health and healthcare disparities first gained significant federal recognition with the release of two Surgeon General's reports in 2000 that showed disparities in tobacco use and access to mental health services by race and ethnicity. These reports were followed with the first major legislation focused on reduction of disparities, the Minority Health and Health Disparities Research and Education Act of 2000, which created the National Center for Minority Health and Health Disparities and authorized AHRQ (Agency for Healthcare Research and Quality) to regularly measure progress on reduction of disparities. Soon after, the Institute of Medicine released two seminal reports documenting racial and ethnic disparities in access to and quality of care. Over the last decade, awareness of disparities has increased at all levels of government and among the general public, although substantial gaps in awareness remain, particularly among the public.

Life expectancy in the United States continues to increase over the years. For the emerging majority people, this is not always the case because of health disparities, chronic illnesses, and other factors, including substance abuse, lower socioeconomic status, and key concerns related to birth, such as lower birthweight and higher infant and maternal mortality (Carratala & Maxwell, 2020).

According to Thomson (2011), "Urbanites are also at above-average risk of violence, accidents, polluted air and water and shortages of green space and nutritious food—all with potentially unhealthy consequences, especially for the poor." Many urban communities are plagued with insufficient resources, crumbling schools, housing that is substandard, and other environmental and social factors that create enormous stress and unhealthy living conditions.

Health and Health Disparities

The Institute of Medicine's (IOM) report, *Unequal Treatment: Confronting Racial and Ethnic Disparities in Health Care*, significantly raised the level of awareness and attention given to minority health and health disparities. According to the report, in 1999, Congress requested that the IOM (1) assess the extent of racial and ethnic disparities in health care, assuming that access-related factors such as insurance status and the ability to pay for care are the same, (2) identify potential sources of these disparities, and (3) suggest intervention strategies (Smedley et al., 2003).

Health disparities have a variety of contributing factors or determinants. Socioeconomic status, insurance coverage, poverty, environment, commercial, language barriers, disability, educational level, and gender are some of the determinants that can impact health disparities. The gaps in health status and mortality between White people and emerging majority people (particularly African American and Hispanic people) have been well documented, and much hard data about these discrepancies has been collected (Drescher-Burke, 2010). When compared with White people, African American people have higher rates of diabetes, infant mortality, and many other conditions; they are sicker and also have a higher mortality rate (Drescher-Burke, 2010).

Health disparities frequently refer to disparities in health care, including differential access to screening and/or treatment options, or unequal availability of culturally or linguistically knowledgeable and sensitive health personnel (Adler & Stewart, 2010). It is conceivable that health policy and public health funding decisions can be made depending upon the perspective and definition approach used by the legislators and decision makers. How one defines *health disparities* or *health equity* can have important policy implications with practical consequences (Braveman, 2006).

Much of the discrepancy in health care can be accounted for by social factors; namely, lower income and lower rates of health insurance are associated with worse health. However, even after controlling for socioeconomic conditions, White people enjoy better health and have lower mortality rates (Drescher-Burke, 2010). The causes of health disparities are varied and not always clear, but most researchers agree that disparities are a reflection of social and economic inequities and political injustice (Whitman et al., 2011). While there probably is some overt racism, many physicians (who are usually White) and other healthcare providers harbor unconscious biases toward racial groups different from their own (Drescher-Burke, 2010). Researchers have suggested that as a result of systematic and historical differential treatment, African American people have a low level of trust in the medical establishment, causing them to seek medical care and undergo recommended medical procedures less often (Drescher-Burke, 2010).

The Office of Disease Prevention and Health Promotion's Healthy People 2030 program (U.S. Department of Health and Human Services, n.d.) states the following:

> A person's community can have a major impact on their health and well-being. Healthy People 2030 focuses on ways organizations, businesses, schools, and residents can help build healthier communities. It is useful to review the Healthy People 2030 initiative to gain insight regarding health conditions, health behaviors, population groups, settings and systems and social determinants of health.

In terms of both urban and **suburban communities**, local interventions and policy are key, particularly in terms of health and safety risks (*Neighborhood and built environment*, n.d.). As per Healthy People 2030, particularly in terms of creating neighborhoods and environments that promote health and safety:

> Interventions and policy changes at the local, state, and federal level can help reduce these health and safety risks and promote health. For example, providing opportunities for people to walk and bike in their communities—like by adding sidewalks and bike lanes—can increase safety and help improve health and quality of life. These kinds of amenities are usually found in suburban communities.

Determinants of Health

Access to affordable healthy foods is one determinant of health. As Thomson (2011) states, "The concept of food deserts has been around for about 20 years and has been gaining currency in tandem with rising public consciousness of the effect—for good or ill—of eating habits on health."

As Ritter and Graham (2017) assert, "Socioeconomic status is one of the most important predictors of health. Socioeconomic status is typically measured by educational attainment, income, wealth, occupation, or a combination of these factors". These factors have a large impact on the social conditions in which individuals live. The Centers for Disease Control and Prevention (2016) provides a useful overview of the social determinants of health: "Conditions in the places where people live, learn, work, and play affect a wide range of health risks and outcomes." These conditions are known as **social determinants of health (SDOH)**. We know that poverty limits access to healthy foods and safe neighborhoods and that more education is a predictor of better health. We also know that differences in health are striking in communities with poor SDOH, such as unstable housing, low income, unsafe neighborhoods, or substandard education. By applying what we know about SDOH, we can not only improve individual and **population health** but also advance health equity. The CDC "views population health as an interdisciplinary, customizable approach that allows health departments to connect practice to policy for change to happen locally" (CDC, 2020).

Rose (2013), drawing from the article "Health Disparities Across the Lifespan: Meaning, Methods, and Mechanisms" by Adler and Stewart (2010), describes the health status gap that exists between socioeconomic groups in the United States:

> Racially, ethnically and socioeconomically, there are significant differences, essentially stemming from the reality that those who had education less than the others had the worst health. Considering levels of education, even if one had average levels of education, they were not as healthy as those individuals who had high levels of wealth and education. Along racial and ethnic lines, Black and Hispanic people indicated fair or poor health, as compared to White people. Poverty is indicated as a clear factor in terms of health as five times as many adults who are poor, as compared to the wealthiest individuals, report that their health is either fair or poor.

Poverty

Ritter and Graham (2017) describe the additional health challenges faced by those living in poor urban environments:

> Members of minority cultures are more likely to live in poor neighborhoods. These neighborhoods often have poor performing schools, high crime rates, substandard housing, few healthcare providers and pharmacies, more alcohol and tobacco advertising, and limited access to grocery

stores with healthy food choices. These social determinants of health can accumulate over the course of a life and can be detrimental to physical and emotional health.

According to Ritter and Graham (2017), "Poverty is higher among certain racial and ethnic groups and is a contributing factor to health disparities because poverty affects many factors, including where people live and their access to health care". Higher socioeconomic status is generally associated with better health. The effects of higher socioeconomic status can include improved access to health-enhancing resources, improved access to health care, and a greater likelihood of living in a healthier neighborhood (Ritter & Graham, 2017). Despite improvements, differences persist in healthcare quality among racial and ethnic minority groups. People in low-income families also experience poorer quality care (Barakat & Konstantinidis, 2023).

Ritter and Graham (2017) explain the effect that one's neighborhood has on health:

> There is little doubt that neighborhood characteristics are important elements associated with health. Residents of socially and economically deprived communities experience worse health outcomes on average than those living in more prosperous neighborhoods. Neighborhoods may influence health through relatively short-term influences on behaviors, attitudes, and healthcare utilization, thereby affecting health conditions that are more immediate. Neighborhoods also can influence health on a long-term basis through "weathering," whereby the accumulated stress, lower environmental quality, and limited resources of poorer communities experienced over many years negatively affects the health of residents.

Environmental Determinants

When referring to environment, there are key factors, namely, socioeconomic, sociopolitical, and sociocultural; of course, there is the physical environment, which includes air, water, chemicals, waste, vectors, and habitat alterations (Shi and Singh, 2019). In general, the latter may not be problematic but what happens when air is polluted, water is contaminated, and chemicals are toxic? There are also disease vectors and safety hazards that must be considered. In terms of environmental and commercial determinants of health, these are some of the issues to be discussed, along with potential remedies. The key topic in this area is **environmental justice**. According to the Environmental Protection Agency (EPA), environmental justice is defined as follows (Carlson, 2023):

> The fair treatment and meaningful involvement of all people regardless of race, color, national origin, or income, with respect to the development, implementation and enforcement of environmental laws, regulations and policies. It will be achieved when everyone enjoys the same degree of protection from environmental and health hazards, and equal access to the decision-making process to have a healthy environment in which to live, learn and work.

The various ways that environmental injustice occur are as follows:

- Geographic inequity—environmental hazards situated in close proximity to certain groups or populations
- Procedural inequity—disproportionate burdens on certain groups by way of enforcement of environmental regulations
- Social inequity—the inability of certain groups to participate in decision-making around environmental matters and the balance of power, per discrimination.
- Environmental racism—disproportionate environmental impact on groups or communities because of their racial or ethnic status

There are many examples of environmental injustice. One concrete and current example taking place involves water quality in Flint, Michigan. The problem began 10 years ago. According to news reports (Quarishi, 2024):

> The Environmental Protection Agency (EPA) says lead in the water in Flint, Michigan, is lower than federal safety limits specify. It's been a decade since the city, attempting to save millions of dollars, inadvertently exposed more than 100,000 people, including vulnerable children, to lead seeping from aging pipes—and many residents still don't trust what's coming out of their faucets and showers.

Beyond the devastation from the contamination of the water in Flint, Michigan, there is a lack of trust of those who are supposed to ensure environmental justice, namely the EPA in this scenario. In U.S. communities where people are experiencing poverty, various types of EPA violations pertaining to water are often found. Beyond water pollution, there are drought conditions and industrial occurrences that impact the water supply (Carlson, 2021). Environmental injustice is not a new problem. Per Borunda. (2021):

> Research on environmental injustice began in the late 1970s, after residents of a Black middle-class neighborhood in Houston, Texas, found out that the state was going to permit the siting of a solid-waste facility in their community. One question loomed large in the residents' minds: Why was it being placed here and not in the white neighborhoods nearby?

Borunda points out further that this led to a review of data by a sociologist named Robert Bullard. He reviewed the data and found that "14 of the city's 17 industrial waste sites—accounting for over 80 percent of the city's waste tonnage—were situated in Black neighborhoods, though only 25 percent of Houston's population were Black."

This led to other similar findings throughout the United States and ultimately, a movement to attempt to rectify the problem. As with all health disparities impacting Black and Brown people throughout the United States, there is a tendency to prolong the discussion of the details including where it is happening, who is doing it, how it is impacting the communities, and beyond. Although this is laudable and necessary, what is most important is to find a remedy as quickly as possible once the problem has been identified.

The EPA recently announced, via a press release, an effort to address environmental injustice. It involves a first-of-its-kind clearinghouse of information that can be accessed by the public for federal and non-federal resources. Per the EPA Press Office (2024):

> "The Environmental Justice Clearinghouse is a transformative resource guide built to help us accomplish our agency-wide environmental justice goals," [said] Theresa Segovia, Principal Deputy Assistant Director for the Office of Environmental Justice and External Civil Rights. "Having an online, easily accessible library of information will ensure that resources from across the country are at the fingertips of all environmental justice stakeholders and advocates. And it will only be made stronger with suggestions from the American people."

Clearly, given that the problem of environmental justice was initially identified in 1970, it has taken an incredibly long time for such a clearinghouse to be implemented, and it does not solve the problem. In terms of health disparities, it seems that merely stating that it is a step in the right direction will not suffice. There is no doubt that bigger steps need to be taken swiftly as lives continue to be at stake in communities where environmental injustices continue to take place.

Remedies and Environmental Justice

There are many remedies that must be taken into consideration. Earth Justice (2021) lists some examples:

> One potential remedy is to modernize homes in an effort to improve indoor air quality. This would include the provision of incentives, by Congress/government, for more energy efficient appliances. This is already happening at some levels with the Energy Star Program (EPA), which is a combination of government and manufacturer efforts providing tax credits for consumers/businesses based on their buying decisions (Energy Star, n.d).

Another potential remedy pertains to drinking water. There is no disagreement, in any circles, about the need for clean water. There must be clean drinking water in every community. This requires modernization of all aspects of the delivery of water in every community, no matter the socioeconomic status.

An additional and the final potential remedy to be discussed here is the removal of toxic chemicals in environments where there are people and life of all species. This seems to be common sense and has to happen because it is not the case in well-to-do communities, as lower socioeconomic status is a factor. The bottom line is that environmental justice must be at the forefront of public health initiatives. Impacted communities must be part of the discussion and leading the process as they will know best how they are being harmed and what remedies are needed.

REMEDIES

- More government initiatives to modernize homes to improve indoor air quality, especially in low-income communities where there is public and low-income housing.
- The government at every level must ensure clean drinking water for all in EVERY community.
- The government must ensure the removal of toxic chemicals in environments where there are people and life of all species.
- Involve communities impacted by environmental justice in ALL initiatives relevant to remedying environmental injustice.

Commercial Determinants of Health (CDOH)

According to the World Health Organization (2023), "**commercial determinants of health (CDOH)** are the private sector activities that affect people's health, directly or indirectly, positively or negatively." Commercially, there are factors that impact health. Some examples of these factors as examples in terms of food per the World Health Organization (WHO) are breast milk substitutes, processed foods, and sugar-sweetened beverages and beyond. Tobacco is another culprit. Hence, CDOH is an important issue to discuss in terms of achieving health equity. According to Lacy-Nichols et al. (2023):

> Tackling the [CDOH] is necessary for progress on health equity and will determine whether or not the health-related targets of the SDGs [Sustainable Development Goals] are met.

Weight Loss Drugs

Currently, prescription weight loss drugs are commercially produced products that must be considered in terms of CDOH as they are becoming increasingly popular in the United States and beyond. There are varying opinions on the level of side effects from these drugs on a continuum of mild to moderate to serious. Additionally, these drugs may be very expensive and it is not necessarily the case that insurance will cover them.

According to the Mayo Clinic (2022), there are six weight loss drugs approved by the Food and Drug Administration (FDA) for long term use:

- Naltrexone/bupropion (Contrave)
- Liraglutide (Saxenda)
- Orlistat (Xenical, Alli)
- Phentermine-topiramate (Qsymia)
- Semaglutide (Wegovy)
- Setmelanotide (Imcivree)

One of these drugs, **semaglutide** (which is the generic name for the tradename drugs **Ozempic** and **Wegovy**) belongs to a class of pharmaceuticals known as glucagon-like peptide-1 (GLP-1) receptor agonists. It is taken as an injection (self-injection) with potential side effects, per the Mayo Clinic (2022), which also points out that "Semaglutide also is used to help control type 2 diabetes" and that it has a range of side effects, which include "nausea and vomiting, diarrhea, belly pain, headache and tiredness." The FDA (U.S. Food & Drug Administration, 2020), per clinical trials that led to the approval of this drug, indicates that there are more potential serious side effects, in addition to those mentioned above, per the following statement:

> OZEMPIC may cause serious side effects including low blood sugar, inflammation of the pancreas, complications of diabetes-related retina disease (diabetic retinopathy) and allergic reactions. In animal studies, mice and rats that received OZEMPIC were more likely to develop a certain kind of thyroid cancer. It is not known whether this may occur in humans.

Details that led to the approval of ozempic are provided by the FDA (U.S. Food & Drug Administration, 2020):

> The FDA approved OZEMPIC based on evidence from seven clinical trials of 4087 patients with type 2 DM. The trials were conducted at 536 sites in 33 countries, including Canada, Mexico, Russian Federation, Ukraine, Turkey, India, South Africa, Japan, Hong Kong, multiple European countries, Argentina, and the United States.

Data from another trial was also considered, which was described as follows (U.S. Food & Drug Administration, 2020):

> The FDA also considered data from one separate trial of 3297 patients with type 2 DM who were at high risk for cardiovascular events. This trial was conducted in 20 countries in Europe, Russian Federation, Turkey, Brazil, Israel, Malaysia, Brazil, Mexico, Thailand, Taiwan, Canada, and the United States.

FDA approvals, as pointed out by Hathaway et al. (2024), ultimately led to Semaglutide (Ozempic; Novo Nordisk) being approved by the U.S. FDA in December 2017 to treat type 2 diabetes (T2D) and in December 2022 to treat obesity (typically at higher doses, such as Wegovy [Novo Nordisk]).

Prescription weight loss drugs are currently a hot topic with celebrities, such as Oprah Winfrey touting her own personal use and stating the following in a *People* magazine article (Leonard, 2023): "The fact that there's a medically approved prescription for managing weight and staying healthier, in my lifetime, feels like relief, like redemption, like a gift." Although Winfrey is entitled to her opinion, as everyone is, based on her life story, are weight-loss prescription drugs a gift? Maybe they are for her, in her opinion, but is this the case for people who may be influenced by her words about these drugs? After all, she is one of the most significant influencers in the United States and perhaps the world. Winfrey will not state publicly which of the weight loss drugs she is taking, nor does she discuss side effects, either personally or based on discussions with physicians. Are these weight loss drugs a public health concern? If not thus far, should they be?

The following is noted in the discussion section of a research paper by Sodhi et al. (2023):

> This study found that use of GLP-1 agonists for weight loss compared with use of naltrexone/bupropion was associated with increased risk of pancreatitis, gastroparesis, and bowel obstruction but not biliary disease. Given the wide use of these drugs, these adverse events, although rare, must be considered by patients who are contemplating using the drugs for weight loss because the risk-benefit calculus for this group might differ from that of those who use them for diabetes.

Additionally, a correlational study conducted by Hathaway et al. (2024) found a potential risk of non-arteritic anterior ischemic optic neuropathy (NAION), which specifically causes visual impairment. There were 16,827 patients in this study who did not have a history of this opthamalogic problem, Their findings in summary were:

> This matched cohort study of 16,827 patients revealed higher risk of NAION in patients prescribed semaglutide compared with patients prescribed non–glucagon-like peptide receptor agonist medications for diabetes or obesity. They also state: "Our main finding is that pre-scribed semaglutide is associated with an increased risk of NAION." It is important to note that they offer a statement regarding causality by indicating that this study did not necessarily indicate causality and that a larger, retrospective study is needed that is multi-centered with other specific elements/options (e.g., population-based cohort study, a prospective, randomized clinical study, or a post-market analysis of all GLP-1 RA drugs).

Recently, the artist Macy Gray, who was hospitalized from Ozempic side effects, stated, "I took Ozempic. I can't go to the bathroom. I was up all night" (JoVonn, 2024). She further complained that she felt at a loss of breath and was taken to the hospital. Gray shared why she started taking Ozempic (JoVonn, 2024):

> "I've gained a lot of weight over the past couple of years, and this is right about the time when everybody started talking about this Ozempic. So I thought, I'm not taking [the weight] off the right way. Let me see if I can get one of these."

Ultimately, exploring popular weight loss drugs relative to CDOH is criti-cal particularly because there is a tremendous incentive for the manufacturers of these drugs and investors to continue promoting and offering them. Specifi-cally, as one significant example, is described by Rice (2023): "Danish drugmaker Novo Nordisk has entered a new chapter in its 100-year history—thanks to its newfound success with two products: Ozempic and Wegovy." The title of Rice's article says it all, which is "How Ozempic and Wegovy turned Novo Nordisk into a $400 billion company." Given the definition of CDOH mentioned earlier, there is no doubt that weight loss drugs fall under the category of a CDOH, and hence, remedies and further study are in order.

REMEDIES

Stop organizations from prioritizing profits over the health of people. According to Lee and Freudenberg (2022), there are categories that must be considered, which include behavioral change, regulation, fiscal policy strategies, citizen and consumer activism, and litigation/legal remedies. These approaches involve:

- Educating the public on necessary behavioral change efforts that reduce/ eliminate their participation in harmful product usage and activities offered by commercial entities.
- Regulation of markets that may be involved in harmful commercial practices
- Participation by consumers to reduce actions by corporations including activism
- Soliciting the help of attorneys to proceed with litigation or other legal remedies to end unsavory practices of commercial entities in terms of health.
- Ensuring that every potential consumer/patient using prescription weight loss drugs is informed of all possible side effects, from mild to serious, as well as about the details and outcomes of clinical trials and the profit margins for companies who make them.
- Removal of influencers/celebrities from the discussion of prescription weight loss drugs in all forms of media, including social media and corporate media platforms, so that patients can have informed discussions with their healthcare providers about the facts associated with these drugs, without celebrity marketing, based, on their usage and pharmaceutical input (including commercials, samples, etc.) in that discussion
- Consumers should litigate if they are harmed by weight loss drugs if they were prescribed without informed consent about the potential side effects.

Access to Care and Community-Based Providers

According to the Kaiser Family Foundation (Ndugga et al., 2012), some populations are at a distinct disadvantage in accessing health care in the United States:

> Hispanics, Blacks, and American Indians/Alaska Natives as well as low-income individuals all are much more likely to be uninsured relative to Whites and those with higher incomes. Low-income individuals and people of color also face increased barriers to accessing care, receive poorer quality care, and ultimately experience worse health outcomes.

Nash et al. (2016) defines population health as the (1) distribution of health outcomes within a population, (2) health determinants that influence this distribution, and (3) policies and inventions that affect those determinants. Population health outcomes can be improved by focusing on these determinants. Determinants of health include individual behavior, social influences, physical environment, medical care, public health policy, and intervention.

The limited availability of healthcare providers in some communities can serve as an impediment to health care, as the Kaiser Family Foundation (2008) explains:

> Despite efforts since the 1970s to increase the number of health professionals in medically underserved areas, members of racial/ethnic minority groups are still underrepresented in the healthcare workforce

and are more likely than Whites to live in neighborhoods that lack adequate health resources. For example, 28% of Latinos and 22% of African Americans report having little or no choice in where to seek care, while only 15% of Whites report this difficulty. African Americans and Latinos are also twice as likely as Whites to rely upon a hospital outpatient department as their regular source of care, rather than a doctor's office where opportunities for continuity of care and patient-centered care are greater. This is a result of many factors, including the higher rates of uninsured and the limited availability of primary care physicians in some communities of color.

These disparities in healthcare availability, accessibility, and affordability lead to distinct problems in underserved populations.

Overall Remedies

Comprehensive efforts must be made to address and resolve the fundamental and historic social and economic issues that continue to plague urban communities where people are experiencing poverty—especially emerging majority communities—as compared to the lack of these concerns in affluent suburban communities. Some key remedies include: access to good and strong schools; housing; jobs; transportation; social services; caring and high-quality healthcare providers and institutions; healthy food options; clean and safe environments with parks; and living environments free of toxic waste. Violence of any and all forms in the urban community is a major concern that must be resolved with strong leadership and cooperation of all, including the community, community leaders, elected officials, public safety, law enforcement, and policy makers. Meaningful strides must be made in closing the health gap. Finally, health disparities must remain a local to national priority that gets the support and resources necessary to make a marked difference. As the U.S. population grows and continues to become represented by more people of color, it is in the nation's best interest to elevate health disparities to a prominent and significant priority.

Ultimately, there should also be a focus on stress reduction in all communities but particularly in urban environments where experiences can be more intense.

The Science of Happiness (Evidence-Based)

Seeking and experiencing happiness is a measure to reduce stress. On April 24, 2018, Laurie Santos, a professor of psychology at Yale University, offered a lecture—*Psychology and the Good Life*—based on evidence-based research that focused on the highlights of key aspects of happiness (Hathaway, 2018). This lecture was adapted into a course called *The Science of Well-Being* that went on to become the most popular course in the university's history (Yale Online, n.d.). Some of the top insights from the Science of Well-being course include:

1. Happiness matters for performance (mental health matters).
2. Make time for social connections—talking to people in real time.

3. Helping others makes people happier than we expect.
4. Make time for gratitude every day.
5. Healthy practices (e.g. exercise, sleep, etc.) matter more than we expect.
6. Being in the present moment and savoring the good things (eg., meditation) are helpful.
7. Give yourself the gift of self-compassion (e.g., mindfulness, common humanity, self-kindness).
8. Become wealthy in time, not in money—time affluence is good; time famine is not good.

These are perhaps some steps that individuals suffering from some of the atrocities mentioned in this chapter can take as they await and/or are involved in initiatives from public health, government (local to national) healthcare providers and beyond to implement remedies to the problems rather than simply offering continuous research, which leads to problem-centered distribution of information. The emphasis of all research and action must be remedy-centered to actually solve problems.

WRAP-UP

This chapter focused on health disparities and healthcare disparities by explaining the difference between these terms in relationship to racial and ethnic groups in urban communities as compared to suburban communities. Suburban communities, for the most part, are not experiencing most of the issues mentioned here, with the exception of the weight loss drugs, perhaps, given that they are costly and some are not covered by health insurance. Hence, key areas of exploration for urban communities include socioeconomic status, determinants of health, poverty, access to quality healthcare services, providers that serve urban communities, and other key issues. Remedies are provided that will be helpful in reducing/eliminating health inequities with an emphasis on why this must be a national priority in the United States, as the nation continues to become more diverse based on rapidly increasing numbers of people of color, hence emerging majorities. Happiness is discussed as a potential remedy in that it promotes stress reduction, which is useful for all parties involved.

Chapter Problems

1. Explain the current concerns regarding weight loss drugs mentioned in this chapter.
2. Describe key points made by Healthy People 2030 in this chapter.
3. Explain commercial determinants of health.
4. What is environmental justice?
5. Why is it important for health disparities to remain a local to national priority?

References

Adler, N. E., & Stewart, J. (2010). Health disparities across the lifespan: meaning, methods, and mechanisms. *Annals of the New York Academy of Sciences, 1186*, 5–23. https://doi.org/10.1111/j.1749-6632.2009.05337.x

Barakat, C., & Konstantinidis, T. (2023). A Review of the Relationship between Socioeconomic Status Change and Health. *International Journal of Environmental Research and Public Health, 20*(13), 6249. https://doi.org/10.3390/ijerph20136249

Borunda, A. (2021). *The origins of environmental justice—and why it's finally getting the attention it deserves.* National Geographic. https://www.nationalgeographic.com/environment/article/environmental-justice-origins-why-finally-getting-the-attention-it-deserves

Braveman, P. (2006). Health disparities and health equity: concepts and measurement. *Annual Review of Public Health, 27*, 167–194. https://doi.org/10.1146/annurev.publhealth.27.021405.102103

Carlson, G. (2023). *Human Health and the Climate Crisis.* Jones and Bartlett Learning.

Carratala, S., & Maxwell, C. (2020, May 7). *Fact sheet: Health disparities by race and ethnicity* [Report]. Center for American Progress. https://www.americanprogress.org/article/health-disparities-race-ethnicity/

Centers for Disease Control and Prevention. (2016). Social determinants of health (SDOH): What to know. http://www.cdc.gov/socialdeterminants/

Dehlendorf, C., Bryant, A. S., Huddleston, H. G., Jacoby, V. L., & Fujimoto, V. Y. (2010). Health disparities: definitions and measurements. *American Journal of Obstetrics and Gynecology, 202*(3), 212–213. https://doi.org/10.1016/j.ajog.2009.12.003

Drescher-Burke, K. (2010). Health disparities in the United States: Social class, race, ethnicity, and health. Donald A. Barr. Reviewed by Krista Drescher-Burke. *The Journal of Sociology & Social Welfare, 37*(1), Article 13. https://doi.org/10.15453/0191-5096.3502

Earth Justice. (2021, November 4). 8 climate justice solutions that Congress must pass with the Build Back Better Act. https://earthjustice.org/brief/2021/build-back-better-act-climate-environment

Energy Star. (n.d.). Federal Tax Credits for Energy Efficiency. Retrieved from: https://www.energystar.gov/about/federal-tax-credits

EPA Press Office. (2024, April 23). *EPA announces online collection of environmental justice resources.* U.S. Environmental Protection Agency. https://www.epa.gov/newsreleases/epa-announces-online-collection-of-environmental-justice-resources

Hathaway, J. T., Shah, M. P., Hathaway, D. B., Zekavat, S. M., Krasniqi, D., Gittinger, J. W., Cestari, D., Mallery, R., Abbasi, B., Bouffard, M., Chwalisz, B. K., Estrela, T., & Rizzo, J. F. (2024). Risk of nonarteritic anterior ischemic optic neuropathy in patients prescribed semaglutide. *JAMA Ophthalmology, 142*(8), 732. https://doi.org/10.1001/jamaophthalmol.2024.2296

JoVonn, J. (2024, September 14). Macy Gray Hospitalized On Television From Ozempic Side Effects, 'I Can't Walk Without Losing My Breath'. *Black Enterprise.* https://www.blackenterprise.com/macy-gray-hospitalized-ozempic/

Kaiser Family Foundation. (2008, October). *Eliminating racial/ethnic disparities in health care: What are the options?* https://www.kff.org/wp-content/uploads/2013/01/7830.pdf

Lacy-Nichols, J., Jones, A., & Buse, K. (2023). Taking on the Commercial Determinants of Health at the level of actors, practices and systems. *Frontiers in Public Health, 10.* https://doi.org/10.3389/fpubh.2022.981039

Lee, K., & Freudenberg, N. (2022). Public Health roles in addressing commercial determinants of health. *Annual Review of Public Health, 43*(1), 375–395. https://doi.org/10.1146/annurev-publhealth-052220-020447

Leonard, E. (2023, December 14). Oprah Winfrey reveals she uses weight-loss medication as a 'maintenance tool': 'I'm absolutely done with the shaming' (exclusive). *People Magazine.* https://people.com/oprah-winfrey-reveals-she-uses-weight-loss-medication-exclusive-8414552

Mayo Clinic. (2022). *Prescription weight-loss drugs: Study the pros and cons of medicines to treat obesity.* https://www.mayoclinic.org/healthy-lifestyle/weight-loss/in-depth/weight-loss-drugs/art-20044832

Nash, D. B., Fablus, R. J., Skoufalos, A., Clarke, J. L., & Horowitz, M. R. (2016). *Population health: Creating a culture of wellness* (2nd ed.). Jones & Bartlett Learning.

Ndugga, N., Pillai, D., & Artiga, S. (2012). *Disparities in health and health care: Five key questions and answers*. Kaiser Family Foundation. https://www.kff.org/racial-equity-and-health-policy/issue-brief/disparities-in-health-and-health-care-5-key-question-and-answers/

Neighborhood and built environment. (n.d.) Healthy People 2030. Office of Disease Prevention and Health Promotion, U.S. Department of Health and Human Services. https://health.gov/healthypeople/objectives-and-data/browse-objectives/neighborhood-and-built-environment

Quarishi, A. (2024, April 26). *Residents still have concerns about Flint's water.* CBS News. https://www.msn.com/en-us/news/other/residents-still-have-concerns-about-flint-s-water/ar-AA1nGaBS

Rice, N. (2023, October 10). *How Ozempic and Wegovy turned Novo Nordisk into a $400 billion company.* CNBC. https://www.cnbc.com/2023/10/10/ozempic-wegovy-novo-nordisk.html

Ritter, L. A., & Graham, D. H. (2017). *Multicultural health* (2nd ed.). Jones & Bartlett Learning.

Rose, P. R. (2013). *Cultural competency for the health professional.* Jones & Bartlett Learning.

Shi, L., & Singh, D. A. (2019). Delivering health care in America: A systems approach (7th ed.). Jones & Bartlett Learning.

Smedley, B. D., Stith, A. Y., & Nelson, A. R. (Eds.). (2003). *Unequal Treatment: Confronting Racial and Ethnic Disparities in Health Care.* National Academies Press. https://doi.org/10.17226/12875

Sodhi, M., Rezaeianzadeh, R., Kezouh, A., & Etminan, M. (2023). Risk of gastrointestinal adverse events associated with Glucagon-Like peptide-1 receptor agonists for weight loss. *JAMA, 330*(18), 1795. https://doi.org/10.1001/jama.2023.19574

Thomson, S. C. (2011). Urban health care: disparities abound. *Health progress (Saint Louis, Mo.), 92*(6), 4–11.

U.S. Department of Health and Human Services (n.d.). Office of Disease Prevention and Health Promotion. Healthy People 2030 (n.d.). Neighborhood and Built Environment. https://health.gov/healthypeople/objectives-and-data/browse-objectives/neighborhood-and-built-environment

U.S. Food & Drug Administration. (2020). Drug trial snapshot: Ozempic. https://www.fda.gov/drugs/drug-approvals-and-databases/drug-trial-snapshot-ozempic

Whitman, S., Shah, A., & Benjamins, M. (2011). *Urban health: Combating disparities with local data.* Oxford University Press.

Yale Online. (n.d.). *The science of well-being.* Yale University, Department of Psychology. https://online.yale.edu/courses/science-well-being

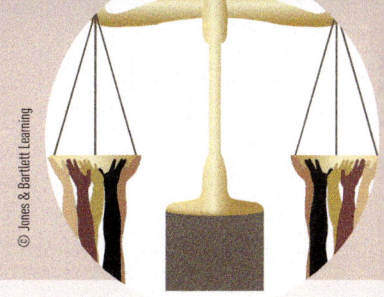

CHAPTER 8

Rural Communities and Health Disparities: Issues, Concerns, and Remedies

KEY TERMS

access to care
health disparity
health equity
Healthy People initiative
Medicaid
Medicare

migrant and seasonal agricultural
 worker (MSAW)
risky behaviors
rural health
Rural Healthy People
Rural Healthy People 2030

LEARNING OBJECTIVES

After reading this chapter, you should be able to do the following:

1. Explain some of the key issues regarding health disparities and rural communities.
2. Delineate health issues that impact migrant and seasonal agricultural workers.
3. List risky behaviors that members of rural communities may participate in.
4. Discuss how socioeconomic status impacts the health status of individuals in rural communities.
5. Identify key Rural Healthy People 2030 objectives.

Introduction

Although health disparities in urban communities are usually the focal point of this issue, there are serious problems unique to rural communities that contribute to the overall health status gap in the United States. According to Healthy People 2030,

health disparity is "a particular type of health difference that is closely linked with social, economic, and/or environmental disadvantage" (U.S. Department of Health and Human Services, n.d.). Additionally, Healthy People 2030 defines **health equity** as "the attainment of the highest level of health for all people" and goes on to explain that "achieving health equity requires valuing everyone equally with focused and ongoing societal efforts to address avoidable inequalities, historical and contemporary injustices, and the elimination of health and health care disparities" (U.S. Department of Health and Human Services, n.d.). Based on these definitions, it is clear that health equities and health disparities are intricately intertwined and that in order to achieve health equity, health disparities must be eliminated.

There are very specific risk factors that contribute to poor health conditions for people living in rural environments, leading to health disparities. According to the Commonwealth Fund, "these geographic disparities are especially stark in the United States, where about 15% of the population, or roughly 46 million people, live in rural areas" (Gunja, 2023). The National Institute of Health (NIH) (2022) states that some of the key issues that affect these communities are heart disease, cancer, lung disease, stroke, obesity, and diabetes, which are the leading causes of death. Other issues are fatal car crashes, deaths by suicide, and drug overdoses.

Additionally, a lack of, or slow, employment growth translates to a lack of health insurance in many instances, unless individuals have reached the poverty level and are eligible for **Medicaid**, or if they are 65 or older and, therefore, eligible for **Medicare**. The other possibility is seeking healthcare insurance through options created by the Affordable Care Act. In terms of unemployment in the United States, according to Dumont (2024), although there have been positive changes to the nation's economy, unemployment issues still exist in rural communities "especially for prime working-age men and those with less than a high school degree." He states further:

> ". . .advances in technological innovation and automation, declines in the extraction of certain energy resources, increases in globalization, and a shift to the "knowledge-based" economy have coincided with dispropor-tionately negative employment outcomes in many rural, or "nonmetro," communities. . ."

Risky Behaviors

According to a Centers for Disease Control and Prevention (CDC) report, to prevent chronic health problems, individuals must engage in certain behaviors, including: not smoking; maintaining healthy body weight; staying active; not drinking too much alcohol; and getting enough sleep. And, according to the CDC, only one in four members of rural communities is following these guidelines. Another health risk for all rural individuals stems from their geographic locations. Rural areas tend to have fewer healthcare providers, pharmacies, and other resources than urban areas. As illustrated in **Table 8-1**, the life expectancy for members of rural communities has been generally lower than for members of urban communities across all racial, ethnic, and gender categories. This continues to be the case.

Table 8-1 Rural Versus Urban Life Expectancy (per 100,000 People)

Life Expectancy	Rural Communities	Urban Counties
All	76.8	78.8
Male	74.1	76.2
Female	79.7	81.3
White	77.2	79.2
Black	72.8	74.2
Native American and Alaska Native	74.8	85.8
Asian and Pacific Islander	84.9	86.9
Hispanic (Ethnicity)	82.2	83.1

Data from Singh, G. K., & Siahpush, M. (2014). Widening rural-urban disparities in life expectancy, United States, 1969–2009. *American Journal of Preventive Medicine, 46*(2), 19–29.

REMEDIES

Rather than dwell on the health problems associated with rural communities, looking toward remedies is a more useful approach. According to the Commonwealth Fund (Gunja, 2023), a key issue in these communities is lack of access to health care due to their geographic location. The Commonwealth explored health issues in rural communities in other countries and came up with the following suggestions as potential remedies to try to assuage the issues. These remedies include the following:

- Universal health care to ensure access to all at no cost as not only are rural communities limited by access to care but the cost factor needs to be eliminated.
- Modify a process in the United States that is used in the United Kingdom to increase **access to care**, which involves placing more pharmacies in rural communities, enabling pharmacists to provide basic information and offer basic primary care. The key aspect of this would be to ensure that pharmaceutical licensure enables such basic care in the United States.
- Utilize telehealth in rural communities, ensuring that training for physicians and reimbursement mechanisms are in place to handle this type of delivery of care.
- Develop incentives and requirements for physicians and other healthcare providers to serve in rural communities. For example, specific scholarship programs could be provided that require rural community service programs or loan forgiveness for doing so.

Migrant Farmworkers

Another group to consider when assessing health disparities in rural communities is people who are **migrant and seasonal agricultural workers (MSAWs)**. Their health status is adversely affected by myriad issues, including hazardous work environments, poverty, low wages, inadequate housing, limited availability of clean water and septic systems, limited access and continuity of care, lack of insurance, and cultural and language barriers (Rural Health Information Hub, 2024).

People who are migrant farmworkers may face an additional challenge in that a significant number are undocumented immigrants and lack authorization to work in the United States (Kandel, 2008). The estimated number of agricultural workers in the United States is approximately 2.5 million, with most residing and working in California (Hansen & Donohoe, 2003), although this number varies. Other estimates have reported that 3–5 million MSAWs and their dependents (including husbands, wives, children, and other family members) live in the United States (Colt et al., 2001). Again, currently, it is difficult to attain a specific number. Larson (2013), citing the definitions provided by the Migrant Health Program of the Bureau of Primary Health Care, United. States. U.S. Code, defines a migratory farmworker as "an individual whose principal employment is in agriculture, who has been so employed within the last 24 months, and who establishes for the purposes of such employment a temporary abode" and a seasonal farmworker as "an individual whose principal employment is in agriculture on a seasonal basis and who is not a migratory agricultural worker" (42 USC CHAPTER 6A, SUBCHAPTER II, Part D: Primary Health Care, n.d.). Essentially, MSAWs provide labor that fortifies the U.S. fruit and labor industry (Mobed et al., 1992).

Health Issues

Mobed et al. (1992) explain some of the health issues that impact people who are MSAWs:

> "Potential farm work-related health problems include accidents, pesticide-related illnesses, musculoskeletal and soft-tissue disorders, dermatitis, noninfectious respiratory conditions, reproductive health problems, health problems of children of farm workers, climate-caused illnesses, communicable diseases, bladder and kidney disorders, and eye and ear problems."

Serious issues continue to exist even in the current times. According to the Rural Health Information Hub (2024), MSAW populations experience serious health problems, including diabetes, malnutrition, depression, substance use, infectious diseases, pesticide poisoning, and injuries from physical stress and work-related machinery.

Because the population of MSAWs is constantly moving, longitudinal studies have been limited. Hansen and Donohoe (2003) point out some of the same issues as those previously stated and also include infectious diseases (including bacterial, fungal, and parasitic infections), heat stress, respiratory conditions, reproductive issues, oral health concerns, cancer, and social and mental health problems. Federal dollars are provided to assist with some of this population's many health issues, with services provided by Federally Qualified Health Centers (FQHCs) and Migrant Health Centers. Migrant Health Centers receive funding from the Health Resources Services Administration, per the Public Health Service Act, Section 330(g). These grants enable the provision of health care to individuals regardless of either their ability to pay or their immigration status and are supposed to provide culturally competent care. The community health centers accept Medicare, Medicaid, and other forms of insurance for MASWs and their families (Rural Health Information Hub, 2024).

The Tragic Health Status of Migrant and Seasonal Agricultural Workers

What is taking place in America regarding people who are MSAWs is a tragedy. Although there is concern expressed regarding undocumented immigrants, including the belief among some people that they should be removed from the United States or made legal citizens (there are a range of opinions), immigration reform has yet to occur. This situation causes political consternation between various factions and is extremely controversial. Many of the people purporting that immigrants must enter the country on a documented status and maintain such clearance fail to acknowledge that there is complicity in employing undocumented migrants. Employers of people who are MSAWs enjoy the fruits of their labor—literally, in some cases—but pay them minimally and do not ensure that they have access to health care. Some people in the United States believe that there must be admission and understanding that people who are MSAWs are a benefit to the United States economy, particularly in terms of the fruit and vegetable industry. People who are MSAWs are grossly underpaid despite the intensity of their labor. For example, one key health issue, birth and neonatal problems, exemplifies the intensity of their labor, as explained by Hansen and Donohoe (2003):

> Prolonged standing and bending, overexertion, dehydration, poor nutrition, and pesticide or chemical exposure contribute to an increased risk of spontaneous abortion, premature delivery, fetal malformation and growth retardation, and abnormal postnatal development. Moreover, low socioeconomic status; frequently young maternal age; and late, little, or no prenatal care increase risks to mother and child.

REMEDIES

Hansen and Donohoe (2003) recommend the following to improve the health status of MSAWs. Many of these potential remedies are applicable to rural communities in general also.

- Create a stronger public health infrastructure.
- Enroll more healthcare providers to work with underserved populations.
- Employ more community outreach workers.
- Train bilingual and bicultural healthcare providers.

(continues)

REMEDIES   *(continued)*

- Encourage alternative healthcare delivery methods (e.g., "healthcare vans").
- Implement more advanced information-tracking systems that can be networked among clinicians.
- Increase preventive health services such as dental care, family planning, accident prevention, and detection and control of chronic diseases.
- Broaden legislation and protection through improved U.S. Department of Labor, Occupational Safety and Health Administration, and Environmental Protection Agency standards to eliminate overcrowded and unsanitary living conditions and workplace hazards and exposures.
- Create a system of universal access to care.
- Improve education, including health literacy, among MSAWs.
- Educate MSAWs about prevention, detection, and treatment at their homes, workplaces, or community centers.
- Include migrant health care in medical, nursing, and dental school curricula (e.g., interactive lectures).
- Improve physician recognition, management, and reporting of pesticide-related illnesses.

Rural Healthy People 2030

The **Healthy People initiative** takes place every 10 years and involves objectives that are identified with the goal being to improve the health of the nation on a measurable basis by keeping track of goals that are set. The problems in rural communities are quite significant and hence there is a companion initiative entitled **Rural Healthy People** (Callaghan et al., 2023). **Rural Healthy People 2030** is in progress now.

The priorities for rural communities, in terms of these objectives, are mental health and mental health disorders, addiction, overweight and obesity, economic stability, drug and alcohol use, workforce, preventive care, diabetes, nutrition, and healthy eating. In a recent study, rural community stakeholders were asked what they thought were the priorities in terms of rural health. The following was the outcome:

> "The analysis finds that for the first time across three decades of Rural Healthy People, a greater proportion of respondents selected "Mental Health and Mental Disorders" and "Addiction" as Healthy People priorities for rural America, than did "Health Care Access and Quality". Even still, respondents *ranked* "Health Care Access and Quality" as the single-most important rural priority (Callaghan et al., 2023)."

Based on these findings, it appears to be imperative that initiatives/remedies to address these issues must be at the forefront. Universal access to care would serve to assist dramatically with access to care concerns. In terms of mental health and mental disorders, increased psychological and psychiatric care would be extremely helpful—with the understanding that stress is most likely a major contributing factor given some of the primary issues mentioned earlier in this chapter, which include unemployment and poverty. Socioeconomic status is a serious social determinant of health. People who experience poverty are often stressed/under duress and, consequently, the anguish/desperation associated with it may lead to other concerns, of which mental health issues may be at the forefront. Mental health concerns also exist in urban communities, but in general, there is more access to mental health care. As indicated by Morales et al. (2020):

> "The reasons underlying this mental health treatment disparity are well documented and include reduced access to providers and limited availability of specialty mental health care in rural areas, lack of trained mental health providers and care coordination in rural medical care, and underutilization of available services."

This can be rectified by the recruitment and offering of more mental health providers in rural communities, along with an array of such services. Other approaches should be considered heavily, which are not western medicine/pharmaceutical (in terms of psychiatrist) oriented. For example, yoga and meditation centers should be made available in community health centers and community outreach centers in rural communities where stress and other mental health concerns are overwhelming. Since rural communities may not have access to mental health care that is needed, a study was conducted in Montana around the use of yoga for students who were experiencing mental health issues (depression and anxiety symptoms). As stated by Davis et al. (2022):

> . . .44% of Montana's population is classified as rural or frontier, meaning they are some of the smallest and most geographically isolated areas in America. Therefore, innovative mental health delivery methods are desperately needed for not only rural Montanans, but other geographically isolated areas in our nation.

The bottom line is that in the process of trying to provide remedies for ongoing problems in the United States, in rural communities specifically and beyond, innovative approaches must be considered. New innovative approaches should be sought, but perhaps revisiting what has existed for thousands of years may be useful with options such as yoga, meditation, and similar approaches in dealing with mental health concerns.

REMEDIES

- The provision of more mental health providers.
- Overall reduction of poverty in rural communities.
- Consideration of non-Western medicine approaches to deal with stress and other mental health issues, such as yoga and meditation, which can be offered in outreach centers in rural communities where stress and other mental health concerns are overwhelming.
- More research is needed to understand and implement remedies in rural communities with an emphasis on diversity and the wide-array of health issues that they experience.

WRAP-UP

There are serious problems that contribute to the health status gap of rural communities as compared to the rest of the United States population. One specific factor that is key to the overall problem is lack of access to care. Additionally, there are **risky behaviors** that must be considered that impact **rural health**, including smoking, heavy alcohol consumption, and lack of regular exercise. Stress, lack of funds, and lack of access to productive, positive exercise facilities and mental health care are the primary reasons for such behaviors. People who are MSAWs have particular health concerns due to their lack of access to care. Specific remedies must be considered to address this population's myriad health problems.

First, research is needed to better describe health disparities between rural and urban areas, emphasizing the fact that rural places are not monolithic, across the United States. Second, research is needed on how trends in rural population health are affecting rural communities. Third, research is needed on the ways in which economic well-being and livelihood strategies interact with rural health. Fourth, we need to better understand the health implications of the physical and social isolation characterizing many rural communities, lack of access to mental health and consider innovative options for the latter, such as yoga, meditation, and other non-Western medicine and pharmaceutical approaches to address these concerns.

Chapter Problems

1. List three specific factors that contribute to poor health conditions for people in rural communities.
2. What are some of the key health concerns for people who are MASWs in the United States?
3. What do you think are the best solutions for improving the health status of people who are MSAWs? Why?
4. How does poverty impact rural health?
5. Describe why innovative approaches should be considered to address mental health issues in rural communities.

References

Callaghan, T., Kassabian, M., Johnson, N., Shrestha, A., Helduser, J., Horel, S., Bolin, J. N., & Ferdinand, A. O. (2023). Rural healthy people 2030: New decade, new challenges. *Preventive Medicine Reports, 33*, 102176. https://doi.org/10.1016/j.pmedr.2023.102176

Colt, J. S., Stallones, L., Cameron, L. L., Dosemeci, M., & Zahm, S. H. (2001). Proportionate mortality among US migrant and seasonal farmworkers in twenty-four states†. *American Journal of Industrial Medicine, 40*(5), 604–611. https://doi.org/10.1002/ajim.1126

Davis, L., Aylward, A., & Buchanan, R. (2022). Trauma-Informed Yoga: Investigating an intervention for mitigating adverse childhood experiences in rural contexts. *Educational Studies, 58*(4), 530–559. https://doi.org/10.1080/00131946.2022.2102495

Dumont, A. (2024, January 19). *Changes in the United States Economy and Rural-Urban Employment Disparities*. Fed Notes, Board of Governors of the Federal Reserve System. https://www.federalreserve.gov/econres/notes/feds-notes/changes-in-the-us-economy-and-rural-urban-employment-disparities-20240119.html

Gunja, M. Z. (2023, July 24). *Rural Americans struggle with medical bills and health care affordability.* The Commonwealth Fund. https://www.commonwealthfund.org/blog/2023/rural-americans -struggle-medical-bills-and-health-care-affordability

Hansen, E., & Donohoe, M. (2003). Health issues of migrant and seasonal farmworkers. *Journal of Health Care for the Poor and Underserved, 14*(2), 153–164. https://doi.org/10.1353 /hpu.2010.0790

Kandel, W. (2008, July). *Profile of migrant farmworkers, a 2008 update* (Economic Research Report No. 60). UnitedStates Department of Agriculture. https://ers.usda.gov/sites/default/files /_laserfiche/publications/46038/ERR-60.pdf?v=59011

Larson, A. C. (2013, May). *Migrant and seasonal farmworker enumeration profiles study.* Oregon Update. https://www.oregon.gov/oha/HPA/HP-PCO/Documents/2013%20Update%20to%20 MSFW%20Enumeration%20Studies%20Report.pdf

Mobed, K., Gold, E. B., & Schenker, M. B. (1992). Occupational health problems among migrant and seasonal farm workers. *Western Journal of Medicine, 157*(3), 367–373.

Morales, D. A., Barksdale, C. L., & Beckel-Mitchener, A. C. (2020). A call to action to address rural mental health disparities. *Journal of Clinical and Translational Science, 4*(5), 463–467. https://doi .org/10.1017/cts.2020.42

Mehta, K., Gabbard, S. M., Barrat, V., Lewis, M., Carroll, D., & Mines, R. (2000). *Findings from the National Agricultural Workers Survey (NAWS) 1997–1998: A demographic and employment profile of United States farmworkers.* United States Department of Labor.

National Institutes of Health. (2022, March). *Health in rural America: Connecting to care.* News in Health. https://newsinhealth.nih.gov/sites/newsinhealth/files/2022/March/NIHNiHMar2022 .pdf

Rural Health. (2024, May 16). *Health behaviors in rural America.* Centers for Disease Control and Prevention. https://www.cdc.gov/rural-health/php/public-health-strategy/public-health -considerations-for-health-behaviors-in-rural-america.html

Rural Health Information Hub. (2024). Migrant and Seasonal Farmworker Health. Retrieved from: https://www.ruralhealthinfo.org/topics/migrant-health

U.S. Department of Health and Human Services. (n.d.). Health Equity in Healthy People 2030. Retrieved from: https://health.gov/healthypeople/priority-areas/health-equity-healthy-people -2030

42 USC CHAPTER 6A, SUBCHAPTER II, Part D: Primary Health Care. (n.d.). https://uscode.house .gov/view.xhtml?hl=false&edition=prelim&req=granuleid%3AUSC-prelim-title42-chapter6A -subchapter2-partD&f=treesort&num=0&saved=%7CNDIgdXNjIDI1NGI%3D%7CdHJlZXN vcnQ%3D%7CdHJ1ZQ%3D%3D%7C20%7Ctrue%7Cprelim

CHAPTER 9

Understanding the Impact of Urban/ Suburban/Rural Education on Urban/ Suburban/Rural Health and Remedies

Edmund Adjapong, PhD and **Courtney Elizabeth Rose**, MEd, EdD

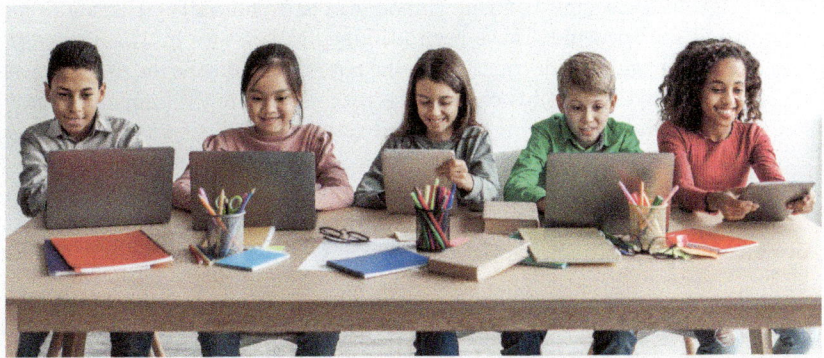

KEY TERMS

achievement gap
Brown v. Board of Education
colorblindness
common school system
cultural capital
cultural incongruence

culturally relevant pedagogy
demographic imperative
health literacy
tracking
Virtual Professional Learning Network
  (VPLN)

LEARNING OBJECTIVES

After reading this chapter, you should be able to do the following:

1. Describe the link between health and education.
2. Understand the history of the development of the public school system that exists in America today.
3. Define "achievement gap" and how it has been used to perpetuate beliefs about particular groups' educational abilities and outcomes.
4. Identify and explain the link between educational achievement and health outcomes.
5. Explain the role of culture as it relates to teaching and learning.

Introduction

The link between education and health is well-known and highly researched. Access to both health care and education are closely tied to, and mitigated by, one's geographic location and socioeconomic status. Those holding higher paying jobs, which is closely linked to educational attainment, have the ability to live and move to locations in closer proximity to better schools, more nutritional food sources, transportation, and health services (Weingart, 2014). Additionally, one's ability to engage in educational processes is closely linked to their health status. Chronic illness and poor nutrition impact attendance rates, concentration, and cognitive skills, all of which deeply impact the degree to which students are able to connect and engage with academic content (Zimmerman & Woolf, 2014). Digging deeper, schools and the curriculum have been identified as key sites in which to engage America's youth with health education in the hopes of improving the nation's health literacy and outcomes. In this chapter, the authors explore the dominant conceptualizations of the academic **achievement gap** and the history of the American schooling system, providing insight into the root causes of the education gap as well as potential and necessary remedies for long-term change toward equitable access to quality educational experiences, and by association, improved health literacy and outcomes, particularly for historically marginalized populations.

Defining Health Literacy

Decades of studies show that higher levels of academic achievement have positive impacts on individuals' health behaviors and health outcomes. Specifically, education fosters the development of cognitive skills, problem-solving abilities, and personality traits, among others, that mediate the relationship between health and education (Ross & Wu, 1995; Zimmerman & Woolf, 2014). Most notably, the hard skills acquired in school (i.e., reading comprehension and argumentation) increases individuals' **health literacy** making it easier for them to understand their health needs, read and interpret instructions, and advocate for their own health needs and those in their families and communities. Previously defined as "the degree to which individuals have the capacity to obtain, process and understand basic health information and services needed to make appropriate health decisions" in the U.S. Department of Health and Human Services' (HHS) Healthy People 2010 and Healthy People 2020 reports, the definition of health literacy was changed and expanded for the Healthy People 2030 report to address both personal and organizational health literacy. Healthy People 2030 is a HHS initiative, which promotes health through the use of data-driven national objectives, and is the fifth iteration of this process. Currently, the HHS defines each as follows (Centers for Disease Control and Prevention, 2024; Healthy People 2030, n.d.):

- Personal health literacy: the degree to which individuals have the ability to find, understand, and use information and services to inform health-related decisions and actions for themselves and others.
- Organizational health literacy: the degree to which organizations equitably enable individuals to find, understand, and use information and services to inform health-related decisions and actions for themselves and others.

The new definitions signal a greater focus on the latter portions of the former definition, developing individuals' capabilities to *use* health information and services to improve health-related decision-making. Exploring the different ways individuals use health-related materials or make health-related decisions, recent research categorizes these behaviors into three levels of personal health literacy:

1. Basic/functional literacy: Basic skills in reading and writing that enable one to read health-related materials or labels (i.e. labels on medication). Individuals with basic health literacy skills often respond well to clearly communicated directives for specific goals and contexts (for example, taking medication, participating in prevention activities and engaging in some behavioral changes).
2. Communicative/interactive literacy: More advanced cognitive and literacy skills which, when combined with social skills, enable one to search for and gather, interpret, and communicate/discuss information as it pertains to the health of themselves and/or loved ones. Individuals with communicative/interactive literacy skills can better distinguish between different sources of information and respond to more interactive structured means (for example, school-based health education, mobile services, and interactive websites).
3. Critical literacy: Even further advanced cognitive skills, which when combined with social skills, enable one to gather and critically analyze information relating to a greater range of health determinants from a wide range of sources. Individuals operating with critical health literacy skills can access and use information to exert greater control over life events and situations through informed decision-making and individual/collective advocacy rooted in a deeper understanding of the social, economic, and environmental determinants of health that extend far beyond the self and are clearly linked to large-scale community and population benefits. (Nutbeam & Lloyd, 2021; Wittink & Oosterhaven, 2018).

American Adults' Health Literacy

In 2003, the U.S. Department of Education's (USDOE) National Center for Education Statistics sponsored and released the National Assessment of Adult Literacy (NAAL), a study on English Literacy among American adults. Assessing a representative sample of 19,000 adults ages 16 and over, including over 1000 people incarcerated in federal and state prisons, the NAAL study provided insight into American adults' literacy performance in three types of literacy: prose (searching, comprehending, and using continuous texts like editorials, news stories, instructional materials, etc.), document (searching, comprehending and using non-continuous texts like job applications, payroll forms, maps, food labels, etc.) and quantitative (identifying and performing computations like balancing checkbooks/bank accounts, calculating a tip, determining the total amount of an order, etc.). Most notably, the NAAL study incorporated a health literacy component, making it the first-ever representative national assessment designed specifically to measure adults' ability to use literacy skills to read and understand health-related information, establishing a baseline for future assessments of health literacy (National Center for Education Statistics, n.d.).

Estimates based on the findings of the 2003 NAAL study show that only 12% of American adults have *proficient* health literacy (which aligns closely with a critical health literacy, as listed earlier) while the majority, around 53%, had *intermediate* (which would likely place them in the communicative health literacy skills). Women demonstrated a higher level of health literacy than men, as did White and Asian/Pacific Islander adults as compared to Black, Hispanic, American Indian/Alaska Native, and multiracial counterparts. Age, English language proficiency, and education all played a significant role as well. Specifically, in terms of education, nearly 49% of adults without a high school diploma had *below basic* health literacy, while only 15% of those with a high school diploma and 3% of those with a bachelor's degree fell in the same category (Kutner et al., 2006).

At the time of writing this chapter, no follow-up to the 2003 NAAL study has been conducted. However, the global Program for the International Assessment of Adult Competencies (PIAAC) was conducted in 2012 and 2014 to gather a representative sample of American adults and includes an exploration of health information seeking behaviors (HISB) in connection with individuals' literacy, numeracy, and problem-solving skills (LNPS). The PIAAC has returned similar results as the NAAL, providing further support to not just develop individuals' literacy skills, but to identify and employ strategies aimed *specifically* at increasing the levels of critical health literacy among the American adult population.

Health Education in Schools

Given the persistence of this data over time and the strong connection between critical health literacy skills and improved health outcomes, many health educators have argued that the best remedy for improving American adult health literacy is to focus on developing these skills with the youth "when life-long health habits are first being formed" (Auld et al., 2020). Calls to integrate health education into American schools/curriculum appear to have started in the early 19th century as leaders and officials in both Education and Public Health argued for the importance of health instruction for children to learn to preserve their lives and the lives of others (Auld et al., 2020). Early initiatives and programs focused primarily on using schools as sites to provide health services, such as health and hygiene checks by school nurses, increasing the cleanliness of schools, and communicating didactic messages, primarily directed at parents, on the importance of taking children for proper treatment of illnesses in the hopes of decreasing the spread of disease. Partnerships between education and health/medical organizations, such as the 1911 joint effort of the National Education Association (NEA) and the American Medical Association (AMA) as well as key reports on the status and effectiveness of health education efforts, such as the 1960s School Health Education Study, continued to highlight and stress the need for concerted and collaborative efforts to develop better personal health-related decision-making and increase the overall health of American citizens.

In the late 1990s and early 2000s, the term "coordinated school health programs" gained popularity in reports from the CDC and other health organizations as they identified eight factors impacting children's health, including health education. However, this term was not embraced by educational organizations and leadership, and in 2014 the CDC partnered with the ASCD (formerly the Association for Supervision and Curriculum Development) to produce the Whole School, Whole Community, Whole Child (WSCC) framework designed to ensure every child is healthy upon *entering* K-12 schooling and receives education about healthy practices and lifestyle choices throughout their schooling years. As with most other curricular decisions, it is largely up to the state and local governments to determine what should be taught as a part of public school health education curriculum. However, many public and private organizations have worked to develop resources, including National Health Education Standards, that state and local districts are highly encouraged to use in the development and selection of curricular materials aimed at improving health literacy (National Consensus for School Health Education, 2022; SHAPE America, 2024). The long history of efforts and available health education resources leaves a question as to what is contributing to the continued and persistent gaps in health literacy and health outcomes. In order to answer this question, it is necessary to understand the issues of equity and access that have directly impacted the experiences of students and educators within the education system.

Mind the Gap

Unfortunately, another similarity between health and education is the gap between the quality of services and outcomes that exists between various groups of the population, often drawn along racial and socioeconomic lines and rooted in historical and systemic practices and policies intended to limit access and opportunity. In the increasingly test-based approach to education, the "achievement gap" has become one of the biggest buzzwords within the field of education. This gap disproportionately affects students in predominantly African American and Latino populations, and in low-income urban areas. Since the inception of the compulsory American schooling system, various laws, mandated policies, curricular designs, and education reform agendas became enmeshed in deficit-based constructions of difference and diversity. These have been used to limit access to educational opportunities and resources for those in historically marginalized and underserved populations (Anderson, 1988; Kliebard, 2004; Nasaw, 1981). Historically, constructions of race, gender, (dis)ability, and social class have been used to establish a cultural norm rooted in the ideals of a White, middle-/upper-class, male-dominated society (Delpit, 1988; Gay, 2000; Irizarry, 2009). Within this framing, perceived social and cultural differences resulted in the continuous labeling of those who deviate from, or are not able to fit within, the "norm" as "socially and/or culturally deprived," in need of fixing, or in some extreme cases, removal from the system altogether.

How Did We Get Here?

Historians in the fields of Education and Sociology explore the development of the **common school system**, which was the precursor to the compulsory public education system currently functioning within American society. Fearing the consequences of granting the right to vote to the "common man," those in power quickly moved to develop a system of education that would work to socialize and civilize the children of the poor whose education was previously the responsibility of the family (primarily the mother) to provide. Using compulsory taxation of the people, the government publicly funded their schools, claiming that it was the only way to guarantee "protection from the rapacity of the unschooled" (Nasaw, 1981). Through various reform movements, proponents of the common schooling system constantly worked to ensure that resources (monetary, material, and human) were used efficiently. This resulted in multiple "reform efforts," which limited access to various components of the curriculum to those it was deemed unnecessary for, particularly as the use of various tests and sorting tools became popular methods to determine one's intellectual capacity and projected future place in society. Thus, social mobility, or the ability for one to "pull themselves up by their bootstraps," was limited for many, thereby reproducing existing social stratification and protecting the elite positions of those in power (Nasaw, 1981).

Within this movement, the education of recently freed Black enslaved people, and poor White people, particularly in the South, became a major area of contention among proponents of the common schooling movement. Fearing both the overeducated *and* uneducated freed Black man, the majority of schools initially designed for this population provided training in service-oriented, and largely manual, labor that continued to limit them to work in the homes, fields, and later, factories of White America (Nasaw, 1981). Therefore, some argue that from its inception, compulsory public education, as it exists today, was never intended for the inclusion of African American people, or other racial/ethnic groups, and the basic infrastructure of American society works to perpetuate the subjugation and exclusion of the majority of members in these groups (Adjapong, 2017).

The Sorting Game

One can trace current practices in the use of testing to the introduction of intelligence quotient (IQ) testing. Initially used in France, the IQ test was brought to the United States as a means of determining the "innate intelligence" of individuals and detecting the "genetically inferior" (Kamin, 1974). Through the use of these tests, intelligence became closely attributed to those of Western European descent with a disproportionate number of poor people and those of Eastern European, Native American, and African descent determined unintelligent. Linking intelligence and genetics in this manner, IQ testing becomes a means of justifying social inequity and the persistent gap between the wealthy and the under-resourced. Even more disturbing, IQ testing is historically linked to the eugenics movement within the United States, in which some states passed laws to sterilize those determined to be "feeble-minded" and Congress passed the Immigration Act of 1924, which restricted immigration from Southern and Eastern Europe (Kamin, 1974).

The "science" behind intelligence quotient (IQ) testing became the basis for segregating students into two tracks: (1) those educated to work in service and manual labor; and (2) those educated for higher education and prestigious careers (Kamin, 1974). Traces of this same system are clearly visible in the **tracking** practices, often labeled "ability grouping" that exists within the American public school system today and acts as a covert way of pushing disproportionate numbers of students of color, particularly Black and Latinx students, out of high-level and college-preparatory courses (Gamoran et al., 1995). In response to arguments of intentionally discriminatory actions, many look to the law to define the circumstances in which test use may be discriminatory or otherwise inappropriate. Under the Equal Protection Clause of the 14th Amendment, landmark cases have been filed intending to show testing practices and policies were intentionally discriminatory and/or act to preserve the effects of prior discrimination.

Presently, these tests are no longer used to justify historical claims of *inferiority* along socially constructed lines of difference such as race, class, or gender. However, they are still widely used to measure student learning, assess learning disabilities and/or giftedness, and explain/predict educational outcomes. Given that the culture of schools is grounded in the social norms of dominant White culture of society, the standard of teaching and learning remains tipped in favor of similar cultural norms. Not surprisingly, there remains an ever-widening gap between the performance of students from low-income and diverse racial/ethnic groups and a simultaneous over-representation of these students in special education and remedial courses. It is through the increased use of test performance as a predictor of future success and the subsequent tracking and labeling practices that are associated with it that lead many students to internalize their scores to a degree in which they essentially embody them in their day-to-day lives.

In many schools, the language of the testing culture becomes entrenched in daily functioning. Students are no longer "learning"; they are trying to "achieve mastery" or at the very least "reach proficiency." Classrooms are covered in posters and charts outlining "what smart and/or good students do" complete with various mnemonic devices to help students memorize and remember them when it all has to come down for state testing. Additionally, in preparation for each subject-area assessment, teachers are often asked to devote a portion of their class time to "differentiated instruction," which involves breaking their classes down to performance-based groups, determined by their scores on tests and quizzes given throughout the school year, to target specific skills and concepts for specific students.

In the case of testing culture, a stigma arises in the form of rewards and consequences based on students' ability to perform on a standardized task on which great value is placed collectively by the group and broader educational systems. Regardless of student, teacher, and family buy-ins, the students' performance on these tests are used to place them in future classes, determine their access to resources and opportunities, and serve as a predictor for future success on the same task the following year. Thus, even the well-intentioned teacher faces a moral dilemma of rebelling against, and resisting the notion of, standardization while also preparing the students to compete within a system that lives and breathes by it. Similarly, any parent/guardian wishing to guide their children to academic success must either concede to these testing practices, hiring tutors, and test prep coaches beginning as early as third grade, or removing their students from the public school system altogether into private schools where testing does not function as a rigid gatekeeper marketed as a tool for accountability, but in actuality, functions to keep many opportunities out of reach for specific populations.

From Achievement Gap to Opportunity Gap

Although the achievement gap itself is discussed very clearly as a matter of inequality between racial groups, dominant narratives in the public conversation attempt to shift the problem out of the sphere of race matters to one of social class and family values. Shifting the dialogue in this manner reframes the issue as inequality of *engagement with and performance in* education. This places the root cause of the problem in the families themselves as factors, such as family structure, parenting styles, and neighborhood characteristics, are used to explain the persistence of unequal levels of academic achievement across racial lines (Burchinal et al., 2008; Dotterer et al., 2012). Beginning in the first few years of a child's life, the burden is placed on single, low-income, working parents (largely mothers and predominantly people of color) to educate themselves on the various types of educational/childcare programs that would better prepare their children for the K-12 experience. Additionally, through research comparing experiences across racial groups within similar social class backgrounds, researchers and scholars find that cultural differences in parenting styles also contribute to the inequalities in school readiness as children from some racially and culturally diverse home environments are deemed unready to engage with the learning environments as compared to their White counterparts (Dotterer et al., 2012).

However, contrary to these views are those presented by scholars and researchers who maintain that it is not inequality of *engagement and performance*, but rather inequality, and more accurately inequity, of *opportunity to access* quality education (Walters, 2001; Ladson-Billings, 2006; Milner, 2012). Running parallel to the aforementioned research, scholars holding this position place the root of the problem in the various systems of society. They present the argument that through legal and political moves, the state intentionally shifted the onus of achieving equity within education from the schools to the people while simultaneously justifying the discriminatory actions of those in powerful positions (Walters, 2001; De Vito, 2007). These researchers and scholars agree that there is a difference in the approaches and values given to the educational experiences of parents living in low-income, urban environments, and their children as compared to their middle and upper class, suburban counterparts. However, they find that it is impossible to discuss these disparities without explicitly exploring matters of race relations (Ladson-Billings, 2006; Milner, 2012).

Similar to the work of those researchers focusing solely on social class, these scholars begin their exploration of the problem in the late fifties and early sixties. However, they explore more closely what was going on within the legal and political spheres of society, highlighting major Supreme Court cases that allowed particular regions to continue to essentially deny the right to education to various racial and ethnic groups (De Vito, 2007). In their initial work of applying Critical Race Theory to education, educational researchers Gloria Ladson-Billings and William F. Tate examine the emphasis on property rights within American society (Ladson-Billings and Tate, 1995). Noting the priority of protecting property in the years leading up to the development of the constitution and the construction of enslaved Black people as such property to White owners, Ladson-Billings and Tate (1995) note the lack of incentive to protect the human rights of Black people, even after the abolishment of slavery. Although many counter this argument by pointing to the various "victories" within civil rights litigation, particularly the widely debated ***Brown v. Board***

of Education decision, educational and legal scholars point to the ambiguity that exists within much of this legislation that often leads to slow progress, and in many cases none at all (Crenshaw, 1988; Ladson-Billings, 2004).

(Mis)Interpreting Brown v. Board of Education

As previously mentioned, increased emphasis and importance on student test scores highlights the variations in performance across both racial and socioeconomic lines, which has come to be known as the "achievement gap." Sociologists and educational researchers hold varying views on the central causes of this gap in student outcomes, however many link it back to the foundations on which the very system was built (Ladson-Billings, 2012). In a country with a long history of racism and racial inequity, the integration of African American students into the educational system may have had adverse effects in terms of psychological well-being and overall acquisition of resources (physical, financial, and human) (Ladson-Billings, 2012; Payne, 2008). Therefore, the central question is whether or not Black students have become more disadvantaged in the decades following the famous *Brown v. Board of Education* decision that found it unconstitutional to segregate schools based on race. Specifically, while the integration of schools was presented as an opportunity to "level the playing field for all students," research points to evidence that it actually resulted in more costs than benefits for students of color within this country, particularly Black students.

Schools and educational curriculum are some of the primary tools used by the governing body of society, particularly in America, in terms of socializing citizens (all members of society must attend and all members spend the majority of their formative years within the walls of schools). Additionally, in societies in which academic success is the predominant path to economic success, it is logical to presume that those with high stakes in the economy want to ensure that their positions are secure (Kingston, 2001). Therefore, in discussing the integration of two groups historically grounded in two very different social and cultural backgrounds, such as African American and White students, it is necessary to explore the manner in which one group's social and **cultural capital** becomes a barrier in a world dominated by the other.

Questions concerning the overall intent and consequences of desegregation of schools per the *Brown* decision have generally focused on comparing the culture of the schools that Black students attended pre-*Brown* with that of racially integrated schools post-*Brown*. While few would suggest that the American education system go back to the overtly segregated circumstances of the pre-*Brown* era, there is a need to address the negative effects that African American/Black students experience due to the common (mis)interpretation of the language used in the decision itself. Gloria Ladson-Billings (2004) summarizes the argument in her comparison of the *Brown* decision to that of a musician landing on a wrong note in the middle of a performance. She uses this image to "convey the problem of good intentions gone awry" as "one wrong note does not destroy or invalidate an entire performance, but it does create a kind of dissonance that is more or less evident depending on one's vantage point" (Ladson-Billings, 2004).

Those advocating for desegregation within the public schools had good intentions of creating an equal playing field, particularly the families of African American students who wanted to ensure that their children received the same level of access to high-quality educational facilities, materials, and experiences. However, in fighting for equal access they unintentionally fueled the belief held by those in dominant circles of society that African American students/students of color are inferior to White students and, some argue, ultimately did more damage than good (Ladson-Billings, 2004; Blanchett et al., 2005; Horsford, 2010). In this regard, existing research asserts that the issues stemming from school segregation were due to systemic and institutionalized racism, which extended beyond the school system itself and permeated throughout society as a whole. Therefore, since these underlying issues were not directly addressed and blame was instead placed on African American people (and other racial/ethnic groups) themselves, long-term change that would benefit these historically marginalized groups would be difficult to achieve (Massey & Denton, 1993; Ladson-Billings, 2004; Blanchett et al., 2005).

Predominantly African American schools in the pre-*Brown* era provided supportive environments in which educators provided students with the skills and knowledge they needed in order to be successful in navigating the racially stratified system in which they lived (Horsford, 2010). Educational historians acknowledge the lower quality of the materials and facilities provided to African American educators, however, the strong levels of care, trust, and understanding between educators, students, and families allowed for African American students to flourish within these racially segregated neighborhood schools. Additionally, the strong presence of African American teachers and administrators during this time provided African American students with role models that could relate to the racism and inequity that the students experienced outside of the school walls (Ladson-Billings, 2004; Horsford, 2010). Thus, at this time, schools and educators held a strong value within the African American community, going to great lengths in order to enrich the curriculum with experiences that would help their students build the same skills that their White counterparts were receiving (afterschool programs and clubs focused on drama, speech, and scholastic accomplishment as examples) (Walker, 2000).

Subsequently, with the passing of the *Brown* decision came a steep decline in the number of African American teachers present in schools, as African American students were bused out to White working-class schools and their neighborhood schools shut down. Environments within these mixed-race schools provided students with an opportunity to learn how to communicate and work with members of other races; however, since the underlying institutionalized racism within society was never addressed, within-school segregation was common practice (Ladson-Billings, 2004; Wells et al., 2005). The post-*Brown* era brought with it the tendency to track more White students into high-level or gifted courses, in some cases as early as Kindergarten (Wells et al., 2005).

Additionally, faced with educating students from diverse racial and cultural backgrounds, it became common to push for a culture built on "**colorblindness**" in which racial and cultural differences were ignored to emphasize similarities between and among students. This practice often left students to navigate the harsh realities of a racially stratified society on their own (Wells et al., 2005). Finally, desegregation found more funds and resources moving out of the African American community and into the White schools in which the students would be integrated. However, due to the policies and systemic practices within housing, banking, and other federal agencies, as well as the various methods in which White schools were able to work around the policies that would force full integration, many African American people could not afford to follow these resources in order to place their students within these schools (Massey & Denton, 1993; Blanchett et al., 2005). In this regard, the newly-integrated schools within the new system appeared colorblind on the surface, but little attention was given to addressing the underlying, lasting consequences of segregation (i.e., Black underachievement and internalized messages of racial inferiority/superiority) (Omi & Winant, 1994), and worked under the assumption that simply placing White and Black students together would be enough to achieve educational equality. In addition to the practices in this section, the testing culture and practices mentioned earlier in this chapter provide a key example of a practice that continues to impact students and educators today, and is one that has long-lasting impacts reaching far back into America's segregated past.

Lasting Impact of Segregation

Placing heavier emphasis on the intangible psychological factors for Black people, in the *Brown* decision the Supreme Court argued that the racially segregated learning environment "generates a feeling of inferiority as to their status in the community that may affect their hearts and minds in a way unlikely to ever be undone" (*Brown v. Board of Education*, 1954). The *Brown* decision presented the foundation for the debate between the colorblind/performance-based approach and the race-/culture-conscious approach. However vague language in the *Brown* decision, which placed the onus on local authorities and courts to determine the best methods of achieving these principles based on contextual factors largely associated with geographical location, exposed the tension around the explicit use of race, and later culture, as a factor in the process.

Desegregation, as it was outlined in *Brown*, is no longer an effective process through which educational equality can be accomplished within American society. As Bell (2002) argues, race-based power hierarchies, built around White over Black conceptions of superiority, are too highly entrenched within the systemic functioning of American society. The myth of *Brown* assumes that simply creating "diverse" learning environments will automatically promote a more welcoming and accepting society, rectifying past discrimination. However, without addressing the underlying assumptions about race, true equality cannot be achieved. The colorblind mentality fails to recognize that although the Constitution aims to protect individuals, its creators did not have *all* individuals in mind, a fact that becomes much more noticeable in the shifting demographic landscape of today's public education system.

Current Demographic Landscape of America's Public Education System

Recent data from the National Center for Education Statistics (NCES) and U.S. Department of Education (USDOE) project that students of color will constitute the majority of the student population, accounting for 56%, as soon as 2024 (U.S. Department of Education, 2016). The national poverty rate for school-age children (ages 5–17) remains around 20%, with recent data showing increases in 41 states between 2000 and 2014 (Kena et al., 2016). The image of the "traditional family" is also shifting with a greater number of students coming from homes headed by single parents, those with different sexual orientations, and a wide variety of other family structures. Additionally, across the nation, there is an increase in homes in which English is not the primary or dominant language spoken, with some schools reporting up to 100 different languages spoken in the early 2000s (Ukpokodu, 2002). By the 2013–2014 school year, 9.3% of public school students were English Language Learners (ELLs) (Kena et al., 2016).

Amid this changing demographic landscape, the K-12 teacher workforce remains largely racially, culturally, linguistically, and socioeconomically homogeneous (Villegas & Irvine, 2010). Statistical data shows the teacher workforce is over 80% White, English-speaking, middle-class, and from suburban or rural communities (Gay, 2000; Lowenstein, 2009). Although research shows evidence that teacher education programs are attempting to diversify their applicant and student pools, projected data suggest the teaching force will remain primarily homogeneous for a long time (Cochran-Smith, 2003a). Explicit attention to the challenges of this **demographic imperative** is critical in order to improve the educational opportunities and outcomes for students who do not fit within the White, patriarchal, middle-class norms.

The demographic implications for education go beyond gaps in numerical representation between students and teachers. Looking beyond the numbers there are also marked differences in the biographies and lived experiences of many teachers and the diverse students in their classrooms. Teachers coming from middle-class, suburban environments who speak only English and teaching in urban environments serving students who are racially, linguistically, and socioeconomically diverse will likely have different cultural frames of reference and perspectives through which to interpret and make sense of the world (Banks et al., 2005). This **cultural incongruence**, or difference in the cultural frames of reference and daily lived realities, can limit these teachers' capacity to function as role models for many of their students or act as cultural brokers/agents for students capable of assisting students in bridging home and school experiences (Villegas & Irvine, 2010).

Perhaps most alarmingly, dominant discourses that frame "diversity" as "deficit" often cause White, middle-class teachers to view cultural diversity as obstacles to be overcome resulting in lowered expectations or fears about working with different cultural and life experiences, particularly in traditionally underserved areas (Banks et al., 2005; Ladson-Billings, 1999; Nieto, 2005). This construction of difference is a discursive practice that remains central to debates within teacher education concerning how to prepare teachers for diverse populations. Data pointing to the "demographic imperative," or persistent, and widening, gap between a student body that is increasingly racially/ethnically, linguistically, and socioeconomically diverse and a teaching force that remains predominantly White, female, middle-class, and English-speaking produces an increased sense of urgency in how to approach teacher education, presenting varied perspectives on the best practices in preparing effective educators for *all* students (Banks et al, 2005; Ladson-Billings, 1999; Lowenstein, 2009; Zeichner, 2003).

Bridging In-School and Out-of-School Selves

In response to the demographic imperative, professional organizations and institutions whose primary missions are concerned with the preparation of teachers have taken official action toward the redesigning of teacher education programs, curriculum and practice. In 1972, the American Association of Colleges for Teacher Education (AACTE) formed one of the first commissions on multicultural teacher education, making three assertions: (1) cultural diversity is a valuable resource, (2) multicultural education is education that preserves and extends the resource of cultural diversity rather than merely tolerating it or making it "melt away," and (3) a commitment to cultural pluralism ought to permeate all aspects of teacher preparation programs in this country (Banks et al, 2002; Cochran-Smith, 2003a). In 1976, the National Council for the Accreditation of Teacher Education (NCATE) added multicultural education and teaching for diversity to its standards.

Subsequently, all institutions seeking accreditation were required to show evidence that they were planning for the incorporation of multicultural content by 1979 and then provided within all teacher education programs by 1981 (Cochran-Smith, 2003b). A prominent thread throughout multicultural teacher education research focuses on this urgent need to (re)structure university-based programs for the development and implementation of more effective multicultural teacher education courses and programs. Looking to existing research documenting the work of successful educators of diverse populations (i.e., Ladson-Billings' *Dreamkeepers*) as well as the damaging discourses and practices impacting the educational experiences of culturally diverse students, scholars contributing to this work identify key components in the transformation of formal teacher education for diversity.

Culturally Relevant/Responsive Education

Literature looking at the larger structural issues in formal university-based teacher education programs highlight the common practice of segregating explicit discussions of culture, race, and diversity to single courses within programs. These courses may be optional and not required for completion of degree programs and send the message that attention to diversity is optional, or only important once other content-specific skills are mastered (Cochran-Smith, 1991; Ladson-Billings, 2000; Villegas & Lucas, 2002). Additionally, detaching these courses from the rest of the curriculum makes it difficult for concepts covered within them to be reinforced enough to make a lasting impact on future practice once teachers enter the classroom (Villegas & Lucas, 2002).

Instead, proponents of critical multicultural and culturally relevant pedagogical practices call for a shift in the design of teacher education programs that integrate issues of cultural relevance and diversity throughout the entire program. Aligning directly to the core tenets of **culturally relevant pedagogy**, Villegas and Lucas (2002) identify six strands necessary in the development of the culturally relevant educator:

1. socio-cultural consciousness;
2. affirming attitudes toward students from culturally diverse backgrounds;
3. commitment and skills to act as agents of change;
4. constructivist views of learning;
5. learning about students; and
6. culturally relevant teaching practices.

Using these six strands can serve "as an organizing framework" through which to build a vision for a program that infuses attention to diversity throughout the curriculum and gives "conceptual coherence to the preparation of teachers for diversity" (Villegas & Lucas, 2002).

Transforming teacher education programs through some of the strategies suggested by Cochran-Smith (1991) and Villegas and Lucas (2002) helps to address some issues that teachers experience as they attempt to take what they have learned back into their K-12 classrooms. Transforming teacher education in this way may encourage preservice teachers to adopt situated pedagogies that more explicitly address issues of race, class, and gender and create more culturally congruent teaching and learning environments for culturally diverse students (Ladson-Billings, 2000). Teachers need opportunities to develop the necessary cross-cultural competency or sociopolitical awareness required in the construction of culturally affirming and meaningful curriculum, instruction, and interactional patterns that are connected to students' prior experiences and culturally-specific ways of learning and knowing (Banks et al, 2005; Gay, 2000; Ladson-Billings, 1999).

Social Media and Education

Technology has transformed human life through improved communication, social networking, the ease to access information, and improved entertainment to name a few. In education, technology is used as a tool to improve student learning and to make content more accessible. While there are many applications of technology in education and within classrooms, limited consideration is given to how technology, specifically social media, can impact teachers' learning and professional development. Many educators in the 21st century use various forms of technology as part of their daily teaching practices and as part of their personal lives. Many teachers turn to a **Virtual Professional Learning Network (VPLN)** found on social media platforms to learn and to grow professionally. A VPLN is a uniquely personalized space where participants can engage in dialogue with a network of individuals from around the world via social media platforms such as X (formerly known as Twitter) to support one another's continuous professional learning. Garrison (2007) describes a VPLN as a synchronous or asynchronous online platform for individuals to collaboratively engage in critical thinking and discussions around specific issues (Trinkle, 2009). VPLNs consist of global virtual learning networks that enable participants to share diverse, global perspectives on teaching strategies and educational issues. VPLNs are mainly found on Twitter with educators and other stakeholders using hashtags to engage in conversation and share materials. While there are shortcomings of traditional professional development for educators, through their participation in VPLNs, they are provided opportunities to meet their specific professional learning needs (Krutka et al., 2017). Some argue that VPLNs provide educators with the opportunity to use social media platforms as a tool to interact with colleagues and experts who share similar interests and concerns while transcending spatial boundaries using an electronic device as simple as a cell phone (Gee, 2004). Further, Twitter chats (of VPLNs) occur often during the same scheduled time each week allowing educators to plan in advance to participate, given their busy schedules or even plan to participate in multiple VPLNs that cater to their multiple specific needs (Conner et al., 2009). Through virtual interactions with colleagues and experts, educators can access and share a variety of tools, including skills, habits, resources, ideas, and information that will support their daily practice (Krutka et al., 2017).

WRAP-UP

Education is widely documented as one of the primary social determinants of health. Education has an effect on income level, healthy eating habits, access to healthier neighborhoods, and can create opportunities for overall better health. Additionally, those in both the education and public health sectors identify schools as key sites to address and improve health literacy *as* healthy habits are beginning to form rather than attempting to change unhealthy habits in adulthood. However, while access to free and public education is a constitutional right, as discussed in this chapter, access to adequate and effective education that caters to students' needs is limited, especially for groups who have historically been marginalized. As a result, access to high-quality and effective health education materials and instruction is also often limited for these groups. To provide equitable access to both adequate opportunities to attain an education and for the development of critical health literacy and the ability to access and advocate for quality health care for all, there must be a restructuring of both systems. There are specific remedies that should be considered to resolve issues pertinent to health education and education with the goal being to improve health literacy for all (**Figure 9-1**).

In education, as with health care, this restructuring requires an explicit acknowledgment and discussion of the historical missteps in law, policy, and practice that have given way to existing discriminatory practices. Recent shifts

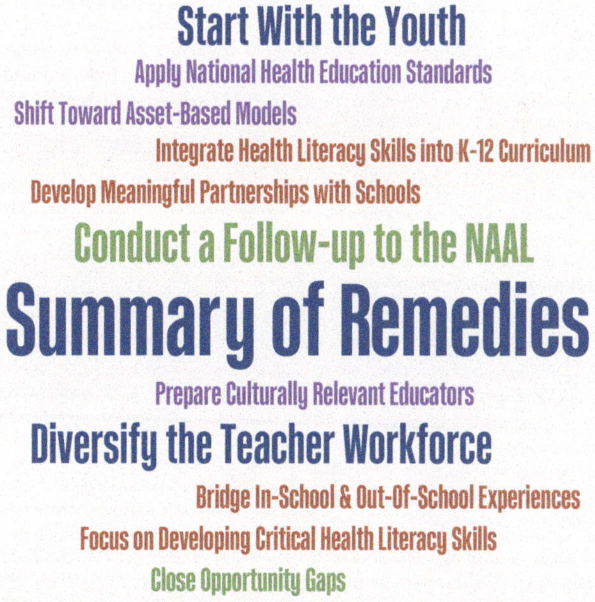

Start With the Youth
Apply National Health Education Standards
Shift Toward Asset-Based Models
Integrate Health Literacy Skills into K-12 Curriculum
Develop Meaningful Partnerships with Schools
Conduct a Follow-up to the NAAL
Summary of Remedies
Prepare Culturally Relevant Educators
Diversify the Teacher Workforce
Bridge In-School & Out-Of-School Experiences
Focus on Developing Critical Health Literacy Skills
Close Opportunity Gaps

Figure 9-1 Specific remedies pertinent to education and health education to improve health literacy for all.

in teacher education and pedagogy/curricular designs center these discussions as issues of race and culture are integral components in the development of culturally relevant educators and their practice. Additionally, finding new ways to incorporate technology and communication styles, instructional materials, and other practices of engagement rooted in youth culture, help to bridge students' personal and academic identities, creating stronger ties to the educational environment. In doing so, it is possible to see a shift from viewing culturally, racially, and ethnically diverse students as being culturally deprived to being culture rich, providing valuable insights, perspectives, and experiences through which to enhance the learning community and to create more welcoming and equitable experiences for all.

Chapter Problems

1. Describe the link between education and health.
2. Define health literacy and why many experts in the education and public health find it necessary to prioritize health education in K-12 schools.
3. The 1954 *Brown v. Board of Education* decision declared segregated schools to be unconstitutional, however the authors discussed the ways in which *Brown* actually resulted in numerous and long-lasting negative results. List and briefly describe at least two negative consequences of *Brown* mentioned in this chapter and their impact on one's educational experience.
4. Describe what culturally relevant pedagogy looks like in practice.

References

Adjapong, E. S. (2017). Bridging theory and practice in the urban science classroom: A framework for hip-hop pedagogy. *Critical Education, 8*(15), 5–22.

Anderson, J. D. (1988). *The education of blacks in the south, 1860-1935*. The University of North Carolina Press.

Auld, M. E., Allen, M. P., Hampton, C., Montes, J. H., Sherry, C., Mickalide, A. D., Logan, R. A., Alvarado-Little, W., & Parson, K. (2020). Health Literacy and Health Education in Schools: Collaboration for Action. *NAM Perspectives, 2020*, 10.31478/202007b. https://doi.org/10.31478/202007b

Banks, J. A., Cochran-Smith, M., Moll, L., Richert, A., Zeichner, K., LePage, P., Darling-Hammond, L., Duffy, H., & McDonald, M. (2005). Teaching diverse learners. In L. Darling-Hammond & J. Bransford (Eds.), *Preparing teachers for a changing world: What teachers should learn and be able to do* (pp. 232–274). Jossey-Bass.

Bell, L. A. (2002). Sincere fictions: The pedagogical challenges of preparing White teachers for multicultural classrooms. *Equity & Excellence in Education, 35*(3), 236–244. https://doi.org/10.1080/713845317

Blanchett, W. J., Mumford, V., & Beachum, F. (2005). Urban School Failure and Disproportionality in a Post-Brown Era: Benign Neglect of the Constitutional Rights of Students of Color. *Remedial and Special Education, 26*(2), 70–81. https://doi.org/10.1177/07419325050260020201

Brown v. Board of Education, 347 U.S. 483 (1954). https://www.archives.gov/milestone-documents/brown-v-board-of-education

Burchinal, M., Nelson, L., Carlson, M., & Brooks-Gunn, J. (2008). Neighborhood characteristics and child care type and quality. *Early Education and Development, 19*(5), 702–725. https://doi.org/10.1080/10409280802375273

Centers for Disease Control and Prevention. (2024, October 16). What is health literacy? Centers for Disease Control and Prevention. https://www.cdc.gov/health-literacy/php/about/index.html

Cochran-Smith, M. (1991). Learning to Teach against the Grain. *Harvard Educational Review, 61*(3), 279–311. https://doi.org/10.17763/haer.61.3.q671413614502746

Cochran-Smith, M. (2003a). Learning and unlearning: the education of teacher educators. *Teaching and Teacher Education, 19*(1), 5–28. https://doi.org/10.1016/S0742-051X(02)00091-4

Cochran-Smith, M. (2003b). Standing at the crossroads: Multicultural teacher education at the beginning of the 21st century. *Multicultural Perspectives, 5*(3), 3–11. https://doi.org/10.1207/S15327892MCP0503_02

Conner, J., Pope, D., & Galloway, M. (2009). Success with less stress. *Educational Leadership: Journal of the Department of Supervision and Curriculum Development, 67*(4), 54–58.

Crenshaw, K. W. (1988). Race, reform, and retrenchment: Transformation and legitimation in antidiscrimination law. *Harvard Law Review, 101*(7), 1331–1387.

Delpit, L. (1988). The silenced dialogue: Power and pedagogy in educating other people's children. *Harvard Educational Review, 58*(3), 280–299. https://doi.org/10.17763/haer.58.3.c43481778r528qw4

De Vito, D. (2007). The gap between the real and the ideal: The right to education amid fiscal equity legislation in a democratic culture. *Ethics and Education, 2*(2), 173–180. https://doi.org/10.1080/17449640701610111

Dotterer, A. M., Iruka, I. U., & Pungello, E. (2012). Parenting, race, and socioeconomic status: Links to school readiness. *Family Relations: An Interdisciplinary Journal of Applied Family Studies, 61*(4), 657–670. https://doi.org/10.1111/j.1741-3729.2012.00716.x

Gamoran, A., Nystrand, M., Berends, M., & LePore, P. C. (1995). An organizational analysis of the effects of ability grouping. *American Educational Research Journal, 32*(4), 687–715. https://doi.org/10.2307/1163331

Garrison, D. R. (2007). Online community of inquiry review: Social, cognitive, and teaching presence issues. *Journal of Asynchronous Learning Networks, 11*(1), 61–72.

Gay, G. (2000). *Culturally responsive teaching: Theory, research, and practice.* Teachers' College Press.

Gee, J. P. (2004). *An introduction to discourse analysis: Theory and method.* Routledge.

Healthy People 2030. (n.d.). *Health Literacy in healthy people 2030.* Office of Disease Prevention and Health Promotion. https://health.gov/healthypeople/priority-areas/health-literacy-healthy-people-2030

Horsford, S. D. (2010). Black superintendents on educating Black students in separate and unequal contexts. *The Urban Review, 42*(1), 58–79. https://doi.org/10.1007/s11256-009-0119-0

Irizarry, J. G. (2009). Representin': Drawing from hip-hop and urban youth culture to inform teacher education. *Education and Urban Society, 41*(4), 489–515. https://doi.org/10.1177/0013124508331154

Kamin, L. J. (1974). *The science and politics of I.Q.* Lawrence Erlbaum.

Kena, G., Hussar, W., McFarland, J., de Brey, C., Musu-Gillette, L., Wang, X., Zhang, J., Rathbun, A., Wilkinson-Flicker, S., Diliberti, M., Barmer, A., Bullock Mann, F., & Dunlop Velez, E. D. (2016, May). *The condition of education 2016* [NCES 2016-144]. National Center for Education Statistics. https://nces.ed.gov/pubs2016/2016144.pdf

Kingston, P. W. (2001). The unfulfilled promise of cultural capital theory. *Sociology of Education, 74,* 88. https://doi.org/10.2307/2673255

Kliebard, H. M. (2004). *The Struggle for the American Curriculum, 1893-1958.* Routledge.

Krutka, D. G., Carpenter, J. P. & Trust, T. (2017). Enriching Professional Learning Networks: A Framework for Identification, Reflection, and Intention. *TechTrends 61,* 246–252. https://doi.org/10.1007/s11528-016-0141-5

Kutner, M., Greenburg, E., Jin, Y., & Paulsen, C. (2006, September). The health literacy of America's adults: Results from the 2003 National Assessment of Adult Literacy [NCES 2006-483]. National Center for Education Statistics. https://nces.ed.gov/pubs2006/2006483.pdf

Ladson-Billings, G. (1999). Chapter 7: Preparing teachers for diverse student populations: A critical Race Theory perspective. *Review of Research in Education, 24*(1), 211–247. https://doi.org/10.3102/0091732X024001211

Ladson-Billings, G. (2000). Fighting for our lives: Preparing teachers to teach African American students. *Journal of Teacher Education, 51*(3), 206–214. https://doi.org/10.1177/0022487100051003008

Ladson-Billings, G. (2004). Landing on the wrong note: The price we paid for Brown. *Educational Researcher, 33*(7), 3–13. https://doi.org/10.3102/0013189X033007003

Ladson-Billings, G. (2006). From the achievement gap to the education debt: Understanding achievement in U.S. Schools. *Educational Researcher, 35*(7), 3–12. https://doi.org/10.3102/0013189X035007003

Ladson-Billings, G. (2012). Through a glass darkly: The persistence of race in education research and Scholarship. *Educational Researcher, 41*(4), 115–120. https://doi.org/10.3102/0013189X12440743

Ladson-Billings, G., & Tate, W. F. (1995). Toward a critical race theory of education. *Teachers College Record, 97*(1), 47–68. https://doi.org/10.1177/016146819509700104

Lowenstein, K. L. (2009). The work of multicultural teacher education: Reconceptualizing white teacher candidates as learners. *Review of Educational Research, 79*(1), 163–196. https://doi.org/10.3102/0034654308326161

Massey, D. S., & Denton, N. A. (1993). *American apartheid: Segregation and the making of the underclass.* Harvard University Press.

Milner, H. R. (2012). Beyond a test score. *Journal of Black Studies, 43*(6), 693–718. https://doi.org/10.1177/0021934712442539

Nasaw, D. (1981). *Schooled to order: A Social History of Public Schooling in the United States.* Oxford University Press, USA.

National Center for Education Statistics. (n.d.). Health Literacy Component of the 2003 National Assessment of Adult Literacy. National Assessment of Adult Literacy (NAAL). https://nces.ed.gov/naal/pdf/HealthLiteracyFactSheet.pdf

National Consensus for School Health Education. (2022). *National health education standards: Model guidance for curriculum and instruction* (3rd Ed.). https://www.schoolhealtheducation.org/wp-content/uploads/2024/02/National_Health_Education_Standards_Guide-02.21.2024.pdf

Nieto, S. (2005). Schools for a New Majority: The Role of Teacher Education in Hard Times. *The New Educator, 1*(1), 27–43. https://doi.org/10.1080/15476880490447797

Nutbeam, D., & Lloyd, J. E. (2021). Understanding and Responding to Health Literacy as a Social Determinant of Health. *Annual Review of Public Health, 42*, 159–173. https://doi.org/10.1146/annurev-publhealth-090419-102529

Omi, M., & Winant, H. (1993). On the theoretical concept of race. In C. McCarthy, & W. Crichlow (Eds.), Race Identity and Representation in Education (pp. 3-10). Routledge.

Payne, C. M. (2008). *So much reform, so little change: The persistence of failure in urban schools.* Harvard Educational Publishing Group.

Ross, C. E., & Wu, C.-l. (1995). The links between education and health. *American Sociological Review, 60*(5), 719–745. https://doi.org/10.2307/2096319

SHAPE America. (2024). 2024 National health education standards educator kit. In *National Health Education Standards.* https://www.shapeamerica.org/ItemDetail?iProductCode=NSHESEK

Trinkle, C. (2009). Twitter as a professional learning community. *School Library Monthly, 26*(4), 22–23.

Ukpokodu, N. (2002). Breaking through preservice teachers' defensive dispositions in a multicultural education course: A reflective practice. *Multicultural Education, 9*(3), 25–33. https://www.proquest.com/docview/216309385?fromopenview=true&pq-origsite=gscholar&sourcetype=Scholarly%20Journals

U.S. Department of Education. (2016). *The state of racial diversity in the educator workforce.* Office of Planning, Evaluation and Policy Development, Policy and Program Studies Service. https://eric.ed.gov/?id=ED571989

Villegas, A. M., & Irvine, J. J. (2010). Diversifying the teaching force: An examination of major arguments. *Urban Review, 42*, 175–192. https://doi.org/10.1007/s11256-010-0150-1

Villegas, A. M., & Lucas, T. (2002). Preparing culturally responsive teachers. *Journal of Teacher Education, 53*(1), 20–32. https://doi.org/10.1177/0022487102053001003

Walker, V. S. (2000). Valued Segregated Schools for African American Children in the South, 1935-1969: A review of common themes and characteristics. *Review of Educational Research, 70*(3), 253–285. https://doi.org/10.3102/00346543070003253

Walters, P. B. (2001). Educational Access and the State: Historical continuities and discontinuities in racial inequality in American education. *Sociology of Education, 74*, 35. https://doi.org/10.2307/2673252

Wells, A. S., Holme, J. J., Revilla, A., & Atanda, A. K. (2005). How desegregation changed us: The effects of racially mixed schools on students and society. Teacher's College, Columbia University. https://www.researchgate.net/publication/254430527_How_Desegregation_Changed_Us_The_Effects_of_Racially_Mixed_Schools_on_Students_and_Society

Weingart, T. (2014, April 29). At the intersection of health and education: One community's story. *VCU News.* https://news.vcu.edu/article/At_the_intersection_of_health_and_education_One_communitys_story

Wittink, H., & Oosterhaven, J. (2018). Patient education and health literacy. *Musculoskeletal science & practice, 38,* 120–127. https://doi.org/10.1016/j.msksp.2018.06.004

Zeichner, K. M. (2003). The adequacies and inadequacies of three current strategies to recruit, prepare, and retain the best teachers for all students. *Teachers College Record the Voice of Scholarship in Education, 105*(3), 490–519. https://doi.org/10.1111/1467-9620.00248

Zimmerman, E., & Woolf, S. H. (2014, June 5). *Understanding the relationship between education and health* [Discussion paper]. Institute of Medicine. https://nam.edu/wp-content/uploads/2015/06/BPH-UnderstandingTheRelationship1.pdf

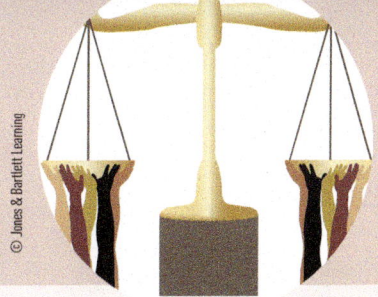

CHAPTER 10

Women and Health Disparities: Issues, Concerns, and Remedies

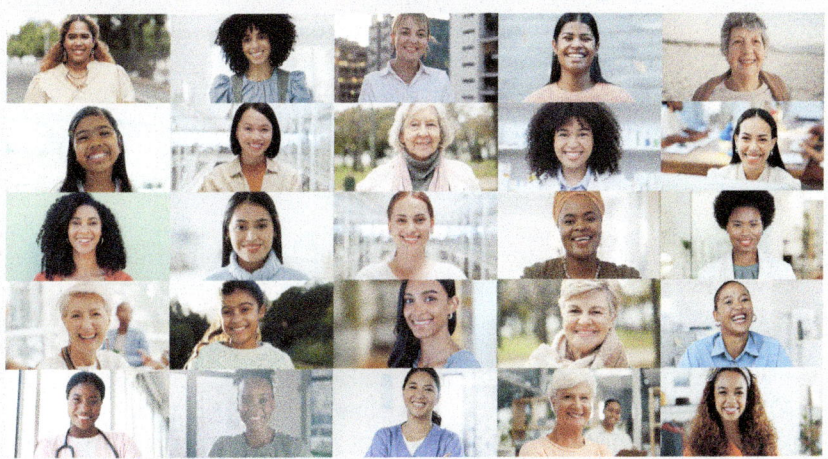

KEY TERMS

Aid to Families with Dependent
  Children (AFDC)
diabetes
family wage
Healthy People 2030
hypertension
infant mortality rate (IMR)

low birth weight (LBW)
mass incarceration
maternal mortality rate (MMR)
morbidity rates
Temporary Assistance for Needy
  Families (TANF)

LEARNING OBJECTIVES

After reading this chapter, you should be able to do the following:

1. Discuss key factors that impact the health status of women.
2. Identify specific illnesses that are more prevalent in women.
3. Explain potential solutions for closing the health status gap between emerging majority women and White women.
4. Describe important aspects of women's health per Healthy People 2030.

Introduction

In considering the health status of women in the United States, key factors that must be taken into consideration include race/ethnicity and socioeconomic status. These factors are quite complex, relating to neonatal care, birth outcomes, and increased prevalence of certain diseases. Moreover, the quality and accessibility of care to women vary drastically from one social setting to another, with particular hardship experienced by women who live in low-income areas and incarcerated women. This chapter will explore some of these concerns with an emphasis on remedies with insight from **Healthy People 2030**, which is an initiative that promotes health through the use of objectives and is the fifth iteration of this process.

Race

In exploring race in terms of women's health, cultural norms are significant. Often, Black women, for example, are burdened by poverty, lack of access to care, and limited education. Poor diet is also a critical factor for some. However, it is important to recognize that not all Black people, including Black women, are poor. U.S. Senator Bernie Sanders, who was a candidate in the United States presidential primary race of 2016, was chided for making this generalization. He stated at the Democratic debate in Flint, Michigan, on March 16 of that year, "When you're White … you don't know what it's like to be poor." He later corrected this statement, as the reality is that in terms of sheer numbers, there are more poor White people than poor Black people in the United States. Although poverty rates are higher for Black and Hispanic groups, over 19 million White Americans, 41% of the poor, live below the poverty line. Often overlooked, they're spread across rural and suburban areas, especially Appalachia and the Midwest, and affect women similarly (Yen, 2013). Hence, poverty is not limited to emerging majorities of any race or ethnicity, although there is disproportionality, which lends to the health status gap. This insight can be applied to women, as a specific group.

For women who live in communities with predominantly low incomes, there is an increased risk of poor health conditions. Women generally experience illnesses such as cancer, heart disease, stroke, and diabetes, particularly when their income and access to care are limited. Black women are disproportionately impacted. Nevertheless, a report released by the Kaiser Family Foundation (James, 2009) offers the following insight:

In states where disparities appeared to be smaller, this difference was often due to the fact that both White women and women of color were doing poorly. It is important to also recognize that in many states (e.g., West Virginia and Kentucky) all women, including White women, faced significant challenges and may need assistance.

This is validated by the Office of Women's Health which indicates that the Centers for Disease Control and Prevention (CDC) lists the following as the leading causes of death for women in the United States:

- Heart disease
- Cancer
- Stroke
- Chronic lower respiratory disease (CLRD)
- Alzheimer's disease

For most of these issues, namely, heart disease, cancer, and stroke, African American women have the highest rates/the greatest risk of dying from them (Women's Health, 2024).

This is generally the case with socioeconomic status as a key contributing factor as exemplified by the fact that White women who experience poverty and who live in rural areas often have significant issues regarding health and access to care.

Socioeconomic Status and Women's Health

In exploring the socioeconomic status of women, a specific example that is very relevant to the health status gap is African American women who experience mental health issues. Low income and educational levels are associated with lower socioeconomic status overall and correlate with low self-esteem and poor self-concept (Murthy & Smith, 2010). The poor mental health status of some Black women is a reflection of their low socioeconomic status, and racism is also a contributing factor (Murthy & Smith, 2010). Depression is also a key factor. In caring for mental health issues, there is limited help that would be culturally supportive in terms of same-race practitioners, as there is a lack of significant numbers of Black medical practitioners, particularly in the relevant disciplines. Furthermore, in Black communities in general, mental health is stigmatized for Black women, who are seen as the "rock" of the family—essentially the strength and caretaker of pressing issues, including health. Hence, seeking treatment for mental health issues is not the norm.

Additionally, Black women are often at risk for obesity and overweight (Braithwaite et al., 1992). This has been true over an extended period of time including the present. It is important to point out that the notion of obesity as an issue and as a disease is a construct that did not always exist. In many instances, Black women are trying to adhere to norms and body types that are not their own, and more akin to what society is indicating as best, with White women being designated as the ideal prototype with a "thinness is in" mentality. Black women often have very different body types, cultural norms around body shapes, and attitudes associated with their bodies that are different from what the larger society says is best. Nevertheless, culturally, using the guidelines associated with obesity as normative, there are a number of reasons for the outcome of some Black women being classified as obese. One key contributing factor is soul food, which is often prepared with pride and satisfaction for the immediate and extended family (Counihan & Esterik, 1997). Soul food is prepared with a great deal of seasoning, especially salt, with numerous fried dishes and is not a healthy approach to eating. As discussed previously in this text, soul food emerged from slavery as the refuse from the White slaveholders and was often the only sustenance available to the enslaved people. This type of food contributes to obesity for some Black women and their families. Additionally, there are social constructs among various racial and ethnic groups. For Black women, specifically, strength and resilience can often be attributed to a larger size, with dieting sometimes considered a "White thing" (Hill, 2009). It is important to point out that many Black people do not eat soul food. This type of generalization would be incorrect at many levels. It can be a cultural norm for some, but not all Black people, and in some cases, it is eaten but modified substantially with a healthier lean, including less salt and less frying of dishes.

Diabetes and Hypertension

In continuing to explore the health status of Black women, as an example, there are particular diseases that are quite prevalent among this group. Black women have higher rates of **hypertension**, as compared to other groups, and the onset is normally early in their lives. Critical factors may include racism (Braithwaite et al., 1992). Discrimination and racism are known to cause anger, frustration, and psychosocial stress. These problems can lead to elevated blood pressure with the ensuing result of hypertension. Beyond racism, there are other factors, as is the case for many other women, including work stress, raising children, sometimes as single parents, income concerns, bills, caregiving, and beyond. Socioeconomic status must be considered seriously, as financial stress leads to hypertension (Braithwaite et al., 1992). One relief for stress is exercise. Unfortunately, Black women have the highest rate of physical inactivity when compared to other racial groups (Eyler et al., 1998). One of the reasons for lack of exercise is time limitation, as many Black women are single parents, although not all by any stretch of the word. Hence, personal physical activity may be a low priority. Another health outcome is disproportionately high rates of cardiovascular disease, including hypertension, but also heart disease and stroke (Braithwaite et al., 1992). Lack of exercise and diet-related issues (poor diet or food that should be prepared more healthfully, namely soul food as discussed earlier) are some but not all of the contributing factors to obesity and **diabetes**. If you consider these issues historically, not much has changed from the past to the present, which is why it is imperative to not solely dwell on what the problematic issues are, but rather the remedies.

Cancer

Cancer is a major issue for the Black population in the United States, in terms of survival rates. Black people experience the lowest survival rate and highest death rate from cancer as compared to any other racial/ethnic group. The main reasons are lack of access to care, mistrust of providers, and cultural barriers. The mistrust stems from numerous scenarios in which Black people were mistreated and abused in the United States by healthcare providers and used as guinea pigs for research and beyond (Katz, 2008). Indignities such as the Tuskegee experiment have deeply damaged Black people's faith in the medical establishment. Many Black people in the United States are aware of these atrocities and, consequently, will not go to the doctor for preventive care (Braithwaite et al., 1992). Therefore, Black women are less apt to undergo mammograms and other types of screenings because of distrust of healthcare providers (Musa et al., 2009).

Given the racial discrimination discussed here and the low socioeconomic status and related financial stress, the resulting psychological duress leads to increased incidence of breast cancer (Taylor et al., 2007). Although the emphasis of the preceding discussion is on Black women, there is no doubt that emerging majority women in general, beyond Black women, who are also poor, experience serious health issues that contribute to the health status gap between emerging majorities, poor people in general, and the White population in the United States. White women experiencing poverty have similar outcomes without the impact of racism as a contributing factor.

Birth Outcomes

To help ensure that women experience healthy birth outcomes, the Centers for Disease Control and Prevention (CDC) recommends certain protocols for pregnant women. However, socioeconomic status may impact their ability to adhere to such guidelines for the following reasons:

- Health literacy: Women of low socioeconomic status may not have access to, or understand, the information provided by the CDC and beyond regarding important steps toward a healthy pregnancy and delivery.
- Socioeconomic status: Poor women may not have access to healthy food to meet the needs of the mother and child during pregnancy.
- Lack of access to care: Low-income mothers may not have insurance to see an obstetrician throughout their pregnancy. Even though Medicaid may be available, these women may not know how to access the program or may access it very late in the pregnancy, precluding an opportunity to get proper medical guidance.

Key health indices relevant to birth outcomes include low birth weight (less than 2500 grams), **infant mortality rate (IMR)**, and **maternal mortality rate (MMR)**. **Low birth weight (LBW)** refers to the weight of the baby at the time of birth and determines if the baby has a healthy start to life. This measure offers some predictability regarding future **morbidity rates** (incidence of disease) and health outcome relative to maternal risk. The IMR indicates the number of infants who die during their first year of life. The IMR is based on the number of infant deaths per 1000 live births. It is an extremely important measure, as it is commonly used as an indicator of the general health of a population. Per the Central Intelligence Agency (2009), the maternal mortality rate refers to the annual number of female deaths per 100,000 from any cause aggravated by pregnancy or its management, excluding accidental or incidental causes. The rates of these indicators are higher for emerging majority women and White women of low socioeconomic status.

However, Dr. Michael Lu, Obstetrician and Gynecologist at University of California, Los Angeles and Associate Administrator of the Maternal and Child Health Bureau of the Health Resources and Services Administration (HRSA), believes that for many women of color, racism over a lifetime, not just during the 9 months of pregnancy, increases the risk of preterm delivery. To improve birth outcomes, Dr. Lu argues, "we must address the conditions that impact women's health not just when they become pregnant but from childhood, adolescence and into adulthood" (California Newsreel, 2014). He also points out that racism is stressful and that stress is impactful to health at many levels, producing wear and tear on the body systems, including hormonal, metabolic, and inflammatory functions, and over time, this damage may create an overload on the organs and systems, disabling optimal functionality (California Newsreel, 2014).

Unfortunately, women will carry these burdens into their pregnancies, impacting the physiology of the pregnant mother and the fetus. Steps that have been taken thus far to increase access to health care for low-income women, particularly those of color, have done very little to decrease prematurity, low birth weight, infant mortality, and morbidity rates. Dr. Lu points out further that trying to cram the positive aspects of care (nutrients and vitamins) into less than 9 months of prenatal care does not reverse all of the cumulative shortcomings and inequities throughout one's life before pregnancy. This is expecting too much of health care in a short time (California Newsreel, 2014).

Potential Causes Impacting Overall Socioeconomic Status of Women

In a radio interview with Dr. Richard Wolff, who hosts *Economic Update* on WBAI, a listener-supported radio station in New York City, Dr. Harriet Fraad was interviewed by Dr. Wolff. Dr. Wolff is a Professor Emeritus of economics at the University of Massachusetts, Amherst, where he taught economics from 1973 to 2008. Previously, he taught economics at Yale University (1967–1969) and at the City College of the City University of New York (1969–1973). In 1994, he was a Visiting Professor of economics at the University of Paris, France, at Sorbonne (Paritan Valley Community College, 2020). Dr. Fraad, a graduate of Teachers College, Columbia University, is a mental health counselor/psychotherapist with a practice in New York City and a frequent collaborator with Dr. Wolff. She is also Dr. Wolff's wife.

Dr. Fraad's (2016) analysis of the current status of women in the United States is intriguing and provides insight regarding the current socioeconomic status of some women. In her discussion on air with Dr. Wolff, which took place on March 25 (Fraad, 2016), she explains that there are a significant number of unmarried women in the United States and attributes this situation largely to the decline of the **family wage**. The family wage is deemed as the amount of income for a family to live on, in terms of meeting basic needs. She attributes the loss of the family wage in the United States to the outsourcing of jobs to other nations, where United States corporations may pay workers lower wages. These outsourced jobs were primarily, before outsourcing, designated for U.S. men. Industry jobs, including heavy machinery work and factory jobs, she points out, were the main jobs lost. Consequently, the concept of a man and woman marrying, moving to the suburbs, having a family, and him supporting them (the family wage) while the wife stayed home and took care of the kids, was also lost.

Additionally, Fraad (2016) notes that due to the feminist movement, prior to outsourcing, and the need for women to work to supplement the family income as a result of outsourcing and women's desire to work outside of the home, there are many women in the workforce. Her perspective is that, with other factors withstanding, outsourcing led to unemployment and lower-wage jobs, particularly for men who were formerly blue-collar workers. Also, for those men and women who went to college, it is often necessary to factor in student loan debt and the impact that loan repayment has had on the socioeconomic status of young people. Additionally, she emphasizes that many families moved to, or are considering moving to, the city, due to loss of wages and their homes, in many cases with renting as their only option, which is often expensive.

Ultimately, Fraad's point is that this change in, or loss of, the family wage has gravely impacted women, as now working is no longer optional but mandatory. Lower-wage jobs are now more commonplace and, consequently, women and men who choose not to marry, which is often the case, currently are choosing to cohabitate. Many women also find themselves, by choice or circumstances, single mothers. This situation has resulted, per Fraad, in the transformation of children's lives. Single mothers end up with only one income. There is a need to be home with children, but if mothers are working, they cannot be. Finding appropriate people to watch their children is a challenge for single mothers with low income. Hence, many children are "latch keyed" (left home alone when they return home from school, unsupervised by parents/adults). Fraad (2016) points out that as an unfortunate result, children may become victims or abused.

This is an interesting and controversial analysis presented by Fraad (2016) and leaves out some key points that may necessitate deeper consideration from the vantage point of many single mothers who vehemently disagree that raising their children alone places them at a disadvantage. Nevertheless, the issue is somewhat different for emerging majority women, particularly those who are Black and poor. According to Korhonen (2023): "In 2022, there were about 4.15 million Black families in the United States with a single mother. This is an increase from 1990 levels, when there were about 3.4 million Black families with a single mother." She further explains that:

> Single parenthood occurs for different reasons, including divorce, death, abandonment, or single-person adoption. Historically, single parenthood was common due to mortality rates due to war, diseases, and maternal mortality. However, divorce was not as common back then, depending on the culture … In countries where social welfare programs are not strong, single parents tend to suffer more financially, emotionally, and mentally. In the United States, most single parents are mothers. The struggles that single parents face are greater than those in two parent households.

For the purposes of this chapter, it is worth pointing out that Fraad does not discuss race in her analysis.

Welfare and Welfare Reform

The family wage has always been a difficult scenario for Black women, as under the **Aid to Families with Dependent Children (AFDC)** welfare program, Black men were not permitted to live in the homes of Black women and their children or the benefits would be withdrawn.

Often, Black men and women were unable to find work, so social services/welfare benefits were their only option. (Here, we must make it clear that Black people were not the sole recipients of welfare at any time in United States history.) As Kindred (2003) explains, "More white women of childbearing age received AFDC than Black or Hispanic women, but Black and Hispanic women received AFDC in disproportionate numbers." Marchevsky and Theoharis (2000) provide further insight into the AFDC program:

> AFDC had its roots in the mother's pensions programs instituted by most states in the 1910s and 1920s. These programs sought to reinforce women's domestic role and keep mothers out of the workplace by giving "deserving mothers" a small subsidy. "Deserving mothers" were largely defined as white mothers, and these programs were instituted to protect white married or widowed women.

Initially known as ADC (Aid for Dependent Children), its name was changed to AFDC in 1950. The purpose of the program was to allow mothers to stay home with their children, and indeed, they were required to do so (Marchevsky & Theoharis, 2000). Kindred (2003) explains the workings of the program:

> AFDC, as a federally mandated program, was designed to be a federal–state partnership, intended to provide cash assistance to needy children. The federal law required states to provide cash assistance to all eligible families. Each state administered the program and established the income eligibility level and the benefit level available to families within the state, in keeping with federal limitations. The federal government monitored the states' administration of the program and matched the state funds provided.

Further, Kindred (2003) explains the program's outcomes:

> According to the Census Bureau, about 14 million people were receiving AFDC in 1995. This included 3.8 million mothers ages of 15 to 44 years; 500,000 mothers age 45 and over; 300,000 fathers living with dependent children; and 9.7 million children. Nearly half of women on AFDC have never been married. The average mother on AFDC gave birth at age 20, compared to age 23 for women not on AFDC. The average AFDC family has 2.6 children, compared to 2.1 children for families not on AFDC … More white women of childbearing age received AFDC than black or Hispanic women, but black and Hispanic women received AFDC in disproportionate numbers. About 63.5 percent of AFDC recipients lived in private market housing; only about 9 percent lived in public housing.

Temporary Assistance for Needy Families (TANF), enacted in 1996, replaced the AFDC, which provided cash assistance to families with children experiencing poverty. TANF cash assistance can play a critical role in supporting families during times of need (Center on Budget and Policy Priorities, 2022). TANF followed shortly after as a temporary measure with the aim of moving those who had been receiving welfare to work. It also had the added component of "family values" in that one of its aims was to encourage poor people to marry.

This reform is considered controversial. Those who were against it deemed it punitive for the poor, while others found it a necessary measure to stop dependency. No matter one's perspective, the reality is that it did not respond to "the real demographics of poverty—the inadequate labor market, a lack of childcare and health benefits, urban divestment from social services and poor communities" (Marchevsky & Theoharis, 2000). Welfare rolls had to be decreased by at least 50% by the year 2000 with a 5-year limit on cash benefits. Also, 80% of states' welfare recipients were required to find work within 2 years. The options were to find a job, work for the public sector (workfare), or lose their benefits (Marchevsky & Theoharis, 2000).

The bottom line is that programs to assist people experiencing poverty, particularly women who experience poverty and their children, are based on the poverty level. Kindred (2003), citing researchers in the field, explains how the government goes about defining poverty:

> To assess the number of persons living in poverty, the government uses a poverty index by which it sets thresholds that take into account total family income and family size; the thresholds are adjusted annually for inflation. According to this measure, "for example, the 1995 poverty threshold for a single individual was $7,929, while for a family of four (two adults, two children), the threshold was $15,455, and for a family of six (two adults, four children) the threshold was $20,364." In 1998, the official poverty threshold for a family of four was $16,660. According to the official poverty measure "more than 20% of the nation's 67 million children are poor".

Women and children are severely impacted by poverty in the United States. Until this problem is addressed, health disparities will persist. As welfare reform has caused a grave impact, further problems have ensued that are specifically impacting emerging majorities, particularly Black women. One specific example is mass incarceration.

Mass Incarceration and Black Women

Mass incarceration is a serious issue in the Black community. It is a contributing factor to the disruption/destruction of the Black family, leading to the lack of availability of Black men for Black women to marry, thereby leaving Black women alone to raise their children.

However, the mass incarceration of Black people does not pose a problem to the Black family solely in regard to Black women being left to raise children alone.

The reality is that Black women are also disproportionately imprisoned. The American Civil Liberties Union (2007) provides the following insights:

> Women of color are significantly overrepresented in the criminal justice system. Black women represent 30% of all incarcerated women in the United States, although they represent 13% of the female population generally. Hispanic women represent 16% of incarcerated women, although they make up only 11% of all women in the U.S.

Mass incarceration is an atrocity beyond belief. Often, there is lack of consideration regarding how such a process of imprisoning people, in vast numbers, impacts health. However, when families are destroyed, under such tragic circumstances, the stress related to the loss of loved ones and the economic fallout of such is beyond comprehension in terms of family devastation. Mass incarceration has been likened to a public health epidemic. *The New York Times* (The Editorial Board, 2014) offers the following thoughts:

> When swaths of young, mostly minority men are put behind bars, families are ripped apart, children grow up fatherless, and poverty and homelessness increase. Today 2.7 million children have a parent in prison, which increases their own risk of incarceration down the road.

Failure to deal with the debilitating effects of poverty, as well as the implementation of practices that contribute to it, such as mass incarceration, will not serve to close the health status gap but to widen it, particularly for emerging majority women. However, similar to any of the concerns that are impacting the overall health of women, it is more important to focus on the remedies rather than the problems. It is clear what the problems are. They are researched and understood. The remedies must be at the forefront of all efforts.

To that end, recently, in terms of remedies, Wes Moore, the Governor of Maryland took a step to make a dent in the mass incarceration issue. Since mass incarceration disproportionately impacts Black people and other emerging majorities, Governor Moore announced, just prior to Juneteenth, a holiday commemorating the abolition of slavery in Texas in 1865, a new initiative. In an executive order, Moore pardoned 175,000 former incarcerated persons who were convicted for possession of cannabis or drug paraphernalia (misdemeanors only in both categories). As stated by Moore (The Office of Governor Wes Moore, 2024):

> Today, we take a big step forward toward ensuring equal justice for all. But this won't be our last effort. We must continue to move in partnership to build a state and society that is more equitable, more just, and leaves no one behind.

The Attorney General of Maryland, Anthony G. Brown, added to that point indicating that (The Office of Governor Wes Moore, 2024):

> The enforcement of cannabis laws has disproportionately and overwhelmingly burdened communities of color. Opportunities were denied because those who were convicted faced steep obstacles to jobs, education, and housing.

The purpose of this big step, which is the largest pardon for cannabis charges (misdemeanor) of any state in the country, is to move closer to equity in the United States in terms of justice. In Maryland, as is the case for many states in the United States, cannabis is now legal. But many individuals remain incarcerated. In terms of women, mass incarceration must end to lessen the destruction of families, reducing their presence in the criminal justice system, and increasing the pool of men available for marriage, particularly in terms of Black women.

Emerging Majority Providers

Other remedies must include an increase in the number of emerging majority medical providers. Unfortunately, on July 1, 2012, the government disallowed the option of federal subsidized loans for graduate students. Essentially, this means that interest accrues on student loans while individuals are pursuing graduate/professional studies, including medicine. This course was deemed necessary as the Congressional Budget Office indicated it was either the end of subsidized loans or the end of the Pell Grant. Pell Grants are funds that are made available to low-income students for colleges (Hopkins, 2012). The Pell Grant time frame was also reduced from 9 to 6 years, which means less availability of those funds to graduate students. Hence, the outcome is insurmountable debt for future physicians and other healthcare professionals and the need to take out unsubsidized loans to fund their studies, as the options for merit scholarships and other competitive funds, are limited.

To make matters worse, the interest rates on the loans are very high, at 7.9% under the Grad PLUS program. Hence, individuals, particularly those most in need of funding to pursue their education—emerging majorities—may opt out of pursuing degrees in the health professions, due to the high cost and tremendous debt for doing so. Overall, there was a projected shortage of 45,000 primary care doctors and 46,000 specialists by 2020 (Ollove, 2014). This was clearly a problem, and continues to be the case, given the increase in the number of people with health insurance resulting from passage of the Affordable Care Act (ACA) in March 2010. Although more access to care is positive, there must be a sufficient number of culturally competent healthcare providers to meet the demand. The ACA also includes the addition of extra fees and equipment for private practicing physicians. This expense has driven many out of private practice and into hospitals as employees (Gottlieb, 2013), contributing still further to the physician shortage.

The impact of this scenario on the overall population, and women in particular, is dreadful. To improve the health status of women of color who experience a low socioeconomic status, who are not at parity in terms of health with their White counterparts who are experiencing affluence, preventive care is essential. Preventive care involves lifestyle changes, good diets, exercise regimens, and optimal health care or viable healthcare alternatives. Ideally, preventive care is the optimal focus. However, given the shortage of physicians and the pressures, timewise, associated with seeing more patients, how is it possible to accomplish that goal? Patients now have less time with their providers, and preventive care requires significant time, effort, and information distribution through effective communication.

Many physicians, and other healthcare providers in the United States, have major concerns about income, increased paperwork/documentation associated with ACA requirements, repayment of student loans, mass patient influxes, and other woes that occur in such a strenuous environment. These pressures lead to a bottom-line approach rather than an approach focused on reducing health disparities. For emerging majority women experiencing poverty in particular, who are in dire need of optimal health care before, during, and after pregnancy (if they have children), as one example, this is a major problem that must be resolved. There is no doubt that the patient-doctor relationship has an impact on disparities in medical care (Street et al., 2008).

REMEDIES

Some of the remedies, broadly speaking, for women in terms of achieving optimal health/health equity include the following:

- Establishing economic parity between men and women in the United States.
- Eliminating racism and discrimination in the United States, specifically as directed toward emerging majority women.
- Ensuring that women are taken care of before pregnancy, throughout the duration of their lives, not just during pregnancy.
- Educating healthcare providers and researchers about the culture, history, and socioeconomic status of women in an effort to improve birth outcomes for all.
- Providing culturally competent care for diverse groups, recognizing that these groups have diverse histories, languages, cultures, religions, beliefs, and traditions that impact women's health outcomes.
- Recognizing the importance of health literacy in improving the health status of women and their families, as women are usually the caregivers of health for their households/families.
- Improving the United States poverty crisis and unemployment concerns in terms of women's health overall, ensuring access to health care and other necessary resources.
- Ending mass incarceration in the United States, thus enabling the rebuilding of families of color, particularly Black families, and the elimination of significant stress on low-income communities related to such.

Healthy People 2030 and Women

Healthy People 2030 has made health literacy a central focus. One of the initiative's overarching goals demonstrates this focus: "Eliminate health disparities, achieve health equity, and attain health literacy to improve the health and well-being of all" (*Priority areas*, n.d.). Additionally, given the myriad health concerns experienced by women, Healthy People 2030 has set specific objectives to improve women's health. There are many of these objectives for women, too many to list here. However, a sample of some definitely sheds light on the effort to resolve issues rather than letting them remain stagnant or become worse. Specifically, in terms of childbirth, one Healthy People 2030 goal is "Prevent pregnancy complications and maternal deaths and improve women's health before, during and after pregnancy" (*Pregnancy and childbirth*, n.d.). The focus of Healthy People 2030 is not to just indicate problems but to offer goals and insight as to the importance of achieving said goals. Specifically the initiative points out the following (*Pregnancy and Childbirth*, n.d.):

> Some women have health problems that start during pregnancy, and others have health problems *before* they get pregnant that could lead to complications during pregnancy. Strategies to help women adopt healthy habits and get health care before and during pregnancy can help prevent pregnancy complications. In addition, interventions to prevent unintended pregnancies can help reduce negative outcomes for women and infants.

Given that pregnancy and the ensuing problems and joys associated with it are critical aspects of women's health, it is extremely positive that the Healthy People 2030 objectives prioritize such an important matter for women, along with so many other significant issues, including health literacy. Healthy People 2030 should not be limited to those in the health field, in terms of availability, review, and accomplishments. It should be part of all aspects of society with insight provided to the public in all forms of media, with the public observing and participating toward progress. In terms of getting the word out, every woman in the United States should be made aware of all of the Healthy People 2030 objectives and where the nation stands toward their progress as without the input and participation of women in the goals that pertain to them, achieving the said goals will be more challenging. The most important remedy is ensuring that women participate in achieving the goals that pertain to them.

WRAP-UP

Race, ethnicity, socioeconomic status, and diet are some of the factors associated with health disparities among women. Some key health issues to focus on in regard to women are diabetes, hypertension, cancer, and birth outcomes. Poverty must be emphasized in exploring the health status of women, along with issues that contribute to the problem, such as loss of the family wage and mass incarceration. Solutions toward closing the health status gap for women, particularly emerging majority women and all women experiencing poverty, must be sought.

Ultimately, the U.S. medical system must be willing to tailor its efforts to meet the needs of emerging majority women, women experiencing low socioeconomic status, and White women who are experiencing poverty and to ensure their access to care in culturally competent environments to offer a comfort level, culturally and beyond. One step toward this outcome would be ensuring more emerging majority participants in healthcare workforces, from staff to clinicians. Furthermore, there must be recognition of the myriad problems impacting all women, beginning with poverty, and the impact of these conditions on women's overall health and the health of their children and their families at large. Issues of racism and discrimination must not be ignored as a factor contributing to the poor health of emerging majority women, particularly of Black women, who are impacted disproportionately. It must be clear that Hispanic is not a race but rather an ethnicity; thus, Black Hispanic (Spanish-speaking) women must be included in the category with Black women in general when considering the numbers related to health, or lack thereof, of Hispanic people.

Chapter Problems

1. Explain the difference between Temporary Assistance for Needy Families (TANF), Aid for Dependent Children (ADC), and Aid to Families With Dependent Children (AFDC).
2. How are student loans contributing to the shortage of healthcare practitioners?
3. What is mass incarceration, and what recent step was taken in the state of Maryland towards equal justice?
4. List and explain three potential solutions that may positively impact the goal of closing the health status gap for women in the United States.
5. What is the family wage?

References

American Civil Liberties Union. (2007, December 12). Facts about the over-incarceration of women in the United States. https://www.aclu.org/documents/facts-about-over-incarceration-women-united-states

Braithwaite, R., Taylor, S., & Treadwell, H. (Eds.). (1992). *Health issues in the Black community* (p. 55). Jossey Bass.

California Newsreel. (2014, October 23). *How racism impacts pregnancy outcomes* [Video]. YouTube. https://www.youtube.com/watch?v=xUUJIG0-SlA

Center on Budget and Policy Priorities. (2022, March 1). *Policy basics: Temporary Assistance for Needy Families* [Report]. https://www.cbpp.org/research/family-income-support/policy-basics-an-introduction-to-tanf

Central Intelligence Agency. (2009). *The world factbook*. https://www.cia.gov/the-world-factbook/

Counihan, C., & Esterik, P. (Eds.). (1997). *Food and culture: A reader* (p. 272). Routledge.

Eyler, A. A., Baker, E., Cromer, L., King, A. C., Brownson, R. C., & Donatelle, R. J. (1998). Physical activity and minority women: a qualitative study. *Health education & behavior: the official publication of the Society for Public Health Education, 25*(5), 640–652. https://doi.org/10.1177/109019819802500510

Fraad, H. (2016, March 28). *Economic update: How capitalism changes intimacy and family* [Radio broadcast]. Democracy at Work. https://www.democracyatwork.info/eu_how_capitalism_changes_intimacy_and_family

Gottlieb, S. (2013, March 14). The doctor won't see you now. He's clocked out. *The Wall Street Journal.* https://www.wsj.com/articles/SB10001424127887323628804578346614033833092

Hill, S. A. (2009). Cultural images and the health of African American women. *Gender and Society, 23*(6), 733–746.

Hopkins, K. (2012, March 14). Grad students to lose federal loan subsidy. *Yahoo Finance.* https://finance.yahoo.com/news/grad-students-to-lose-federal-loan-210007086.html

James, C. V., Salganicoff, A., Thomas, M., Ranji, U., Lillie-Blanton, M., & Wyn, R. (2009, June). Putting women's health care disparities on the map: Examining racial and ethnic disparities at the state level. Kaiser Family Foundation. https://www.kff.org/wp-content/uploads/2013/01/7886.pdf

Katz, R. V., Green, B. L., Kressin, N. R., Kegeles, S. S., Wang, M. Q., James, S. A., Russell, S. L., Claudio, C., & McCallum, J. M. (2008). The legacy of the Tuskegee Syphilis Study: assessing its impact on willingness to participate in biomedical studies. *Journal of Health Care for the Poor and Underserved, 19*(4), 1168–1180. https://doi.org/10.1353/hpu.0.0067

Kindred, K. P. (2003). Of child welfare and welfare reform: The implications for children when contradictory policies collide. *William and Mary Journal of Women and the Law, 9*(3). Retrieved from http://scholarship.law.wm.edu/cgi/viewcontent.cgi?article=1169&context=wmjowl

Korhonen, V. (2023). Number of Black families with a single mother in the United States from 1990 to 2022. *Statista.* https://www.statista.com/statistics/205106/number-of-black-families-with-a-female-householder-in-the-us/

Marchevsky, A., & Theoharis, J. (2000). "Welfare reform, globalization and the racialization of entitlement". *American Studies, 41*(2/3), 235–265. http://www.jstor.org/stable/40643238

Murthy, P., & Smith, C. (Eds.). (2010). *Women's global health and human rights* (p. 148). Sudbury, MA: Jones & Bartlett Learning.

Musa, D., Schulz, R., Harris, R., Silverman, M., & Thomas, S. B. (2009). Trust in the health care system and the use of preventive health services by older black and white adults. *American journal of public health, 99*(7), 1293–1299. https://doi.org/10.2105/AJPH.2007.123927

Ollove, M. (2014, January 3). Are there enough doctors for the newly insured? *KFF Health News.* https://kffhealthnews.org/news/doctor-shortage-primary-care-specialist/

Paritan Valley Community College. (2020, February 27). Lecture, Discussion to Focus on Economic Dimensions of Everyday Life [Press release]. https://www.raritanval.edu/general-information/newsroom/lecture-discussion-focus-economic-dimensions-everyday-life#:~:text=Wolff%20is%20Professor%20of%20Economics,)%2C%20I%20l%20(Sorbonne

Pregnancy and childbirth. (n.d.). Healthy People 2030. U.S. Department of Health and Human Services. https://health.gov/healthypeople/objectives-and-data/browse-objectives/pregnancy-and-childbirth

Priority areas. (n.d.). Healthy People 2030. U.S. Department of Health and Human Services. https://health.gov/healthypeople/priority-areas

Street, R. L., Jr, O'Malley, K. J., Cooper, L. A., & Haidet, P. (2008). Understanding concordance in patient-physician relationships: Personal and ethnic dimensions of shared identity. *Annals of Family Medicine, 6*(3), 198–205. https://doi.org/10.1370/afm.821

Taylor, T. R., Williams, C. D., Makambi, K. H., Mouton, C., Harrell, J. P., Cozier, Y., Palmer, J. R., Rosenberg, L., & Adams-Campbell, L. L. (2007). Racial discrimination and breast cancer incidence in US Black women: the Black Women's Health Study. *American journal of epidemiology, 166*(1), 46–54. https://doi.org/10.1093/aje/kwm056

The Editorial Board. (2014, November 26). Mass imprisonment and public health. *The New York Times.* https://www.nytimes.com/2014/11/27/opinion/mass-imprisonment-and-public-health.html

The Office of Governor Wes Moore. (2024, June 17). Governor Moore signs nationally historic executive order pardoning 175,000 Maryland cannabis convictions [Press Release]. https://governor.maryland.gov/news/press/pages/governor-moore-signs-nationally-historic-executive-order-pardoning-175000-maryland-cannabis-convictions.aspx

Women's Health. (2024, December 11). Leading causes of death in females. Centers for Disease Control and Prevention. https://www.cdc.gov/womens-health/lcod/females.html

Yen, H. (2013, September 17). Four in five in USA face near-poverty, no work. *USA Today.* https://www.usatoday.com/story/money/business/2013/07/28/americans-poverty-no-work/2594203/

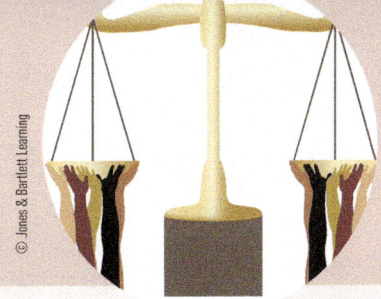

CHAPTER 11

Men and Health Disparities: Issues, Concerns, and Remedies

Patti R. Rose, MPH, Ed.D and **Annie Daniel**, PhD

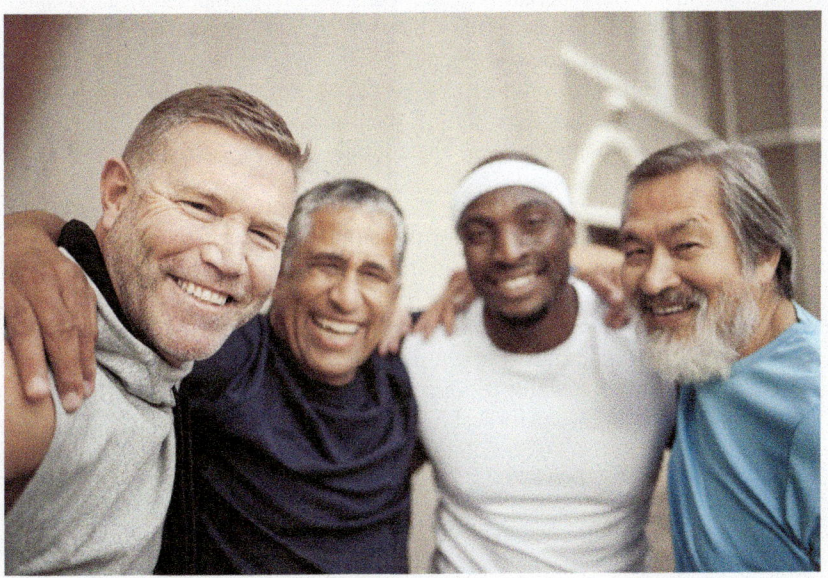

KEY TERMS

Healthy People
Healthy People 2030
Men's Health Network
patriarchal society

pescatarian
prostate cancer
Tuskegee Syphilis Study
watchful waiting

LEARNING OBJECTIVES

After reading this chapter, you should be able to:

1. Understand why men's health is not considered to the same degree as women's health in the United States.
2. List at least three leading causes of death for men in the United States.
3. Identify key reasons why men, in general, do not go to the doctor.
4. Explain whether or not it is recommended in the United States that men screen for testicular cancer.
5. Discuss options as potential remedies to guide men toward healthy lives.

Introduction

In 2020, the fifth iteration of the Healthy People initiative, **Healthy People 2030**, was released, strengthening the focus on social determinants and health illiteracy (Office of Disease Prevention and Health Promotion, 2020a). "Every ten years, the U.S. Surgeon General has released **Healthy People**, a set of health promotion and disease prevention targets to evaluate the nation's health and to guide the nation's resources for the coming decade" (Office of Disease Prevention and Health Promotion, 2020b). This is a laudable effort but, interestingly, beyond Healthy People, men's health is not focused upon as much in the United States as compared to women's health. In fact, according to Nuzzo (2020), there are no national offices to address men's health issues, even though men have worse health outcomes and a shorter life expectancy than women. The question is why? Nuzzo further states the following as possible reasons:

> …a general underappreciation for the number of issues that affect men more than women. Recognition of these issues might be enhanced if the relevant epidemiological data were collated into one source, something that has rarely been done. Another factor that might underlie the lack of progress on men's health issues in the United States is that few attempts have been made to quantify the different amounts of attention given to the fields of men's and women's health.

Nuzzo (2020) also points out:

> … [N]otions of "patriarchy" and "male privilege" are rampant in the media and in academic journals. These concepts, and the *ethos* surrounding them, are not only misguided, but they are likely detrimental to the health of men. They direct attention away from men's health issues, and as generalizations, they do not accurately reflect the lives of many males. For example, what power does a homeless man hold? What aspects of performing manual labor or collecting garbage are privilege?

These questions would clearly inspire significant dialogue in many circles and prompt one to consider what are the key health issues experienced by men, and more importantly, what are the remedies?

Healthy People 2030

Interestingly, as stated by Semlow et al. (2021):

> Of the 355 objectives in Healthy People 2030, there are 30 objectives that explicitly mention women, females or maternal health, but only four objectives that specifically mention men: one regarding **prostate cancer**, one regarding family planning, and two regarding sexually transmitted infections.

According to Healthy People 2030 (*Goal: Improve health and well-being for men*, n.d.), some key men's health issues include lung cancer, heart disease, and prostate cancer. According to Murphy et al. (2017), "for males, life expectancy changed from 76.2 in 2016 to 76.1 in 2017." The authors also point out that for males, life expectancy increased 1.3 years from 73.5 in 2021 to 74.8 in 2022. This increase in life expectancy for men shows improvement, with hopes that this progress will continue.

In considering leading causes of death further, per Healthy People 2030 (*Goal: Improve health and well-being for men*, n.d.):

> Prostate cancer is the most commonly diagnosed cancer and the second leading cause of cancer deaths in American men. Death rates from prostate cancer are much higher in some groups than others. Research shows that closely monitoring prostate cancer is an effective way to reduce the prostate cancer death rate in men who are diagnosed early.

One approach to monitor prostate cancer is entitled **watchful waiting**, which is "one form of expectant management for prostate cancer that may be effective for men with limited life expectancy and slow-growing, low-risk disease" (Johns Hopkins Medicine, n.d.). The Centers for Disease Control and Prevention (CDC) also indicates accidents (unintentional injuries) as a leading cause of death for men as well as cancer (beyond prostate cancer) in the top three (*Goal: Improve health and well-being for men*, n.d.). See **Table 11-1** that lists some leading causes of death among men.

Table 11-1 Leading Cause of Death Among Men

Leading Causes	Deaths	Population
Diseases of heart (I00-I09,I11,I13,I20-I51)	386,766	165,283,553
Malignant neoplasms (C00-C97)	319,336	165,283,553
Accidents (unintentional injuries) (V01-X59,Y85-Y86)	151,629	165,283,553
Cerebrovascular diseases (I60-I69)	71,819	165,283,553
Chronic lower respiratory diseases (J40-J47)	69,004	165,283,553
Diabetes mellitus	57,557	165,283,553
Intentional self-harm (suicide)	39,273	165,283,553

(continues)

Table 11-1 **Leading Cause of Death Among Men**   *(continued)*

Leading Causes	Deaths	Population
Alzheimer disease (G30)	37,475	165,283,553
Chronic liver disease and cirrhosis (K70,K73-K74)	34,340	165,283,553
Nephritis, nephrotic syndrome and nephrosis (N00-N07,N17-N19,N25-N27)	30,178	165,283,553
Parkinson's disease (G20-G21)	24,503	165,283,553
Influenza and pneumonia (J09-J18)	24,060	165,283,553
Septicemia (A40-A41)	20,977	165,283,553
Essential hypertension and hypertensive renal disease (I10,I12,I15)	20,237	165,283,553

Excerpted from Centers for Disease Control and Prevention, National Center for Health Statistics. National Vital Statistics System, Mortality 2018–2022 on CDC WONDER Online Database, released in 2024. Data are from the Multiple Cause of Death Files, 2018–2022, as compiled from data provided by the 57 vital statistics jurisdictions through the Vital Statistics Cooperative Program. Accessed at http://wonder.cdc.gov/ucd-icd10-expanded.html on May 20, 2024 9:43:22 PM.

In general, according to various research sources, men show a great deal of hesitancy toward going to the doctor. For example, the following is noted in an online survey conducted by Cleveland Clinic (2019):

> ...[A]mong approximately 1,174 U.S. males 18 years or older, Cleveland Clinic found that 72 percent of men would rather do household chores, like cleaning the bathroom or mowing the lawn, than go to the doctor.

There are myriad reasons for this expressed by men, including lack of time to do so, not interested in guidance about their diet and how to live, and avoidance of potential bad news about their health. Additionally, the patriarchy plays a role in this non-health care seeking behavior and men. As noted by Almendrala (2016) in a news article:

> Men experience very strong, clear messages about how they're supposed to display their masculinity and hide their vulnerability, and pretty much everything about going to a doctor's office goes against these rigid gender role norms, said professor Glenn Good, an expert on masculinity and the psychology of men at the University of Florida.

This attitude toward not seeking health care is nuanced on a racial basis. For example, per Powell et al. (2016):

> Men's tendency to delay health help-seeking is largely attributed to masculinity, but findings scarcely focus on African-American men who face additional race-related, help-seeking barriers.

In understanding the issues associated with the health of Black men, as an example of race-related help seeking barriers, it is imperative that we review a significant historical occurrence about Black men and health care in the United States. One overarching event, as also mentioned in the chapter pertaining to African American people in general, sets the tone for Black men, their relationship with and their ability to trust healthcare providers and researchers in health care. This event was the **Tuskegee Syphilis Study**. In 1978, Allan Brandt wrote an article entitled "Racism and Research: The Case of the Tuskegee Syphilis Study." In this article, Brandt reviewed the U.S. Public Health Service's 1931 experiment in Macon County, Alabama, in which the study was:

> ... to determine the natural course of untreated, latent syphilis in black males. The test comprised 400 syphilitic men, as well as 200 uninfected men who served as controls. The first published report of the study appeared in 1936 with subsequent papers issued every four to six years, through the 1960s.

This study was particularly atrocious that during the course of the study, in the early 1950s, penicillin became available and the men in the study who had syphilis did not receive it (Brandt, 1978). Furthermore, the United States Public Health Service (USPHS), who was responsible for the study, prevented the men from getting penicillin. This horrendous experiment continued until 1972. As stated by Brandt (1978):

> A committee at the Center for Disease Control decided in 1969 that it should continue. In 1972, The Department of Health, Education and Welfare halted it. Seventy-four of the subjects were alive; twenty-eight, but perhaps more than 100, had died from advanced syphilitic lesions. In August 1972, HEW appointed an investigatory panel which issued a report the following year. They found the study "ethically unjustified," arguing that penicillin should have been provided to the men.

As a result of the Tuskegee Syphilis Study, and other heinous medical studies/experiments on Black people, even today there is a mistrust of the healthcare profession among Black people, including Black men. Since the Tuskegee study focused on Black men, it caused a significant level of mistrust for them. Therefore, it is important that as we study the disparities of male health in general to recognize that Black males have a history of mistreatment in the healthcare system in the United States. This is a great hurdle, among others, that needs to be overcome in order to improve the health of Black men, who may need to seek health care. For too long, very little research and data on the health of Black men has existed. The Black Men's Health Project was created to call attention to the health crisis confronting African-American men in the United States and gather valuable data and insights through a Black Men's Health Survey.

Remedies

To improve men's health, it is believed, by some, that it is important to raise awareness about preventive screenings and regular health care for men of all ages. Interventions to reduce smoking and drinking and promote healthy behaviors can help prevent health challenges and improve men's health (*Goal: Improve health and well-being for men*, n.d.). However, some men, may seek alternative/complementary options, as opposed to seeing a doctor who is strictly Western medicine oriented. Exploring options should be encouraged if men choose to do so with guidance from sources who may understand varying approaches based on culture, insight, and personal decision-making. There is no cookie-cutter answer for all men. Guidance often changes in western medicine. For example, it is important to note that the United States Preventive Services Task Force recommends against screening for testicular cancer in men. This recommendation applies to adolescent and adult men who don't have symptoms of testicular cancer (*Reduce the prostate cancer death rate—C-08*, n.d.). Hence, preventative approaches, contrary to the beliefs of some, are not the approach for all men. This type of message, pertaining to options, is perhaps an approach that will lead to more men exploring varying possibilities to strive for/maintain optimal health.

Additionally, per LaCount (2023), one suggestion for men to maintain good health is to eat healthy food including fruits, vegetables, whole grains, lean protein, and healthy fats while avoiding processed foods, added sugars, and saturated fats. These seem like common sense approaches, but bringing this detail to the forefront, without the assumption that men already know this, is important. Exercise is also recommended to ensure a raised heart rate, sweating, strength training, and beyond. Exercise can also help with stress and other mental health concerns, which are prevalent among men. Yoga and other approaches, such as meditation or breathing exercises and participating in activities that bring joy, as an addendum to exercise help ease stress. Smoking should be avoided and alcohol consumption should be limited. Rest (adequate sleep each night) and managing stress levels are always helpful. Additionally, there is an organization devoted to men's health entitled the **Men's Health Network**. Per the "About" section of their website (Men's Health Network, n.d.) the following is noted:

> This organization Men's Health Network (MHN) is a national non-profit organization whose mission is to reach men, boys, and their families where they live, work, play, and pray with health awareness and disease prevention messages and tools, screening programs, educational materials, advocacy opportunities, and patient navigation.

Some of their remedies for men's health are as follows (Giorgianni et al, 2013):

- *Primary and secondary education*—Boys should be educated about health and wellness during this point in their educational experiences.
- *Higher education*—There should be curriculum offerings that focus on men's health including psychosocial, environmental, and skills relevant to varying lifestyles.
- *Education and training*—In terms of training for clinicians and other health professionals, a focus in the curriculum should include detailed information on an extensive basis about men's health.
- *The media*—In all aspects of the media, there should be advertisements that ensure that there is a focus on boys and men as the target audience to incentivize them to consider health and wellness as a core aspect of their manhood.
- *Outreach*—Efforts should be made to reach out to men by varying health organizations in the public sector, health foundations, and stakeholders (public and private) to develop programs that focus on education and screening for boys

and men, per their choice. Organizations and groups that sponsor lifestyle programs that attract boys and men should begin to incorporate health and wellness related participation in the programs with the goal of showing how health is part of masculinity.

REMEDIES

- Raise awareness about preventive screenings and regular health care for men of all ages.
- For those engaged in Western medicine approaches, complementary options based on individual decision making should be explored.
- Per Healthy People 2030 (*Goal: Improve health and well-being for men*, n.d.), the development and implementation of interventions to reduce smoking and drinking and promote healthy behaviors also can help prevent diseases and improve men's health.
- Suggest to men that to maintain good health, eating healthy food, including fruits, vegetables, whole grains, lean protein, and healthy fats, while avoiding processed foods, added sugars, and saturated fats, is necessary (LaCount, 2023).
- Recommend exercise ensuring a raised heart rate, sweating, and strength training; and exercise to help with stress and other mental health concerns prevalent among men by including yoga and other approaches, such as meditation or breathing exercises as options.

Insight into Men's Health

In an effort to gain insight about men's health, including problems and ideas toward remedies, an interview was conducted with Dr. Eduard Tiozzo, who is an Assistant Professor in the Department of Physical Medicine and Rehabilitation at the University of Miami Miller School of Medicine. He also serves as the lifestyle medicine curriculum Director and Research Director for their residency program. His educational background includes a doctoral degree in exercise physiology and a master's degree in clinical and translational investigation. Outside of work, Dr. Tiozzo tries to live a balanced life. He has been a pescatarian for over a decade and is an avid swimmer. As a member of Swim Fort Lauderdale, he competes in pool events (winning multiple national medals and national team championships with his team) and open water events (including a 10k in Bermuda, a 5k in Barbados, and an Alcatraz swim). He is a dual citizen of the United States and Croatia.

Interview with Dr. Eduard Tiozzo

Dr. Rose: First of all, what is your perception of men's health in the United States? Our interview is strictly related to the United States, unless I ask otherwise.

Dr. Tiozzo: Men's health. What is my perception? I think in general, we all can do more about prevention, rather than management, of health issues. So I think that that's where we have a way to go ... focus more on prevention. What is it that we can do to stay healthy, be healthy, rather than avoid getting conditions or diseases? If that makes sense.

(continues)

Interview with Dr. Eduard Tiozzo   *(continued)*

Dr. Rose: Can you elaborate on prevention because it means a lot of things to a lot of people. Prevention for some people might mean going to the doctor before an illness. When you say prevention, what are you referring to?

Dr. Tiozzo: I think you're healthy, just living a healthy lifestyle. When I say prevention, I mean the first two things that come to my mind are to be more physically active and to eat healthy or healthier than we do. And I think by doing those things, as maybe the core principles of a healthy lifestyle, I think we can achieve a lot more than we currently are, as far as our health.

Dr. Rose: Okay, and could you give me an example when you say, eat healthy? Because that, too, has a lot of different meanings for different people. What do you mean specifically by eating healthy?

Dr. Tiozzo: I think if you set 10 people in a room and ask them that same question, I think they most likely will give you different answers. I think we're still debating what eating healthy is and needs, whether it's intermittent fasting, reduced caloric intake, the paleo or keto diet or a high protein diet. Basically, I would say, if you analyze or look into those "blue zones" where we have a higher percentage of centenarians, people older than 100, and analyze their lifestyle habits, when it comes to diet, specifically, I think you can describe their diet as predominantly plant based, with a high intake of vegetables and fruit, nuts, fish, and low in meat consumption. That doesn't mean that they're vegetarians or vegans, just low in meat consumption and consuming healthy fats. So basically, very close or similar to a Mediterranean diet. I think there is a good amount of research basically showing that when they analyze different diets, the Mediterranean diet consistently has been shown as a very healthy dietary option for various health outcomes.

Dr. Rose: That's very interesting. Let's discuss longevity. The lifespan for men is lower than that of women. In this chapter, I'm interviewing you to solely discuss health pertaining to men. So what you just described, is this relevant specifically to men? Do you think that men should partake in the Mediterranean diet, as one example, as their approach towards a healthy lifestyle?

Dr. Tiozzo: I think so. I don't think there is a difference between men and women as far as how they should incorporate their healthy lifestyle behaviors. I think what works for women works for men and vice versa, pretty much, with maybe some slight differences, right? But I think the approach should be the same, and the benefits are there for both sexes.

Dr. Rose: Okay, great. And why do you think, based on your research, if you're aware of what I just said about the longevity issue between men and women, that men are experiencing a shorter life span than women in the United States?

Dr. Tiozzo: Well, to be honest. I haven't checked that lately, but I think part of it is risky behavior that men tend to engage in more than women. That's also part of that equation, isn't it?

Dr. Rose: What would you say are the risky behaviors you refer to because I always like for people to define terms that they're using? Can you just give me a couple of examples of risky behaviors that you think men participate in, that women don't, that contribute to a shorter lifespan, per your perspective?

Dr. Tiozzo: I'll make one parallel, because I'm currently doing a good amount of research on spinal cord injury. So the statistics are that men, overwhelmingly, have a higher rate of spinal cord injury than women, and that's coming from sports and car accidents injuries and gunshot wounds, as far as risky behaviors.

Dr. Rose: Unintentional injuries are indeed one of the top three health issues for men, so you are spot on.

Dr. Tiozzo: I think you can also add maybe smoking and alcohol consumption. I'm pretty positive the rates are higher in men versus women.

Dr. Rose: Okay. At this point, I'm going to go to the next area that I want to discuss. As I mentioned to you, this is a very forward-thinking piece of work that I'm working on here. I think that Healthy People 2030, and the CDC and NIH, as examples, and similar entities have explored what the problems are, but we really want to get into remedies, because we can talk about the problems forever. I think that in the healthcare field we are very well versed in the problems, but the question is, what do we do about it? How can we fix the problems associated with men's health? We have a lot of room to come up with ideas to help men in terms of longevity. What in your mind, as a Professor and Researcher, do you think are some of the approaches that we can take to deal with men's health as health professionals, as public health practitioners, etc., just off of the top of your head? What do you think based on your professional work?

Dr. Tiozzo: I think education. I don't think we educate our general public audience, men included, when it comes to health and healthy lifestyles. I think that sometimes we even confuse the public, right? You know, there's one piece of research, that says that an average American feels that it's easier for him or her to do taxes versus to describe what healthy eating is, which we just discussed, right? Because, you know, one day we can say, "Eggs are bad for you," and then 10 years later we say, "Well, eggs are actually good for you." So we go back and forth when it comes to certain food items. We had a crusade and war on fats, right? There was a whole push from the government to reduce the fat intake in our diet. And if you still go to any store there is fat-free or fat-reduced, milk and yogurt, etc., So we did that. We reduced the fat intake in our diet, and yet our cardiovascular disease (CVD) rates went up. So now we're claiming, "Well, it's really not fat, it's more sugar that's getting us in trouble." So I think unintentionally, obviously, we oftentimes confuse people as to what is healthy, what they should be doing. But just overall, I think we need to educate people more. I've yet to see a commercial that says, "If you want to lower your risk for high blood pressure or for high cholesterol, the risk for stroke or cardiovascular disease, you should accumulate 150 minutes of physical activity per week or more," right? There is no such commercial. We're bombarded by pharmaceutical commercials about drugs. Yes, part of it is education, and they raise awareness about certain diseases. When we talk about men, there is erectile dysfunction with commercials about it. The studies indicate that the drugs remove a stigma, so men are more likely to go and see a physician about their drug because it's advertised on TV. But I think for the most part, we know where the intention of those commercials are, and it's pretty much to push for greater sale of drugs, of medications, but when it comes to healthy lifestyles, we don't use media to educate people. And so when you ask people what the guidelines for physical activity are, a large majority, I would have to check the percentages, but a large majority do

(continues)

not know what the physical activity guidelines currently are and how much physical activity they should accumulate per day or per week,

Dr. Rose: For men specifically, let's talk about that, because education is the key. You mentioned the media in terms of commercials and so forth. If we want to educate men about health, ranging from boys, because when I speak of men, I'm speaking of boys too, from cradle to the grave. If we want to speak about men, how do you think we can reach them?

Dr. Tiozzo: Social media … just any kind of media. I'm sure there's some kind of statistics as to what kind of media men are engaged by more than women, and maybe targeting a specific media type, whether it's TV or print or social media right? But I don't know if that answers your question.

Dr. Rose: I agree that we have to recognize that there are differences between men and women in the way that we function and do things. We're very different. This monolithic approach that is often used to say, just educate everyone the same way is not working because we can see the difference in terms of longevity and health issues and so forth, which are not exactly the same. If we can begin to think about ideas, by just going back a little bit, headway can be made. In the United States, in terms of health, there used to be an emphasis on men. The clinical trials were for men and etc. But because of the **patriarchal society** (ruled by men) that we live in, women had to step forward and say, hey, what about us? We need help. And so consequently, national entities were put in place to deal with women's health, but there is no such thing for men—not on a governmental basis. So with that being said, men have, due to the system that they created, ultimately put themselves in a situation where attention is no longer placed on them. And so this chapter is sort of a men's advocacy chapter. This chapter only because I also have a chapter on women's health. The question is, how do we reach men now so that we can improve their health? Speaking to you as a Professor and Researcher, but also a man, an athlete, a health-centered person, how do we reach men about their health, including education as you mentioned before and beyond.

Dr. Tiozzo: That's a very good question. How do we reach men? I think we reach men by addressing more specifically men, and not just overall American adults, right? One of the solutions might be—I don't know the statistics I will have to read about it because I don't do that line of research, but my guess is that men tend to see physicians for regular checkups, maybe less than women.

Dr. Rose: Yes, you're right.

Dr. Tiozzo: There is that mentality, "I don't need to see a physician," right? "I'm fine." So perhaps there is some room to see physicians, even if you actually don't have any symptoms or pain. I think it's been advertised for women about mammograms and breast cancer risk. I would say more awareness for colorectal cancer may be helpful. But that's again, for both men and women, not just men specifically, right? I think we're a country of extremes when it comes to everything, politically, economically, and maybe when it comes to health issues, right? So for decades we neglected women's health issues, and now maybe we're getting into another extreme where men are being maybe left behind a bit. So, we go from one extreme to another. We can't seem to find a happy medium, right?

Dr. Rose: If I'm correct in interpreting what you're saying correctly, your point is that we need targeted efforts toward men now in addition to women.

Dr. Tiozzo: Yes

Dr. Rose: All right, great. You are absolutely right. The research and the data show that men do not, for the most part, go to the doctor. They don't want to go because they don't want to hear potentially bad news and so forth. I do cover that in this chapter, so I'm going to go on to the next question, which is a little bit personal. Can you tell me a little bit about your personal health choices and activities? Do you consider yourself to be a healthy man, and if so, how do you achieve it?

Dr. Tiozzo: I do. I really have come to the point where I really consider myself lucky for having obtained the degree that I did in exercise physiology, because it really gave me knowledge and skills, just tools overall, to be able to live what I consider is a healthy lifestyle. What I think works for me. When it comes to physical activity, obviously, as an Exercise Physiologist, that's my focus and my passion. But also, when it comes to diet I'm personally a pescatarian. I have been for about, I want to say, over 10 years now.

Dr. Rose: Okay, tell me a little bit about being a **pescatarian**.

Dr. Tiozzo: It's basically not consuming animal meat. I do consume other animal products, like occasionally I may have cheese or eggs and milk, not so much, but no meat, even no chicken or poultry, because sometimes when I say to people, I don't advertise it, but if people ask me, I share it. When I say I don't eat meat, then oftentimes people say, well, does this mean you don't eat chicken too? For some people, they don't consider chicken to be meat. They consider maybe red meat as meat, but chicken, not necessarily.

Dr. Rose: Yes, perhaps, because chicken falls under the category of poultry.

Dr. Tiozzo: But yeah, so pescatarian would be no meat of any kind, just fish.

Dr. Rose: It seems like when you speak of your healthy lifestyle, the first thing that you mentioned is diet. What else would you say contributes to your leading a healthy lifestyle?

Dr. Tiozzo: I think that overall, I mean being raised and born in Croatia and having Italian roots, I'm very familiar with the Mediterranean diet, which is high in fruit and vegetable intake and also includes healthy fat, fish, nuts, and grains.

Dr. Rose: Do you participate in exercise, and if so, what kind?

Dr. Tiozzo: I would say two-thirds of my exercise routine is swimming, and then maybe one-third is resistance training activities and stretching and yoga.

Dr. Rose: Obviously you're doing so at a very high level. For the average man, who is working every day, for example, let's say from 9–5 in any type of job that is time consuming and so forth, which type of exercising do you think is a good idea in order to stay healthy? How could that particular form of exercise be fit into a man's lifestyle? How do you fit it in?

Dr. Tiozzo: Well, I still compete. So that's a motivation for me. I have a goal. I have a competition in a couple of months. So that's a great motivator to get up at 5 a.m. even on mornings when I don't want to do that because I have that goal ahead of me and I want to accomplish it, whether it's winning something or breaking your personal best or whatever the goals are. For someone who doesn't compete, and just wants to incorporate physical activity to promote fitness and health, my suggestions are to take something that you enjoy doing, because you're more likely to do it. For me, that's swimming. For me, there's something very therapeutic when I swim. I can go in the pool with my mind, busy and you know, my brain running

(continues)

100 miles an hour, but after the swim workout, when I get out, I'm just sort of centered. I feel centered. That's probably the best way to explain my state after swimming. Whatever people's preferences are whether it's walking, jogging, doing yoga, cycling … there's not much hiking here in Florida, but maybe gardening. It's about what you like to do. Whatever you enjoy. That would be my recommendation, because, again, you're more likely to stick to it and have that type of physical activity as part of your lifestyle, as part of who you are.

Dr. Rose: That's a very good point. Perhaps in marketing to men about their health, what you're saying is about enjoying life and incorporating exercise into that. I have just a couple more questions for you. One is a little bit more academic. What do you think should be the primary areas of research around men's health? Where should we be focusing?

Dr. Tiozzo: My focus would be longevity and healthy brain. Obviously, as we live longer, there's a high risk that we will die of a certain condition or disease and lately, we've been reading more about the risk of dementia and Alzheimer's, right? What is it that we can do to alleviate those risks with a healthy lifestyle? I don't think we have a clear answer to that question. To what extent is nature versus nurture, genes versus environment, our choices throughout life that we make relevant? To what extent can men achieve a healthy brain at a later age?

Dr. Rose: What are your thoughts about the healthcare system in the United States as it is currently designed? Is it meeting the needs of men in this country?

Dr. Tiozzo: That's a tough one. I think the quality of health care is there, but I think everything around it is lacking or not there. It's driven by administration; it's driven by profit and money. So you barely have any meaningful contact with your healthcare providers/physicians anymore. It's like an assembly line. There is also insurance, the underinsured, hidden charges and overcharges because we really don't have sort of a menu where you walk into a physician's office and you know how much you will be charged. There's no price list. There's nothing. You're just constantly being surprised and bombarded by the bills, and you have to figure out what they are and you have to fight the insurance and administration when you're overcharged, or where there is a hidden fee, or when there is a test being provided that wasn't really needed. That's my biggest frustration. As a man and as an individual, every time, in this country, when I need to see a healthcare provider, a physician or anyone else, I really do get anxious because I don't know what's going to happen financially, as far as how much cost I'll have to face with that single visit, because I just feel very vulnerable. Even though I do have health coverage, I still know that there's going to be a substantial amount of money to pay. So, I think overall, the quality of care that we have here is great. We're pioneers when it comes to medical industry and treatment but everything around it is just kind of messy.

Dr. Rose: Okay. If you had one suggestion, bearing men in mind at this point, who have to go to the doctor, for whatever reason. If this is the way the system is, then why would they want to go and participate in it? If you have one big suggestion, what would it be to try to fix this?

Dr. Tiozzo: That's a very, very good question. Where would I start? I would remove co-pays and deductibles.

Dr. Rose: Are you saying that because co-pays and deductibles are part of the whole managed care system? Are you speaking of the removal of managed care? Do you think that would make it better, or keeping managed care and just remove the co-pays and deductibles?

Dr. Tiozzo: I think removing them [deductibles and co-pays] because as just one example, if you're self-employed your insurance rate is probably close to $1,000 here in Florida, and that health coverage gives you nothing but one annual a year, and your deductible is $10,000 right? Unless you have a severe medical issue, an accident or surgery, you're really not covered, because every time you step into an office, clinic or hospital, you have to pay out of pocket, right? You're a hard-working individual. That may be the only plan that you have. It doesn't give you much. So that's one part of the equation. Maybe another part of the equation, when it comes to men's health, is to have, specifically, a men's health clinic where men can go and their concerns and health issues can be addressed in those clinics.

Dr. Rose: Very interesting. I love talking to people about this, because we all have the remedies. We just don't have a venue to discuss them. But both of those are great ideas. Just to give you an example, without going into a lot of detail, there is a key example of what you suggest, in play, such as the health savings account (HSA). If you have a deductible, each paycheck, a certain amount of money is provided by your employer/you, pre-tax from your check. A debit card may be provided or the funds can be deposited into your account for medical expenses before the deductible is met. But even if the deductible is not eliminated, are there creative approaches to deal with the deductible so that people don't have anxiety before they go to the doctor, which may be at least one reason why many men do not go. I think those are both great ideas. Also, the idea of a men's health clinic is another good one, but they do exist. To what extent and their efficiency may be a good area for research.

Dr. Tiozzo: Yes. For sure.

Dr. Rose: We are now at our last question. Many of my books include detail about culture, race, nationality, etc., and how that comes into play in terms of health. Given that you are from Croatia, your lifestyle in your country, not just you specifically, but the lifestyle of Croatian men, sans food, because you've already told us about food, how does it differ in terms of health, than for American men?

Dr. Tiozzo: I think in Croatia, we tend to just overall, men included, eat out less, simply because people maybe don't have the means for that over there as much as here. So people cook more and eat homemade food more.

Dr. Rose: Oh, really?

Dr. Tiozzo: I mean, it's kind of a luxury to go out and people indulge in that, maybe occasionally, but not daily or weekly as some people do here, right? I think also, the way our cities are designed in that towns and cities are very walkable, and you can get around by using public transportation. You can get by without necessarily having a car. So as a result, people tend to be more active in Croatia. They just tend to walk more and so maybe those are the two main differences.

Dr. Rose: As far as you know, like here in the United States, is it an issue for men to seek health care and see a physician for any kind of medical issues?

Dr. Tiozzo: I think in Croatia that's even more prevalent because the mentality there, at least when I used to live there—I don't know if that's changed, over

(continues)

the last 18 years—but the mentality over there, even more so for men, is that you only see a physician if you're in pain. If not, you know, what's the point of doing that? So, yeah, I think that's even a bigger issue in Croatia than here.

Dr. Rose: Well, my position, as I have indicated in my book, is that seeing a doctor is not necessarily the panacea of a healthy lifestyle. So it would be very interesting to look at the data to see if in Croatia, since that is the emphasis, if the men are healthier or less healthy than the men in the United States. I mean, it's a very interesting research question. Is the answer that men should go to the doctor more, or that men should lead a healthy lifestyle and the doctor should be relegated to when it's necessary, because there's a problem? This is the age-old question, you know, for public health, but I think now, especially given what you said, we could actually look at the research data to see how men are faring in Croatia.

Dr. Tiozzo: I will tell you that I know that Croatian people are struggling with increasing obesity rates, which is something that we didn't experience when I was growing up. It was never an issue, but it's becoming more of an issue now.

Dr. Rose: I wonder why, given what you just said about the lifestyle and walking and etc., What would be the reason for that?

Dr. Tiozzo: That's good question. I think in every country in Europe and Asia, there is more and more infiltration of fast food. So I think that's part of the equation. I'm sure there's more to it.

Dr. Rose: Thank you so much.

WRAP-UP

Men's health is complicated. Although the United States is a patriarchal society with men largely at the helm in terms of the government, businesses, and financial wealth, their health is often not at the forefront. Also, it seems that many men do not prioritize their own health. Their life expectancy is lower than women's and, in efforts such as Healthy People 2030, there is limited focus in terms of objectives to explore men's health needs thoroughly. In order to improve the health status of men, currently, it is necessary to take steps to enhance their knowledge base, participation, and understanding on a broader basis about what it takes to maintain their health. Some would argue that getting men to go to the doctor more (Western medicine or other options) or at all, is the panacea to ensure healthier lifestyles for them. However, perhaps that is one step for consideration for some men, but other lifestyle factors are critical remedies including eating healthy foods, exercising, managing stress, and other aspects of their mental health. Seeking other medical approaches beyond the western approach may also be an option that men may be open to. Also, effective communication and marketing to boys and men, with important health information focused on their well-being and ensuring that they feel comfortable and knowledgeable about their bodies will be very helpful to include in the compendium of remedies.

Chapter Problems

1. Explain why some men may opt out of going to the doctor/seeking health care.
2. What are some non-medical approaches that men may want to consider in terms of moving toward/maintaining optimal health?
3. Is screening for testicular cancer recommended for all men?
4. What is watchful waiting and its relationship to prostate cancer?
5. Explain the Tuskegee Syphilis Study and discuss whether it was ethical or unethical and its relevance to Black men.

References

Almendrala, A. (2016, June 13). Here's why men don't like going to the doctor. *HuffPost*. https://www.huffpost.com/entry/why-men-dont-go-to-the-doctor_n_5759c267e4b00f97fba7aa3e

Brandt, A. M. (1978). Racism and research: the case of the Tuskegee Syphilis Study. *The Hastings Center Report*, *8*(6), 21–29. https://dash.harvard.edu/server/api/core/bitstreams/7312037c-79d3-6bd4-e053-0100007fdf3b/content

Cleveland Clinic Newsroom (2019, September 4). MeCleveland Clinic Newsroom. Cleveland Clinic Survey: Men will do Almost Anything to Avoid Going to the Doctor. https://newsroom.clevelandclinic.org/2019/09/04/cleveland-clinic-survey-men-will-do-almost-anything-to-avoid-going-to-the-doctor

Giorgianni, S. J., Brott, A., Fadich, A., Rooks, Y., Leonard, B., Henry, A., Davidson, D., Williams, A., Sabbs, D., Lutz, M. D., & Petty, S. D. (2013, May). *Executive summary: Providing for and influencing the care of boys and men in America* (Report). Men's Health Braintrust. https://staging.menshealthnetwork.org/wp-content/library/dialogue2summary.pdf

Goal: Improve health and well-being for men. (n.d.). Healthy People 2030. U.S. Department of Health and Human Services. https://health.gov/healthypeople/objectives-and-data/browse-objectives/men

Healthy People 2030 (n.d.). Health Literacy in Healthy People 2030. U.S. Department of Health and Human Services. https://health.gov/healthypeople/priority-areas

Johns Hopkins Medicine (n.d.). *Watchful Waiting for Prostate Cancer*. Johns Hopkins Medicine. https://www.hopkinsmedicine.org/health/conditions-and-diseases/prostate-cancer/watchful-waiting-for-prostate-cancer

LaCount, B., II. (2023, June 14). Men: Take charge of your health with these pro tips. Vital Record, *News from Texas A&M Health*. https://vitalrecord.tamu.edu/men-take-charge-of-your-health-with-these-pro-tips/

Men's Health Network. (n.d.). Dialogue on Men's Health series of conferences, Providing for and Influencing the Care of Boys and Men in America. https://menshealthnetwork.org/about/

Murphy, S. L., Xu, J., Kochanek, K. D., & Arias, E. (2018). Mortality in the United States, 2017. *NCHS Data Brief, 328*. https://www.cdc.gov/nchs/data/databriefs/db328-h.pdf

Nuzzo, J. L. (2020). Men's health in the United States: a national health paradox. *The aging male: the official journal of the International Society for the Study of the Aging Male*, *23*(1), 42–52. https://doi.org/10.1080/13685538.2019.1645109

Office of Disease Prevention and Health Promotion. (2020a). Healthy People 2030 Is Here! Retrieved from: https://minorityhealth.hhs.gov/news/healthy-people-2030-here

Office of Disease Prevention and Health Promotion. (2020b). *Healthy People 2030 Framework*. https://www.healthypeople.gov/2020/About-Healthy-People/Development-Healthy-People-2030/Framework

Powell, W., Adams, L. B., Cole-Lewis, Y., Agyemang, A., & Upton, R. D. (2016). Masculinity and Race-Related Factors as Barriers to Health Help-Seeking Among African American Men. *Behavioral Medicine, 42*(3), 150–163. https://doi.org/10.1080/08964289.2016.116 5174

Reduce the prostate cancer death rate — C-08. (n.d.). Healthy People 2030. U.S. Department of Health and Human Services. https://health.gov/healthypeople/objectives-and-data/browse-objectives /cancer/reduce-prostate-cancer-death-rate-c-08

Semlow, A. R., Ellison, J. M., Jaeger, E. C., & Griffith, D. M. (2021). Healthy Men 2030: Setting Men's Health Goals as a Tool to Improve the Nation's Health and Achieve Health Equity. *Health education & behavior: The official publication of the Society for Public Health Education, 48*(4), 393–396. https://doi.org/10.1177/10901981211025465

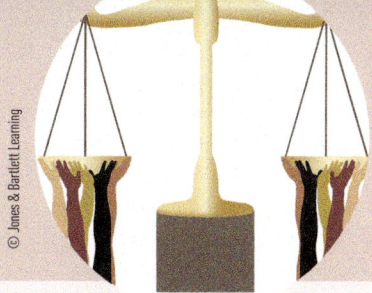
© Jones & Bartlett Learning

CHAPTER 12

Children and Health Disparities: Issues, Concerns, and Remedies

Clarence Cryer, Jr., MPH

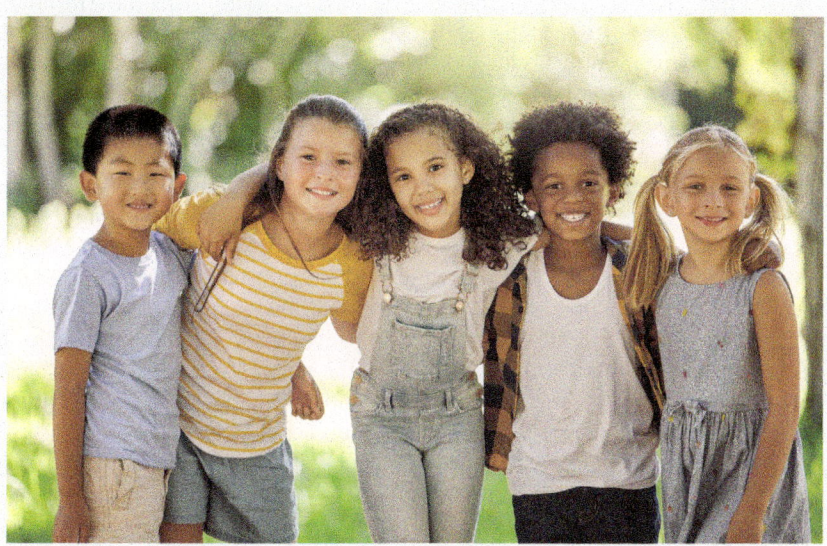

© PeopleImages.com - Yuri A/Shutterstock

KEY TERMS

Agency for Healthcare Research
   and Quality (AHRQ)
childhood obesity
discrimination

Healthy People 2030
National Healthcare Disparities Report
   (NHDR)
social determinants of health (SDOH)

LEARNING OBJECTIVES

After reading this chapter, you should be able to do the following:

1. Identify health conditions with a disproportionate representation of traditional emerging majority and children experiencing poverty.
2. Discuss viable remedies and potential barriers to achieving health equity.
3. Understand the relationship between socioeconomic status/race and health status of the nation's children.
4. Explain the potential impact of changing demographics on the overall health status of the nation's children.

Introduction

In the dawn of the 21st century, the United States is marked by renewed and continued interest in longstanding inequities in the nation's health status. This reaffirmed allegiance to social justice is coupled with deliberate action to illuminate and purge historical imbalances characterized by significant differences in illness and mortality between population subgroups. In 2000, the National Institutes of Health (NIH) founded the National Center on Minority Health and Health Disparities (Institute of Medicine, 2006). The mission of the NCMHD is to lead scientific research to improve emerging majority health and eliminate inequalities. In 2003, the **Agency for Healthcare Research and Quality (AHRQ)** issued its first annual *National Healthcare Disparities Report (NHDR)* (AHRQ, 2014). The *NHDR* was the first national comprehensive effort to measure differences in the quality of, and access to, healthcare services overall and by various populations. The same year, a milestone study of disparities, *Unequal Treatment: Confronting Racial and Ethnic Disparities in Health Care*, was released by the Institute of Medicine (Smedley et al., 2003). The Department of Health and Human Services (DHHS) included the reduction of disparities as a primary goal in its initial Healthy People initiative, Healthy People 2000. This publication of national initiatives for improving the health of all Americans is updated every 10 years. For the next two decades, overarching goals of the program have included health disparities: Healthy People 2010 focused on the elimination and, not just the reduction of, health disparities (U.S. Department of Health and Human Services, 2000a). In Healthy People 2020, the goal was expanded even further. **Healthy People 2030** followed suit with a focus on key issues related to children, including the importance of vision screening, reducing death rates of children aged 1–19, increasing high school graduation rates, reducing suspension rates, reducing mercury exposure, reducing emergency room visits, increasing support around mental health issues, reducing the proportion of children with untreated tooth decay, reducing obesity in children, and beyond. This chapter will focus on potential remedies around two of these issues, namely untreated tooth decay and reducing obesity in children as both are key objectives, among others, identified in Healthy People 2030 (Healthy People 2030, n.d.).

Despite numerous efforts at the turn of the century, disparities in illness and death experienced by emerging majorities and people experiencing poverty, including their children, remain a major obstacle to improving national health. However, the focus of this chapter is not to focus on the obstacles or the problems but rather to consider remedies to solve the problems related to children's health in the United States.

The Health of U.S. Children: Historical Perspective

Per Hooks (2001), love is a key factor in terms of children and is sometimes missing. She states, "although lots of children are raised in homes where they are given some kind of care, love may not be sustained or even present." Hooks also shares a key point from Lucia Hodgson who wrote the book entitled *Raised in Captivity: Why Does America Fail Its Children?* Hooks points out that Hodgson emphasizes the fact that children have no rights and are often victims, as they are abused verbally, physically, starved, tortured, and murdered, without a collective voice. This detail is so macabre that it begs for a discussion toward remedies rather than focus on the depraved reality of the lack of love for children that is too often a reality. Potential remedies and some existing improvements will be discussed in this chapter.

The truth is that compared to their peers in earlier times, the health status of America's nearly 80 million children has generally improved. Collectively, they have a much brighter outlook than did people 18 years and younger during the 19th and 20th centuries. In the 1800s, many children were undernourished, and many did not survive to adulthood, often dying of chronic diseases that are now easily cured or prevented.

At the beginning of the 20th century, infectious diseases, including diarrheal diseases, diphtheria, measles, pneumonia and influenza, scarlet fever, tuberculosis, typhoid and paratyphoid fevers, and whooping cough remained leading causes of child mortality (Guyer et al., 2000). Toward the end of the 1900s, the percentage of child deaths attributable to infectious diseases declined from 61.6% in 1900 to 2% by 1998 (Guyer et al., 2000). During the first decade of the 21st century, there was a shift from infectious disease to unintentional injuries and homicide as leading causes of death. These causes jointly accounted for 47% of all deaths of children and adolescents in 2011 (Hamilton et al., 2013). Today, prevention efforts have led to the elimination/reduction of previously fatal or disabling conditions. Twenty-first-century survival rates for major childhood diseases are high. There have been remarkable declines in mortality from pneumonia and influenza, birth defects, prematurity and low birth weight, respiratory distress syndrome, sudden infant death syndrome, and unintentional injuries (Hamilton et al., 2013). According to the Centers for Disease Control and Prevention (CDC, 2024b):

> Infant mortality is the death of an infant before his or her first birthday. The infant mortality rate is an important marker of the overall health of a society. In 2021, the infant mortality rate in the United States was 5.4 deaths per 1,000 live births.

Since the 19th century, overall life expectancy (**Figure 12-1**) has increased from just under 50 years of age to nearly 80 years in the current century. Infant mortality (deaths to infants during the first year of life, measured as the rate of infant deaths per 1000 live births) has decreased consistently over the past several decades (**Figure 12-2**). Improvements in living conditions, advances in medicine and health

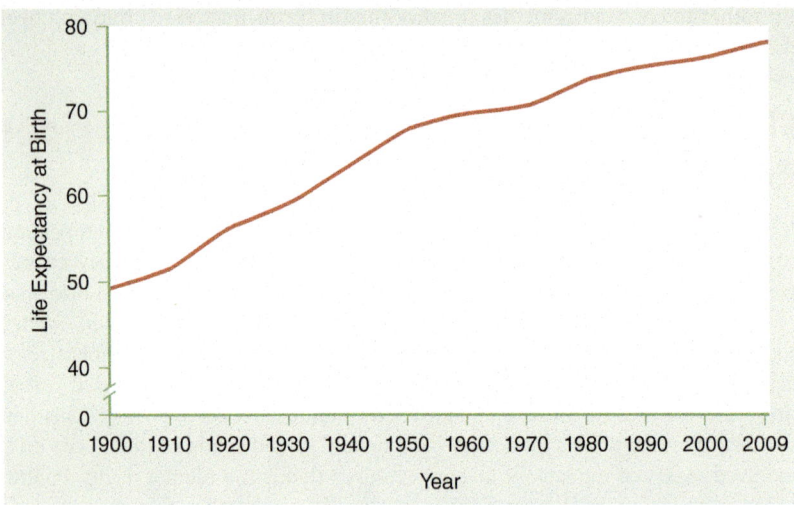

Figure 12-1 Life expectancy at birth in the United States, 1900–2009.

National Institutes of Health (n.d.). *The NIH Almanac: National Center on Minority Health and Health Disparities.* Retrieved from https://www.nih.gov/about-nih/what-we-do/nih-almanac/nih-organization

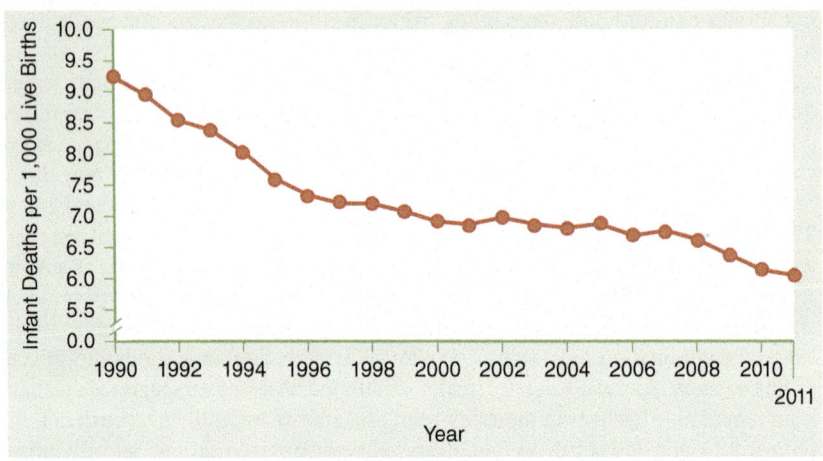

Figure 12-2 U.S. infant mortality rates, 1990–2010, final and preliminary, 2011.

Agency for Healthcare Research and Quality (2003). *National Healthcare Disparities Report.* Rockville, MD: U.S. Department of Health and Human Services, Agency for Healthcare Research and Quality.

care, reductions in smoking during pregnancy, and increased access to, and use of, prenatal care have all been suggested as responsible factors (National Center for Health Statistics, 2010; Singh & Kogan, 2007; Singh & Yu, 1995). According to the CDC (2024a), Life expectancy at birth for the U.S. population in 2022 was 77.5 years, an increase from 76.4 years in 2021.

Life expectancy and infant mortality are vital statistics generally regarded as key indicators of the nation's health. These factors influence policy development as well as research and program funding. In conjunction with better public policies, the nation's rising standard of living, improving nutrition, and income support, programs have also improved circumstances (CDC, 2012). This information is critical to measuring health-related quality improvement and progress toward public health goals for our nation's children.

Issues Relating to Health Disparities

Many dimensions of disparity exist in the United States, particularly in health. If a health outcome is seen to a greater or lesser extent between populations, there is disparity. Despite remarkable improvements in the national health status of children, undeniable challenges remain. The gains have not been evenly distributed. Inequalities have endured for prolonged periods. In fact, the persistence of disparities over time is one of the most arresting features in the history of U.S. health (Satcher et al., 2005). Inequalities have continued (often worsening) despite programs targeting elimination. Over the past several decades, there have been many policy agendas to improve access to societal resources, including medical care. Special initiatives that began in the 1960s, such as the "war on poverty," civil rights legislation, and Medicaid and Medicare have essentially failed. The lack of parity in health for affected groups (including children) has not improved in over 50 years (Williams & Jackson, 2005).

Some children continue to have higher rates of unfortunate health conditions. They also tend to have more barriers to care, poorer quality of care, and unfavorable health outcomes. These differences are best understood within the context of the **social determinants of health (SDOH)**. The World Health Organization (WHO) defines SDOH as the conditions in which people are born, grow, live, work, and age. It is the distribution of money, power, and resources at global, national, and local levels that shapes these unfortunate circumstances (WHO, n.d.).

Likewise, the pervasive (ubiquitous and unwelcomed) influence and effect of disparate health are spread widely throughout various groups of children defined by race and ethnicity. A number of studies reinforcing the impact of race and ethnicity on the health of children indicate that children of color (African American, Native American/Alaska Native, Latino/Hispanic, and Asian American/Pacific Islander people) are more likely than are White children to experience adverse health, growth, and development from birth through adolescence and into adulthood (Children's Defense Fund, 2006).

The disparate issues tied to race not only exist but continue to flourish, owing in part to the conditions from which they emerge: geographic location, education, income, and other sociodemographic variables. Public health research increasingly recognizes that racial/ethnic disparities in health are rooted in these and other social issues (Williams & Jackson, 2005). It follows that disparity in socioeconomic status is a fundamental cause of health inequity in the United States and that health disparities among children are best understood as a combination of the effects of race, ethnicity, and socioeconomic status.

To reiterate, children in Non-White or low socioeconomic status families are prone to poorer health than are children in White or higher socioeconomic status homes across profuse conditions. The profusion of adverse health among poor children and children of color is enumerated in a litany of inequities in morbidity and mortality. This list includes, but is not limited to, incidence, prevalence, and outcomes in infant mortality (Kung et al., 2008), oral health (Paradise, 2012), and childhood obesity (Federal Interagency Forum on Child and Family Statistics, 2015; Wang & Beydoun, 2007) as key examples. A closer look at some of these conditions provides a better understanding of the impact of disparate health on the lives of children.

The Impact of Infant Mortality

Infant mortality is one of the health statistics most frequently used to compare national healthcare systems. It has long been understood as a reflection of how well a society takes care of its most vulnerable citizens and demonstrates the level of commitment to preventing potential adverse consequences of low socioeconomic status. Dramatic declines among all demographic groups represent a major public health success. The preliminary infant mortality rate for 2011 was 6.05 infant deaths per 1000 live births—not significantly different from the 2010 rate of 6.15 deaths per 1000 live births. When viewed over time, however, a clear trend emerges: between 1990 and 2011, infant mortality in the United States dropped 34%. Although the national rate has exponentially declined, disparities in infant mortality remain marked (National Center for Health Statistics, 2010; Singh & Yu, 1995).

In a 2010 publication, the Health Resources and Services Administration, Maternal and Child Health Bureau, reported that during 1935–2007, the infant mortality rate for White infants declined by 3.2% per year, while the rate for Black infants declined by 2.6% per year. As a result of the slower decline in mortality for Black infants, the racial disparity in the infant mortality rate increased between 1935 and 2007 (Singh & van Dyck, 2010). In 1935, the rate for Black infants was 81.9 deaths per 1000 live births, 58% higher than the rate for White infants (51.9 deaths per 1000 live births). In 2007, the Black infant mortality rate of 13.2 was 135% higher than the White infant mortality rate of 5.6 (**Figure 12-3**).

The U.S. infant mortality rate is consistently ranked among the bottom when compared internationally. According to the CDC, the United States has higher rates of infant mortality than any of the other 27 wealthy countries. In 2014, Chen et al. reported that higher infant mortality in the United States is due "entirely, or almost entirely, to high mortality among less advantaged groups" (Chen et al., 2014). In other words, babies born to mothers who are experiencing poverty in the United States are significantly more likely to die in their first year than are babies born to wealthier mothers (**Figure 12-4**).

The Impact of Oral Health

Childhood tooth decay (dental cavities and caries) is one of the most common chronic infectious diseases for children in the United States (Dye et al., 2012). The epidemic affects about one out of five (20%) children aged 5–11 years who have at least one untreated decayed tooth and one out of seven (13%) adolescents aged 12–19 years with at least one untreated decayed tooth (Dye et al., 2015). It is a public health crisis that poses immediate and long-term threats, not just to the teeth of young children but to their overall health and development.

Despite major improvements for the population as a whole, profound disparities persist in children from some races and ethnic groups. In March 2015, the

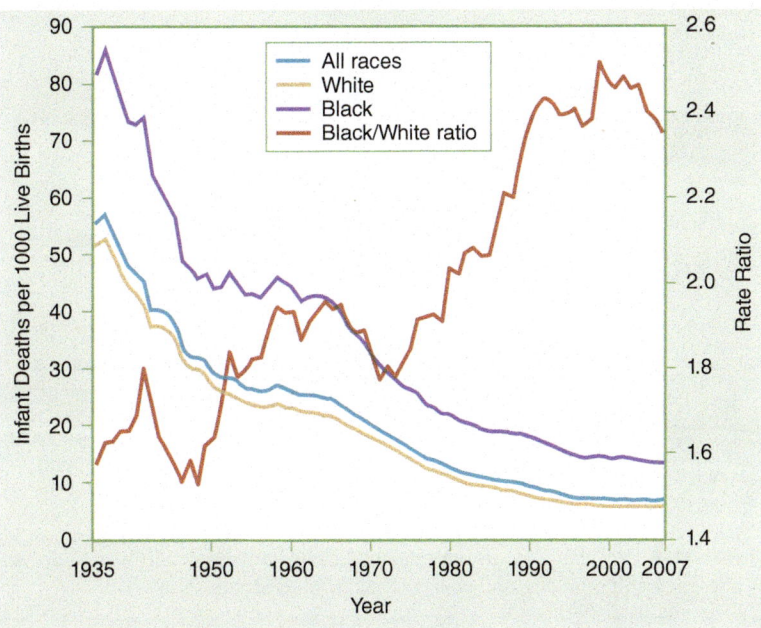

Figure 12-3 Infant mortality rates by race—United States, 1935–2007.

Singh, G. K., & van Dyck, P. C. (2010). *Infant mortality in the United States, 1935–2007: Over seven decades of progress and disparities. A 75th anniversary publication.* Health Resources and Services Administration, Maternal and Child Health Bureau. Rockville, MD: U.S. Department of Health and Human Services.

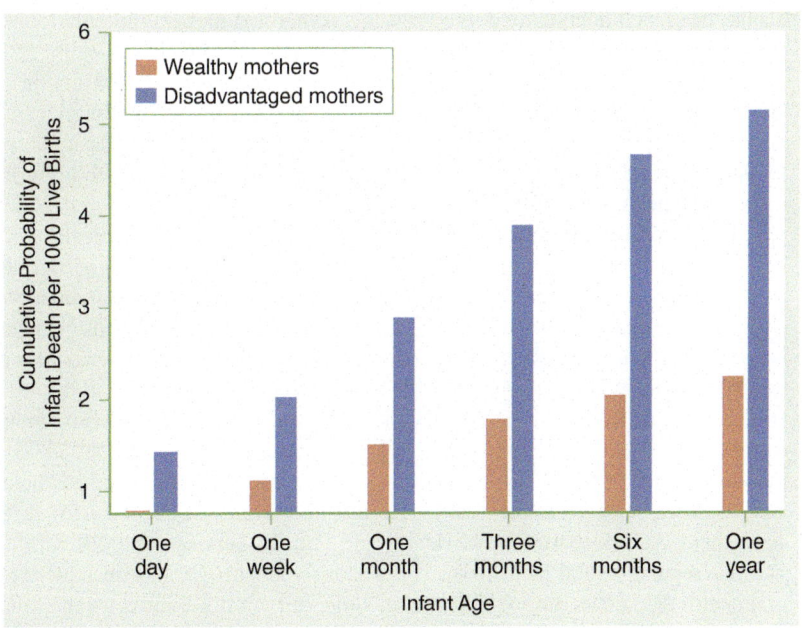

Figure 12-4 A growing income gap in infant mortality.

Data from Chen, A., Oster, E., & Williams, H. (2014, September). Why is infant mortality higher in the U.S. than in Europe? NBER Working Paper No. 20525. Retrieved from http://www.eccbouldercounty.org/wp-content/uploads/2016/07/Infant-Mortality-Brown-University.pdf

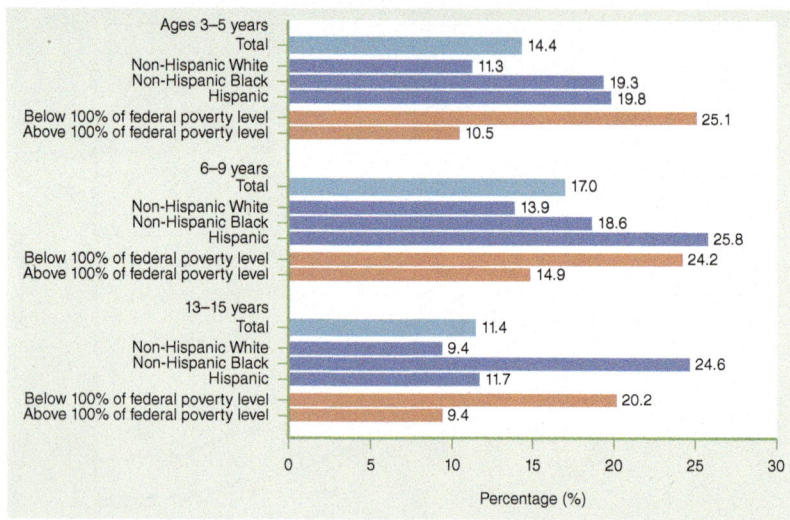

Figure 12-5 Prevalence of untreated dental caries among children and adolescents, by age, race and ethnicity, and poverty level: United States, 2009–2010.

Dye, B. A., Li, X., & Thornton-Evans, G. (2012). *Oral health disparities as determined by selected Healthy People 2020 oral health objectives for the United States, 2009–2010.* NCHS data brief, no 104. Hyattsville, MD: National Center for Health Statistics.

National Center for Health Statistics reported that Black and Latino children are about twice as likely as White children to have untreated tooth decay in primary teeth (Dye et al., 2015). Association between tooth decay and socioeconomic status has been well documented. Studies suggest that it is more commonly found in children who live in poverty or in poor economic conditions (Colak et al., 2013). Furthermore, the burden of untreated dental caries is also concentrated among children whose families are experiencing low incomes. (**Figure 12-5**). The percentage of children and adolescents aged 5–19 years with untreated tooth decay is twice as high for those from lower-income families (25%) as compared to children from higher-income households (11%) (Dye et al., 2015).

Understanding the relationship between oral health and general health underscores the consequences of oral health disparities for children. These inequities are due wholly and in part to complex social and behavioral determinants. Many children, especially those from low-income and traditional emerging majority families, lack basic dental care. The economic factors that often relate to poor oral health include lack of access to health services and an individual's ability to get and keep dental insurance. Oral health has been well established as a fundamental component of general health. Many systemic diseases and conditions have oral manifestations. These manifestations may be the initial sign of clinical dieseases and, as such, serve to inform clinicians and individuals of the need for further assessment (U.S. Department of Health and Human Services, 2000b). Children without regular dental care forfeit this residual benefit. Other consequences of oral health disparities among children include, but are not limited to, the following: children with dental problems are three times more likely to experience pain and to miss school than are children with no oral health problems, and poorer oral health status leads to a greater likelihood of reduced academic performance (Jackson et al., 2011).

Evidence that not all children have achieved the same level of oral health and well-being presents a major challenge. These facts demand the best efforts to address inequities in pediatric oral health.

Remedies

Remedies for children's oral health issues, particularly tooth decay, according to Crider (2023) include encouraging children to brush their teeth often (multiple times per day is optimal), visits to the dentist with consistency, avoidance of sippy cups during sleep, a good diet avoiding snacks that include significant sugar that stick to the teeth or which have a lot of starch, drinking of lots of water, which washes away food debris, and avoiding bacteria exchange with others by sharing utensils and food and drink items.

It is important to be mindful that in order to achieve some of the remedies, availability of resources, health literacy and access to dental care matter. Food choices for children are often based on what is available to them at home. Unhealthy, sugary, starchy processed foods are often cheaper and may be found more abundantly in homes where income is low, as one example. Also, there must be dental insurance if children are to see a dentist consistently. If Medicaid is available, that matter is resolved but other approaches are necessary to ensure access to care with the understanding of why visiting a dentist is necessary.

REMEDIES

Encouraging children to (Crider, 2023):

- Brush their teeth often (multiple times per day is optimal).
- Visit the dentist with consistency.
- Avoid use of sippy cups during sleep.
- Maintain a good diet avoiding snacks that include significant sugar that stick to the teeth or which have a lot of starch.
- Drink lots of water, which washes away food debris.
- Avoid bacteria exchange with others—do not share utensils and food and drink items.

Another specific example of a remedy toward children's oral health concerns, particularly in terms of low-income/underserved communities is a mobile dental unit. One example is the mobile dental unit in Rockingham, North Carolina. The unit was designed to serve children who live in communities where they are underinsured and from families who experience low incomes (Barnes, 2023). There are many examples of these type of units for dental care in communities throughout the United States, often tied to universities, hospitals, Federally Qualified Community Health Centers (FQHCs), and other types of healthcare facilities. These types of programs are very useful and are positive ideas towards resolving a pressing problem for many children in the United States.

The Impact of Childhood Obesity

Childhood obesity, which is defined as a body mass index greater than 30 kg/m^2 and is relative to age and gender, has become a serious public health problem in the United States. The Healthy People 2030 program has an objective specifically

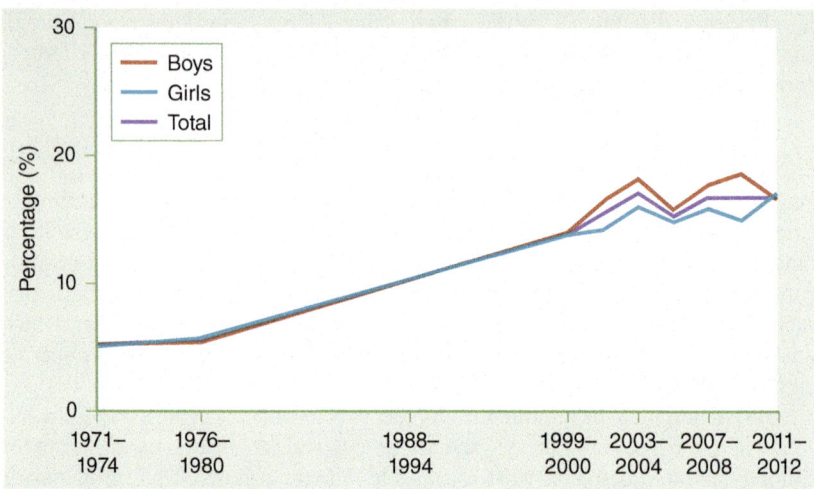

Figure 12-6 Trends in obesity among children and adolescents aged 2–19 years, by sex: United States, selected years 1971–1974 through 2011–2012.

CDC/NCHS. National Health and Nutrition Examination Surveys 1971–1974, 1976–1980, 1988–1994, 1999–2000, 2001–2002, 2003–2004, 2005–2006, 2007–2008, 2009–2010, and 2011–2012; Ogden, C. L., Carroll, M. D., Curtin, L. R., Lamb, M. M., & Flegal, K. M. (2010). Prevalence of high body mass index in U.S. children and adolescents, 2007–2008. *JAMA, 303*, 242–249.

related to childhood obesity, which states "Reduce the proportion of children and adolescents with obesity."

Changes in obesity prevalence from the 1970s show a rapid increase in the 1980s and 1990s, when obesity prevalence among children and teens tripled, from nearly 5% to approximately 15% (**Figure 12-6**).

The available data also show disparities between sociodemographic groups (Wang & Beydoun, 2007; Wang & Lobstein, 2006; Wang & Zhang, 2006; WHO, 2000). The 2015 Institute of Medicine workshop summary, *Examining a Developmental Approach to Childhood Obesity*, scrutinizes disparities in the prevalence of obesity by age and race/ethnicity (**Figure 12-7**). The recent study shows higher rates of obesity during the fetal and early childhood years among Hispanic people and Native Americans. These groups exceed the average rate for all races/ethnicities. Non-Hispanic African American and Non-Hispanic White people have comparatively lower rates, while prevalence exists among Asian American/Pacific Islander people.

Low-income status (below 130% of the poverty level) is also highly associated with overweight/obese status. This finding is confirmed in a recent summary of data from 68 Massachusetts school districts involving 111,799 students in grades 1, 4, 7, and 10. In the 2015 study on the relationship between childhood obesity, low socioeconomic status, and race/ethnicity, researchers found that low socioeconomic status plays a more significant role in the childhood obesity epidemic than does race/ethnicity. In fact, for every 1% increase in low-income status, there was a 1.17% increase in overweight/obese status (Rogers et al., 2015). This pattern was observed across all African American and Hispanic rates in the communities studied.

In the short run, obesity can lead to psychosocial problems (Freedman et al., 2007). In the long term, it often tracks to adulthood. The epidemic has also been associated with other consequences: diabetes, asthma, cardiovascular disease, and cancer. In a 2014 study, the best current estimate of the incremental lifetime per capita medical

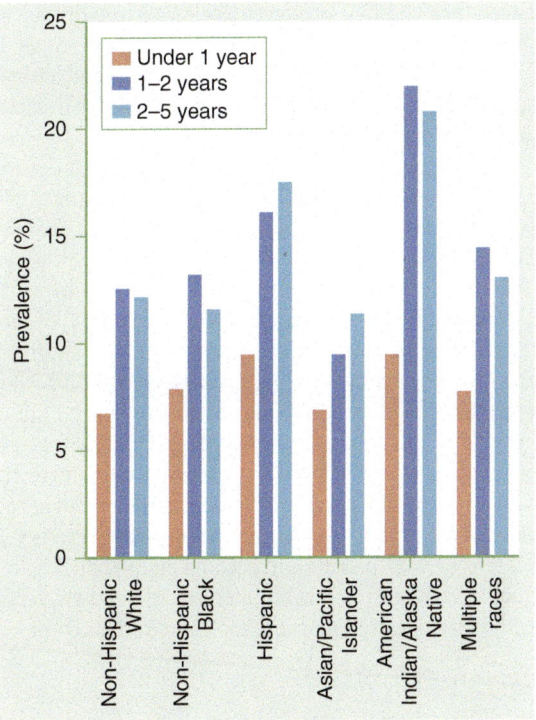

Figure 12-7 Prevalence in obesity, by age and race/ethnicity. Variations in the prevalence of childhood obesity in the United States among different races.

Data from Institute of Medicine (2015). *Examining a developmental approach to childhood obesity: The fetal and early childhood years: Workshop summary.* Washington, DC: The National Academies Press.

cost of a child experiencing obesity in the United States relative to a normal-weight child ranged from $12,660 to $19,630 (Finkelstein et al., 2014). In addition to health costs, there is the social stigma associated with being overweight. It is often as damaging to a child as the physical conditions that frequently accompany obesity.

Remedies for Childhood Obesity

The Harvard School of Public Health, as outlined by Claire McCarthy (2023), recommends an evidence-based treatment approach entitled Intensive Health Behavior Lifestyle Ttreatment (IHBLT), which is:

> … face-to-face, family-based, multidisciplinary counseling on nutrition and physical activity, preferably based in your community and connected to community resources. To make a difference, it should involve at least 26 hours over at least three to 12 months. These programs, unfortunately, are not easily available to most families.

Hence, their other idea is for Pediatricians to step in and see children experiencing obesity regularly and encourage parents to ensure that their children's diets are monitored to reduce the ingestion of sugar-laden drinks. For example, parents should avoid giving their children beverages labeled as "fruit drinks" in favor of 100% fruit juices, and intake of these 100% fruit juices should be limited. Water should be the primary drink for children. Children are also not exercising enough. Children used to spend a great deal of time playing outside and participating in physical activities at school. This has changed as many children spend most of their free time playing video games, engaging in social media, and watching television. According to McCarthy (2023), children should be participating in at least 60 minutes of physical activity each day. This must be accompanied by healthy eating habits.

Healthy People 2030 agrees that a multifactorial approach is necessary to meet the objective specific to reducing obesity in children. To achieve these goals, parents, teachers, and children must understand the importance of proceeding in this direction and there must be affordability in terms of eating healthy, non-processed food. Food prices in the United States have increased radically. Unfortunately, this encourages more eating of processed food, which is unhealthy but cheaper. Hence, remedies are needed at the community/local level, in school systems and policies to bring down inflation at the federal level. Schools must serve healthy meals to children as a start. Perhaps, the provision of information to parents about less screen time for children and the need for them to eat healthy and exercise will go a long way, if information is shared with parents and accompanying policies are put in place at the governmental level, to ensure that children are afforded greater opportunities to experience healthy lifestyles at home, at school, and in their communities.

REMEDIES

McCarthy (2023) recommends:

- Children who are experiencing obesity should be seen by Pediatricians regularly.
- Parents should be encouraged to monitor their children's diets to reduce the ingestion of sugar-laden drinks.
- Water should be the primary drink for children.
- Children should participate in at least 60 minutes of physical activity each day.
- Healthy eating habits must accompany exercise regimens.

Concerns

As racial and ethnic demographics in the United States approach an explosion of diversity, this transformative period is also witnessed in the differences between the people who are experiencing wealth and people who are experiencing poverty. As divides continue to widen faster than ever, ramifications remain unclear. However, without systemic changes, implications for the improved health status of children are bleak. Existing nationwide trends, along with aggravating and mitigating factors, are of primary concern regarding the impact of health disparities on children.

Growth of Emerging Majority Groups

According to U.S. Census data, the nation reached a demographic milestone in July 2011. For the first time, the majority of new members of society (children younger than 1 year) were emerging majority people. These emerging majority people constituted

50.4% of babies born in American society during that period. A year prior, this figure was 49%. In total, 36.6% of the U.S. population were emerging majorities in 2011 (some 114 million people), up from 36.1% in 2010 (Wihbey, 2012).

In 2012, the U.S. Census Bureau compiled updated statistics on changing demographic patterns across the United States. The bureau's findings included the following, as reported by William Frey.

In *Diversity Explosion: How New Racial Demographics Are Remaking America* (Frey, 2015), author William Frey comments, "I think the big thing in the first half of this century will be the diversity boom that we're seeing in this country. It's the part of the population that's going to change everything." Frey explains that the rapid growth of emerging majorities—Hispanic, Asian American, and multiracial people—combined with the slow growth and aging of the White population means that White people will no longer be a majority of the U.S. population. Moreover, "in about ten years we'll have an absolute decline in the nation's White population" (Frey, 2015). With this new generation of emerging majority people, who are having children at a faster rate than White people, the U.S. Census Bureau projects more emerging majority people than White people in the United States by 2044. According to Frey (2020):

> Nationally, the U.S. grew by 19.5 million people between 2010 and 2019—a growth rate of 6.3%. While the white population declined by a fraction of a percent, Latino or Hispanic, Asian American, and Black populations grew by rates of 20%, 29%, and 8.5%, respectively.

This declining growth rate by the White population clearly substantiates the reality that emerging majority people are steadily heading toward a substantiated majority rather than merely emerging.

Implications

From a data-informed perspective, the nation is experiencing a surge in people who are at increased/higher risk of experiencing inequities. The association between income, race/ethnicity, and persistent disparities in health, as related to children in the United States, is well documented. These phenomena continue to evolve in environments not only burdened with explosive costs but proven ill-equipped to manage existing challenges. As current trends continue, so does the need for comprehensive interventions that acknowledge and appropriately respond to the inequities confronting children's health. Until then, concern for widening income gaps and the growth of traditional emerging majorities is not only valid but fraught with discouraging implications.

Race and Ethnicity

Race and ethnicity continue to play a major role relative to health disparities in the United States. This fact underscores a need for closer attention to the next generation's emerging majorities. As seen earlier, people of some racial and ethnic groups have fared worse than have White children with respect to various indicators (e.g., oral health, obesity, and infant mortality). As the nation's populace becomes more diverse and less affluent (as patterns imply), its children will potentially become more susceptible to many health conditions and show higher rates of mortality.

Poverty

Disparities in wealth correlate to disparities in children's health. Poverty, like race and ethnicity, is linked to sustained health disparities. It is also strongly associated with multiple risk factors (e.g., education, housing, access to care) for poor health. Children who experience poverty suffer disproportionately from almost every disease and show higher rates of mortality than those above them. Children experiencing poverty are also more likely to be in fair or poor health than are their White contemporaries (Hughes et al., 2007).

When combined, race and poverty have more severe implications. Poverty factors among the full range of social inequalities to which children from racial and ethnic emerging majority groups in the United States are often exposed. Inequalities in income contribute significantly to disparities in health for children, particularly children from racial and ethnic emerging majority groups (Sanders-Phillips et al., 2009). Poverty and race each involves a myriad of core dynamics. Each has a unique relationship to health outcomes. They are both subject to the positive or negative influence of additional factors critical to the impact of health disparities on children. Two of those factors are *cultural competence* and *discrimination*.

Cultural Competence

The evolving national landscape challenges contemporary mainstream systems to understand and accept differences, engage in self-assessments at individual and organizational levels, and make necessary adaptations to respond effectively. In the face of ongoing change, cultural competence is a major priority. It has been defined as "the ability to [value] understand, appreciate, and interact with persons from cultures and/or belief systems other than one's own, based on various factors" (The OR Briefings, n.d.). It has long been recognized as a "prerequisite to achieving equity in health status" (van Dyck, 2003). This prerequisite is worthy of emphasis. It is an essential ingredient in the recipe for responding to actual and projected demographic changes in the United States. One strategy is to ensure a diverse workforce of public health professionals in the most affected communities. (See Appendices II, III, and IV for cultural competence assessment surveys.)

In recognition of the underrepresentation of people from racial and ethnic emerging majority groups in the public health professions, researchers have concluded that a workforce resembling the society it serves is likely to be more effective in improving health equity in the United States (Duffus et al., 2014). Without a culturally competent infrastructure to appropriately address health disparities among emerging majority populations, elimination of the problem is unlikely. With growing national diversity, the disparity between the racial and ethnic composition of the healthcare workforce and that of U.S. children widens as well. A system that incorporates and promotes awareness of cultural differences without assigning positive or negative values will be better enabled to serve the diverse patient population.

Discrimination

It is a basic principle of public health that all people, including children, have a right to reach their full health potential. The existence of disparities, particularly among children separated by race and income, is compelling evidence that realization of this right is without equity. Whether requisite and necessary environmental changes, such as social and political policy and supportive behaviors, will keep pace with the changing demography remains to be seen.

Historically, **discrimination**, defined as unjust or prejudicial treatment, has played a significant, if not deliberate, role in establishing and maintaining social imbalances in employment, income, housing, education, and health status. In a 2010 study on child and adolescent health, researchers described racial/ethnic discrimination as the foundation for the proximate causes of the social determinants of racial/ethnic disparities in health (Price et al., 2010). Given current demographic changes, implications for the future impact of health disparities on children from racial and ethnic emerging majority groups suggest uncertainty. Despite the proliferation of traditional emerging majority children, an optimistic outlook may be premature. History has shown that neither discrimination nor its consequences are easily eliminated. While the Civil Rights Act of 1964 prohibited discrimination, it did not eliminate discriminatory practices already embedded in the nation's structures and institutions. Subsequent court rulings and changes in statutes have continued for more than 50 years in response to sustained discriminatory treatment. How these and other compelling implications are confronted and managed will prove essential to addressing the impact of health disparities on children. Their resolution is key to successful implementation of comprehensive solutions.

Remedies

The nation's anticipation of health equity for children found tremendous support in the new millennium. Federal agencies, national and local coalitions, and other groups came together in support of this cause. In the United States, the elimination of health disparities in children has been historically addressed by a fragmented network, characterized by a series of knee-jerk reactions often referred to as action plans, initiatives, strategies, programs, interventions, or similar buzzwords. Collective stopgap measures have typically been adopted by the federal or state public health authorities in conjunction with local partners to include, among other parties, community health centers and grassroots organizations. Agencies often operate on short-term, shoestring budgets acquired via intense competition for limited funding. Typically, program longevity is highly dependent upon the availability of financial support. Features have included behavioral interventions (focusing on diet and exercise), screenings (for oral health, obesity, etc.), and public awareness campaigns. This list of popular strategies is not exhaustive but includes common public health promotion and health education programs introduced to priority populations. Various health status analyses suggest that continuing the patchwork methodology is not likely to support the federal vision for health care. Leading performance indicators have demonstrated little improvement over the past several decades. The DHHS vision to eliminate health disparities will remain elusive within the current dystopia. In order for remedies to work, this must change.

The present model for elimination of this nationwide catastrophe is unsustainable due to ongoing challenges. There is a lack of foundation to tackle and overcome aggravating factors. Health disparities occur across a broad range of dimensions, including poverty, discrimination, and other national crises. Reliance on myopic interventions has consistently proven ineffective. In the absence of a magic bullet, a more systemic resolution is in order. It should include the following essential components.

Transformation

A strong and supportive infrastructure of communities and public health systems is essential to the success of any proposed remedy to the national crisis: *health disparities and the impact on the lives of children*. Continued adjustments to our current (failed) system don't work. Starting anew with the development of an overall (all-encompassing) framework is promising. It is a remedy that will require cooperation across industry sectors and governments, and thereby challenge the current boundaries and established norms of operation.

Transforming the current system into one of greater value and functionality will require abandonment of the traditional practices that created barriers to advancing the health of racial and ethnic minorities and the poor. These efforts include unconventional linkages between health care and social service agencies that promote health and well-being within specific geographic areas and among specific populations.

Infrastructure

One integrated/interagency, generalized action plan with individual agency responsibilities centered on shared goals and objectives is in order. Without appropriate physical and organizational composition, sustainability is unlikely. It requires effective, accountable, and inclusive participation at all levels. At times, the United States is one country. At other times, it is a collection of states. For example, every state has its own version of privacy and security. Even some municipalities have weighed in and created their own unique framework. Each framework is the same as a unique language. When one group does not understand the other, communication is impossible. A transformed infrastructure free of fragmentation would provide assistance to patients and families across providers and care settings.

Funding

Most communities and public health systems are committed to doing the right thing, but the finances are not aligned. Public health systems across the country have wonderful plans, all showing positive returns on investment, yet they cannot get the needed funding to see them through. This is a key issue that must be addressed. Sufficient/substantial funding directed towards the children of the United States, health-wise and beyond. Recognition that children are the future of the United States warrants ensuring that their needs are met. Healthy People 2030 has laudable objectives but in order for children to thrive, they must be achieved.

The Impact of SDOH

The SDOH significantly affect health status and are at the core of racial and ethnic disparities. For example, education and income impact access to the resources necessary for health maintenance. Proactively addressing the SDOH must be part of any proposed remedies. A participatory approach (buy-in) to understanding and addressing the issues increases the chances of resolving them over the long term. At the local level, community health assessments (National Center for Chronic Disease Prevention and Health Promotion [U.S.]. Division of Adult and Community Health, 2010a) have helped to articulate what the social determinants are in a particular geographic area. Such a strategy can identify the need for specific, community-based actions. A comprehensive system that identifies these issues would be equipped to readily address and resolve them.

Since discrimination (and its side effects) has been described as the foundation for proximate causes of the social determinants of racial and ethnic disparities (Price et al., 2010), a broad-based strategy for the elimination of health disparities in children must include advocacy for necessary changes or implementations in law, policy, and practices relative to discrimination. Addressing determinants of health related to personal choices/behavior and the social environment is a remedy requiring continued emphasis.

Data Management System

Oversight of data is essential to ensure system effectiveness and should include monitoring and evaluating results over time and the ongoing use of data to develop, implement, and refine solutions. The use of collected information will lead the transformation from documenting health disparities toward eliminating them. Monitoring key performance indicators should occur at regularly scheduled intervals and be reported annually.

Sustainability

Broad-based (comprehensive) strategies for a sustainable system must be implemented in conjunction with appropriate public policy modifications to address social issues that lie at the root of disparities. Effective broad-based systems manage and integrate controlling factors in such a way that optimum health is realized regardless of race, ethnicity, or socioeconomic status. Maximizing quality of care and emphasizing prevention, screening, routine care, and chronic disease management help to cut direct and indirect healthcare costs and reduce financial drains on the system that threaten sustainability.

Education Awareness and Access

A renewed commitment to prevention, with an emphasis on strengthening community-based approaches to reduce high-risk behaviors, will include creating environments that promote wellness and healthy behaviors to prevent and control chronic diseases and their risk factors. Efforts for continued improvement toward access to care must continue. There must be serious steps to ensure health literacy for children and their parents. This can take place in relevant spaces including schools, in pediatrician's offices, community health centers, hospitals, in communities and wherever children are present.

REMEDIES

- End the patchwork methodology currently in place to support the federal vision for health care improvement for children in the United States.
- Implementation of a strong and supportive infrastructure of communities and public health systems is essential to the success of any proposed remedy to the national crisis pertaining to children and health.
- The creation of a transformed infrastructure, free of fragmentation, would provide assistance to patients and families across providers and care settings, with a particular emphasis on children.
- The provision of sufficient/substantial funding directed toward the children of the United States, health-wise and beyond, recognizing that children are the future.
- Meet the Healthy People 2030 objectives for children.
- Maximize quality of care for children and emphasize prevention, screening, routine care, and chronic disease management to help cut direct and indirect healthcare costs and reduce financial drains on the system that threaten sustainability.
- Ensure health literacy for children and their parents.

WRAP-UP

The harsh reality of health disparities among children remains a persistent problem in the United States. It has led to certain groups experiencing worse health outcomes. While these imbalances are commonly viewed through the lens of race and ethnicity, they occur across a broad range of dimensions (such as poverty and education) and reflect a complex set of individual, social, and environmental factors. These disparities limit continued improvement in the nation's overall health status and result in diminished quality of life, loss of income, and other unnecessary costs. The issue becomes increasingly important to address as the nation's children become more economically divided and racially diverse. After decades of increased federal, state, and local focus and initiatives to reduce and/or eliminate health disparities, significant barriers to progress remain.

Although this sounds bleak, the reality is that the increasingly diverse population of the United States is good news and calls for broad and integrated efforts toward resolving the broad-based health issues impacting children, examples of which are presented in this chapter. A forward thinking, positive approach begins with an emphasis/focus on remedies rather than solely focusing on and continually emphasizing the problems. It is time to address the wide range of implications that contribute to disparities pertaining to children, including social and environmental factors, that extend beyond the healthcare system and resolve the issues collective as children are the future of the United States.

Chapter Problems

1. Compared to the health status of children in the 1800s, has the health status of today's children improved or declined? If it has improved, what are the reasons? If not, why not?
2. What role has discrimination played in social imbalance in U.S. society?
3. Explain the problems associated with childhood obesity.
4. Is the infant mortality rate in the United States high or low? Which racial groups are impacted most severely by infant mortality? Why does this disparity exist?
5. What role does poverty play in the health status of children?

References

Agency for Healthcare Research and Quality. (2014). *National Healthcare Quality & Disparities Reports*. https://www.ncbi.nlm.nih.gov/books/NBK578556/

Barnes, B. (2023). Mobile dental unit now open for children in Rockingham County. *WFMY News 2*. https://www.wfmynews2.com/article/news/local/rockingham-county-mobile-dental-clinic/83-36ac2589-d9a3-45ad-af59-58a7be03da67

Hooks, B. (2001). *All about love: New visions*. Harper Collins.

Centers for Disease Control and Prevention. (2012, September 7). National, state, and local area vaccination coverage among children aged 19–35 Months: United States, 2011. *Morbidity and Mortality Weekly Report, 61*(35), 689–696.

Centers for Disease Control and Prevention. (2024a). *QuickStats: Life Expectancy at Birth, by Sex — United States, 2019–2022. Morbidity and Mortality Weekly Report 73*, 293. http://dx.doi.org/10.15585/mmwr.mm7313a5

Centers for Disease Control and Prevention. (2024b). *Infant Mortality*. Maternal Infant Health. https://www.cdc.gov/maternal-infant-health/infant-mortality/index.html

Chen, A., Oster, E., & Williams, H. (2014, September). *Why is infant mortality higher in the U.S. than in Europe?* NBER Working Paper No. 20525. National Bureau of Exonomic Research. https://www.nber.org/papers/w20525

Children's Defense Fund. (2006). *Improving children's health: Understanding children's health disparities and promising approaches to address them*. https://childrensdefense.org/resources/improving-childrens-health-understanding-childrens-health-disparities-and-promising-approaches-to-address-them-2006-report/

Colak, H., Dülgergil, C. T., Dalli, M., & Hamidi, M. M. (2013). Early childhood caries update: A review of causes, diagnoses, and treatments. *Journal of natural science, biology, and medicine, 4*(1), 29–38. https://doi.org/10.4103/0976-9668.107257

Crider, C. (2023, November 27). Treatment options for tooth decay in children. *Healthline*. https://www.healthline.com/health/dental-and-oral-health/treatment-options-for-tooth-decay-in-children

Duffus, W. A., Trawick, C., Moonesinghe, R., Tola, J., Truman, B. I., & Dean, H. D. (2014). Training racial and ethnic minority students for careers in public health sciences. *American journal of preventive medicine, 47*(5 Suppl 3), S368–S375. https://doi.org/10.1016/j.amepre.2014.07.028

Dye, B. A., Thornton-Evans, G., Li, X., & Iafolla, T. J. (2015). Dental caries and sealant prevalence in children and adolescents in the United States, 2011–2012. *NCHS Data Brief*, (191), 1–8.

Dye, B. A., Li, X., & Beltran-Aguilar, E. D. (2012). Selected oral health indicators in the United States, 2005–2008. *NCHS Data Brief*, (96), 1–8.

Federal Interagency Forum on Child and Family Statistics. (2015). *America's children: Key national indicators of well-being, 2015*. U.S. Government Printing Office. https://files.eric.ed.gov/fulltext/ED564158.pdf

Finkelstein, E. A., Graham, W. C., & Malhotra, R. (2014). Lifetime direct medical costs of childhood obesity. *Pediatrics, 133*(5), 854–862. https://doi.org/10.1542/peds.2014-0063

Freedman, D. S., Mei, Z., Srinivasan, S. R., Berenson, G. S., & Dietz, W. H. (2007). Cardiovascular risk factors and excess adiposity among overweight children and adolescents: the Bogalusa Heart Study. *The Journal of Pediatrics, 150*(1), 12–17.e2. https://doi.org/10.1016/j.jpeds.2006.08.042

Frey, W. H. (2015). *Diversity explosion: How new racial demographics are remaking America.* The Brookings Institution Press.

Frey, W. H. (2020). *The Nation is Diversifying even faster than predicted according to new Census Data.* The Brookings Institution. https://www.brookings.edu/articles/new-census-data-shows-the-nation-is-diversifying-even-faster-than-predicted/

Guyer, B., Freedman, M. A., Strobino, D. M., & Sondik, E. J. (2000). Annual summary of vital statistics: trends in the health of Americans during the 20th century. *Pediatrics, 106*(6), 1307–1317. https://doi.org/10.1542/peds.106.6.1307

Hamilton, B. E., Hoyert, D. L., Martin, J. A., Strobino, D. M., & Guyer, B. (2013). Annual summary of vital statistics: 2010–2011. *Pediatrics, 131*(3), 548–558. https://doi.org/10.1542/peds.2012-3769

Healthy People 2030. (n.d.). Reduce the proportion of children and adolescents with obesity — NWS-04. https://health.gov/healthypeople/objectives-and-data/browse-objectives/overweight-and-obesity/reduce-proportion-children-and-adolescents-obesity-nws-04

Hughes, D., Kreger, M., Kushner, K., Pirani, H., & Surie, D. (2007, February). *Reducing health disparities among children: Strategies and programs for health plans.* NIHCM Foundation.

Institute of Medicine Committee on the Review and Assessment of the NIH's Strategic Research Plan and Budget to Reduce and Ultimately Eliminate Health Disparities. (2006). 5. The National Center on Minority Health and Health Disparities. In G. E. Thomson, F. Mitchell, & M. B. Williams, (Eds.), *Examining the health disparities research plan of the National Institutes of Health: Unfinished business.* National Academies Press (US) https://www.ncbi.nlm.nih.gov/books/NBK57051/

Jackson, S. L., Vann, W. F., Jr, Kotch, J. B., Pahel, B. T., & Lee, J. Y. (2011). Impact of poor oral health on children's school attendance and performance. *American Journal of Public Health, 101*(10), 1900–1906. https://doi.org/10.2105/AJPH.2010.200915

Kung, H. C., Hoyert, D. L., Xu, J., & Murphy, S. L. (2008). Deaths: Final data for 2005. *National Vital Statistics Reports, 56*(10), 1–120. https://www.cdc.gov/nchs/data/nvsr/nvsr56/nvsr56_10.pdf

McCarthy, C. (2023, January 23). New pediatric guidelines on obesity in children and teens. Harvard Health Publishing, *Harvard Health Publishing.* https://www.health.harvard.edu/blog/new-pediatric-guidelines-on-obesity-in-children-and-teens-202301242880

National Center for Chronic Disease Prevention and Health Promotion (U.S.). Division of Adult and Community Health. (2010a). *Community Health Assessment and Group Evaluation (CHANGE) action guide; building a foundation of knowledge to prioritize community needs: an action guide.* Centers of Disease Control and Prevention. https://stacks.cdc.gov/view/cdc/5720

National Center for Health Statistics. (2010). *Health, United States, 2009: With special feature on medical technology.* U.S. Department of Health and Human Services.

The OR Briefings. (n.d.). *Cultural competence – Definition and Explanation.* https://oxford-review.com/the-oxford-review-dei-diversity-equity-and-inclusion-dictionary/cultural-competence-definition-and-explanation/

Paradise, J. (2012, June). *Children and oral health: Assessing needs, coverage, and access* (Policy brief). Kaiser Family Foundation's Commission on Medicaid and the Uninsured. https://www.kff.org/wp-content/uploads/2013/01/7681-04.pdf

Price, J. H., McKinney, M. A., & Braun, R. E. (2010). Social determinants of racial/ethnic health disparities in children and adolescents. *The Health Educator, 43*(1), 1–12. https://files.eric.ed.gov/fulltext/EJ942548.pdf

Rogers, R., Eagle, T. F., Sheetz, A., Woodward, A., Leibowitz, R., Song, M., Sylvester, R., Corriveau, N., Kline-Rogers, E., Jiang, Q., Jackson, E. A., & Eagle, K. A. (2015). The Relationship between Childhood Obesity, Low Socioeconomic Status, and Race/Ethnicity: Lessons from Massachusetts. *Childhood obesity (Print), 11*(6), 691–695. https://doi.org/10.1089/chi.2015.0029

Sanders-Phillips, K., Settles-Reaves, B., Walker, D., & Brownlow, J. (2009). Social inequality and racial discrimination: risk factors for health disparities in children of color. *Pediatrics, 124 Suppl 3,* S176–S186. https://doi.org/10.1542/peds.2009-1100E

Satcher, D., Fryer, G. E., Jr, McCann, J., Troutman, A., Woolf, S. H., & Rust, G. (2005). What if we were equal? A comparison of the black-white mortality gap in 1960 and 2000. *Health Affairs (Project Hope), 24*(2), 459–464. https://doi.org/10.1377/hlthaff.24.2.459

Singh, G. K., & Kogan, M. D. (2007). Persistent socioeconomic disparities in infant, neonatal, and postneonatal mortality rates in the United States, 1969-2001. *Pediatrics, 119*(4), e928–e939. https://doi.org/10.1542/peds.2005-2181

Singh, G. K., & van Dyck, P. C. (2010). *Infant mortality in the United States, 1935–2007: Over seven decades of progress and disparities.* Health Resources and Services Administration, Maternal and Child Health Bureau. U.S. Department of Health and Human Services.

Singh, G. K., & Yu, S. M. (1995). Infant mortality in the United States: trends, differentials, and projections, 1950 through 2010. *American Journal of Public Health, 85*(7), 957–964. https://doi.org/10.2105/ajph.85.7.957

Smedley, B. D., Stith, A. Y., Nelson, A. R. (Eds.). (2003). *Unequal treatment: Confronting racial and ethnic disparities in health care.* National Academies Press.

U.S. Department of Health and Human Services. (2000a). *Healthy People 2010: Understanding and improving health.* https://www.cdc.gov/nchs/healthy_people/hp2010.htm

U.S. Department of Health and Human Services. (2000b). *Oral health in America: A report of the Surgeon General—executive summary.* U.S. Department of Health and Human Services, National Institute of Dental and Craniofacial Research, National Institutes of Health.

van Dyck, P. C. (2003). A history of child health equity legislation in the United States. *Pediatrics, 112*(3 Part 2), 727–730.

Wang, Y., & Beydoun, M. A. (2007). The obesity epidemic in the United States--gender, age, socioeconomic, racial/ethnic, and geographic characteristics: a systematic review and meta-regression analysis. *Epidemiologic Reviews, 29*, 6–28. https://doi.org/10.1093/epirev/mxm007

Wang, Y., & Lobstein, T. (2006). Worldwide trends in childhood overweight and obesity. *International Journal of Pediatric Obesity, 1*(1), 11–25. https://doi.org/10.1080/17477160600586747

Wang, Y., & Zhang, Q. (2006). Are American children and adolescents of low socioeconomic status at increased risk of obesity? Changes in the association between overweight and family income between 1971 and 2002. *The American Journal of Clinical Nutrition, 84*(4), 707–716. https://doi.org/10.1093/ajcn/84.4.707

Wihbey, J. (2012, October 25). Census Bureau: Minorities in U.S. growing toward a majority. *The Journalist's Resource.* https://journalistsresource.org/politics-and-government/minorities-in-us-growing-toward-majority-census-bureau/

Williams, D. R., & Jackson, P. B. (2005). Social sources of racial disparities in health. *Health Affairs (Project Hope), 24*(2), 325–334. https://doi.org/10.1377/hlthaff.24.2.325

World Health Organisation. (n.d.). *Social determinants of health.* https://www.who.int/health-topics/social-determinants-of-health#tab=tab_1

CHAPTER 13

Older Adults and Health Disparities: Issues, Concerns, and Remedies

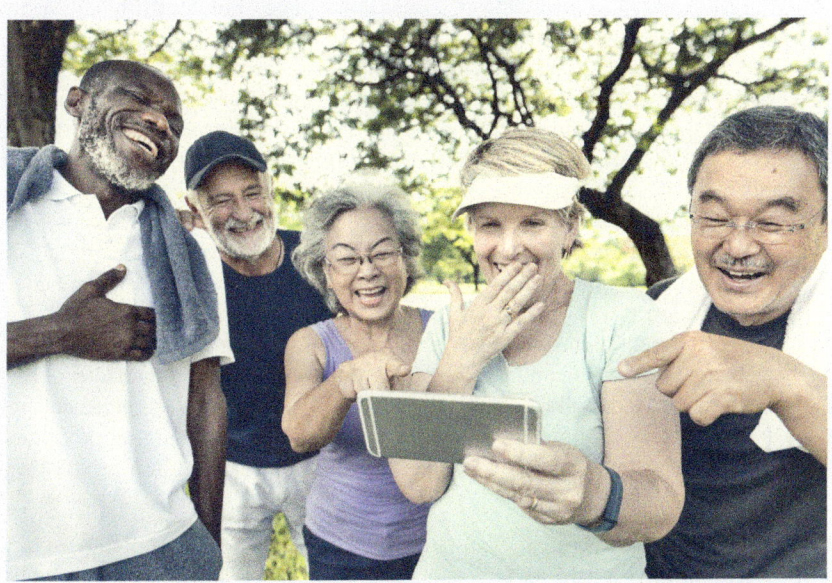

© Rawpixel.com/Shutterstock

KEY TERMS

Confucianism
filial piety
mass incarceration

pharmacodynamics
pharmacokinetics

LEARNING OBJECTIVES

After reading this chapter, you should be able to do the following:

1. Understand selected key issues relevant to health disparities/inequities and the older adult population.
2. List chronic diseases that impact the older adult population.
3. Discuss the impact of mass incarceration of older adults on incarcerated individuals and their families.
4. Explain the term *filial piety* and its relevance to health equity for the older adult population.

Introduction

Respect, obedience, and caring for parents are all key aspects of a concept known as **filial piety**. This is an important part of **Confucianism** and Chinese culture as well as other cultures. However, this notion of providing the utmost care for older adults is not such a familiar concept in the United States, but it is definitely one that warrants serious consideration.

Some fairly recent horrifying incidents illustrate the poor care that older adults receive in the United States. In 2017, during Hurricane Harvey, older adult patients in two Texas nursing homes were left wallowing and suffering in murky, dirty flood-waters when the state did not provide evacuation orders for the facilities (Emily & Branham, 2018). The following year, after Hurricane Irma struck Florida, 11 older adults at a nursing home died when they were left in sweltering heat due to the lack of air conditioning at their facility. Apparently, a tree fell, knocking out the power to the air conditioner and the facility did not have a generator (Kennedy & Slotkin, 2017).

The treatment of older adults in these seemingly extreme examples is woefully inadequate. It is not uncommon for older adults to experience myriad problems. Overall, life for older adults in the United States may involve estrangement from their loved ones, isolation, abuse, over-medication, too many surgical procedures, and more. In fact, abuse of older adults is so pervasive that per the Florida Department of Elder Affairs (2022):

> In honor of World Elder Abuse Awareness Day wear purple on June 15. Why purple? Because purple is the color associated worldwide with dignity and respect, qualities that should be reflected in the way we treat elders. Show the world you care about ending elder abuse, neglect, and exploitation!

Furthermore, in terms of estrangement, many older adults in the United States live alone. According to Robnett et al. (2018):

> Older persons of color are more apt to live alone than older White adults. Specifically, 46% of older Black women lived alone, and older Black men live alone three times more often than older Asian men. However, older men of color were more apt to live with relatives than their White

counterparts. Approximately 14% of Black and Hispanic men of color lived with a relative other than a spouse compared to only 4% of white men doing the same. Older people living alone are three times as likely to live in poverty and less likely to view their economic status as "living comfortably."

Further consideration of the health status of older adults in the United States, per Healthy People 2030 (n.d.-a), is as follows:

Older adults are at higher risk for chronic health problems like diabetes, osteoporosis, and Alzheimer's disease. In addition, 1 in 3 older adults fall each year, and falls are a leading cause of injury for this age group.

Healthy People 2030 further states that "physical activity can help older adults prevent both chronic disease and fall-related injuries." This is one remedy but others must be explored.

Clearly, falling continues to be a significant issue as, per Healthy People 2030 (n.d.-a), falls, the leading cause of injury among older adults, are treated in emergency departments every 13 seconds and claim a life every 20 minutes. In fact, every year, one out of four older adults fall (Older Adult Fall Prevention, 2024); therefore, falls remain a subject of concern for Healthy People 2030 as further analysis and implementation of remedies are necessary.

Other objectives outlined by Healthy People 2030 (n.d.-b) for older adults are as follows:

- Reduce the proportion of older adults who use inappropriate medications.
- Reduce the rate of emergency department visits due to falls among older adults.
- Reduce the rate of hospital admissions for diabetes among older adults.
- Reduce the rate of pressure ulcer-related hospital admissions among older adults.
- Improve cardiovascular health in adults.

Greater efforts are needed to assist older adults to prevent these chronic issues, rather than just treating them after the fact, as they are more apt to use prescription drug treatments to treat chronic problems, compared to other age groups. Treatment currently outweighs efforts to prevent chronic diseases.

Prescription Drugs

The *New York Times* recently published an article entitled "Older Americans Are Awash in antibiotics." As stated by Span (2019) in this piece, "The drugs are not just overprescribed. They often pose special risks to older patients, including tendon problems, nerve damage and mental health issues."

According to Robnett et al. (2018), "advances in medicine and technology have extended life expectancy, and with that, the numbers of drugs used by the average older patient has increased dramatically (p. 58)." Due to the many chronic diseases experienced by the older population, as mentioned earlier, there is a great deal of pain that needs to be quelled, which is quite problematic as this too leads to significant concerns, including misuse and drug dependence/addiction. In short, Robnett et al. (2018) further states:

> Pharmacotherapeutics in the older adult is complicated. This may be the most challenging area of geriatric medicine. The physiologic changes that occur with aging lead to significant changes in both **pharmacokinetics** (i.e., what the body does to a drug) and **pharmacodynamics** (i.e., what the drug does to the body). The variability of these changes relating to chronologic aging adds to the challenge. The need for multiple medications to treat multiple chronic diseases over long periods of time can lead to even more potential complications (p. 272).

Mass Incarceration and Older Adults

According to Gibson (2019), historian Elizabeth Hinton, in her book *From the War on Poverty to the War on Crime: The Making of Mass Incarceration in America*, states that the "The War on Crime and the War on Drugs are two of the largest policy failures in the history of the United States." Hinton also points that "[a] total of 184,901 Americans entered state and federal prisons. Between 1965 and the War on Drugs less than 20 years later, state and federal prisons added another 251,107 inmates."

The number of people incarcerated today in the United States is staggering and the racial and ethnic disparity is glaring. Gibson (2019) states:

> Today, roughly 2 million people are incarcerated in this country, 66% of them African American or Latino. The United States, with 5 percent of the global population but 25 percent of its prisoners, is home to the largest prison system in the world, with an incarceration rate that is five to 10 times that of peer nations.

This unfortunate situation of **mass incarceration** has also impacted older adults in the United States. In general, when one thinks of older adults, mass imprisonment is not necessarily what comes to mind. Based on this, as one ages, there is a tendency toward chronic diseases and other concerns that would seemingly suggest that alternatives should be considered before warehousing older adults behind prison bars, in confinement. This is particularly true if they are not in a physical/mental condition to commit further crimes. The reality is that the opposite is occurring. Chettiar et al. (2012) states the following regarding the types of crimes older adults are likely to commit:

> . . . [M]ost aging prisoners are not incarcerated for murder, but are in prison for low-level crimes. For example, in Texas, 65% of prisoners age 50 and older are incarcerated for nonviolent drug, property, and other nonviolent crimes.

The reality is that if a person commits a crime, there are laws that require his/her imprisonment, but, perhaps, the frailty of age should be taken into consideration, particularly if the person is unable to commit the crime he or she was accused of or any other crimes as the progression of age takes place. Furthermore, "[a]s is the case with the overall American prison population, America's older adult prisoners are overwhelmingly male. Women make up a mere 6% of aging prisoners" (Chettiar, 2012).

This means that many of the women are left without their spouses and children and grandchildren lose their grandfathers in significant numbers, relative to women in the United States, which is similar to the loss that young families experience when men are incarcerated en masse. Since most of the prisoners who are older adults are men, it creates an imbalance in society and an undeniable dismantling of the family, particularly when individuals are supposed to be experiencing their golden years and a sense of respect from society for their wisdom, including mistakes that others can learn from. This is especially true if there were options other than incarceration for older adults who were convicted of nonviolent crimes. Some may argue that if one commits a crime, one must do the time. However, besides the fact that consideration should seriously be given to age and the impact that it has on the body and minds of individuals, incarceration is a tremendously costly endeavor, as many incarcerated people will need special care to tend to their healthcare needs and daily living activities as they age further.

This subject raises the issue of filial piety in regard to older adults. To what extent, based on the nature of the crime, should older adults be forgiven, paroled, or afforded some other options, which take into consideration that they are nearing the end of life? Should they, perhaps, be given the opportunity to impart wisdom, based on their mistakes, rather than languish in prison cells for extended periods of time, including until death? These questions are worthy of consideration in terms of compassion for older adults and ultimate costs to society in a number of ways.

Nursing Homes

Although older adults in the United States have often lived full lives and have made it to their golden years, it is unfortunate that many are relegated to experiences in which they are not dwelling with their loved ones, but rather in nursing homes. Oftentimes, they may not have a choice. In many cases, these older adults are experiencing health issues that may not require hospitalization, but are beyond what their family members can provide for them at home in terms of their activities of daily living (ADL). Nursing homes generally have skilled nurses, occupational and physical therapy, and other services that may be helpful in meeting their needs. In general, the average stay is less than 100 days, as older adults may merely need rehabilitation and when they improve, home may be better for them. Nursing homes are not free, so in addition to the need for care, there is an affordability factor that includes determining if a patient has long term insurance, Medicaid, Medicare, veteran's insurance, or if a patient can afford to pay out-of-pocket. There are assessments and requirements to determine one's eligibility for assistance.

Interview with Dr. Heather Aaron

Insight From a Licensed Nursing Home Administrator and former Deputy Commissioner of Health for the State of Connecticut (Currently the Chief Executive Officer of Whitman-Walker Health Systems Unit in Washington, DC)

In exploring potential remedies to the problems specific to nursing homes in the United States, input from nursing home administrators and public health practitioners is imperative. In the following interview, Dr. Heather Aaron offers insight regarding nursing homes in the United States. This interview has been condensed and edited.

Dr. Aaron has served in the healthcare industry for 35 years. She completed her undergraduate studies at Quinnipiac University in Hamden, Connecticut, where she received a Bachelor of Science degree in health services administration and a Bachelor of Arts in psychology. Dr. Aaron subsequently completed her graduate studies at the Yale School of Medicine, Department of Epidemiology and Public Health, where she received her Master's degree in public health administration, and Antioch University, where she received an EdD in education and professional practice. Dr. Aaron's experience is diverse, including hospital administration, nursing home administration, and the development of independent housing and residential facilities. She has served as a Chief Executive Officer (CEO), Chief Operations Officer (COO), and Chief Financial Officer (CFO) in hospital systems and in the nursing home industry. Dr. Aaron started as an analyst for Harlem Hospital and Bellevue Hospital in New York City, learning in the trenches, while developing a strong knowledge base of healthcare systems.

In 2010, Dr. Aaron relocated to Connecticut and spent nine years as a nursing home administrator, ensuring innovative methods in the delivery of quality care for the under-resourced, older adults, and other marginalized individuals. Her service included the development and implementation of independent housing and residential care housing for nursing home residents.

Dr. Aaron's focus continues to be the social determinants that affect the delivery of quality care and the steps necessary to continue to improve the standards of care for all. She currently serves as the CEO of Whitman-Walker Health System in Washington, D.C.

Interview with Dr. Heather Aaron

Dr. Rose: What is the essential role of nursing homes for older adults?

Dr. Aaron: The essential role of nursing homes is to provide a loving, supportive environment for older adults. As I describe the nursing environment, you will discover that the definition of nursing homes only for older adults is not an absolute today. In many nursing homes, the average age is 65. In some chronic care facilities, residents can be as young as 18 years of age. All nursing homes are regulated by the state and federal government to follow standards of care and are surveyed by the state and federal government to ensure that standards are met. Over the last 12 years, nursing home guidelines have been enhanced by trainings for staff on person centered care to improve the standards of care. The theory behind person-centered care is that residents should have a personalized care plan that is specific to the resident's likes and dislikes. For example, residents take part in their meals and have a variety of choices. Residents' rooms can be personalized. Visiting hours can be extended. Families can stay in the residents' rooms during the end of life stage. Residents can have their choice of music and many more resident-centered choices.

Additionally, nursing homes have varying levels of care. A typical nursing home for older adults is for someone who can no longer take care of themselves without assistance. The residents require assistance with ADL. If the individual cannot be assisted at home, then they have an opportunity for care in a nursing home. Many older adults may have chronic conditions, such as coronary heart disease, diabetes, and high blood pressure and are in a variety of stages of care.

The nursing home will provide the medical care needed. The medical care is led by a medical doctor who is typically a primary care physician. Specialists are called in, as necessary, or appointments are made to transport a resident for specialist care as needed. The nursing homes are staffed for 24/7 care and staffing is regulated by the state department of public health under the umbrella of state and federal regulation. Many nursing homes are short-term rehabilitation facilities. These are typically for those individuals who have had surgery and require rehab services before returning to their homes.

There are many programs with states to assist older adults to stay in their homes with support. Data must be collected and reviewed to validate outcomes. In a perfect world, all should be able to live out their last years with family around for care, as we pass along the stories of our life for the next generation. It is my hope that we will get back to basics and take the responsibility of caring for older adults in a loving home and a gentle environment.

Dr. Rose: Sometimes, there is significant harm that comes to older adults in nursing homes in the U.S. Why do you think this occurs?

Dr. Aaron: Yes, there have been reports of abuse of older adults and it is indeed unacceptable and should not be tolerated. All offenders should be prosecuted to the highest extent of the law. There are several reasons why this happens, including depraved indifference, power, and control. Some would say that is harsh, but taking advantage of someone who cannot fight back is a cowardly, sick act of violence. To address this in the workplace, supervisors must be diligent in their duties and monitor the floor staff and residents' rooms. The facilities must train staff based on proper standards to enable them to be deployed in the most effective and caring manner.

For example, double shifts are not good, because when humans are overly tired, bad care is inevitable. Unfortunately, not all nursing homes follow the standards of care to the letter and not all state public health departments follow federal guidance for oversight. Background checks are of utmost importance to secure the appropriate safe staffing. Supervisors are to work with residents every day and find out their concerns. Lack of complete, appropriate training of staff is a primary variable in the abusive care of older adults. More training and proper supervision will decrease the incidence of inappropriate care.

Dr. Rose: Describe what you believe is an optimal nursing home setting, in an ideal scenario.

Dr. Aaron: The optimal nursing home would have joy, beauty, and tranquility. The staffing would be: five CNAs (certified nursing assistants) for every 30 residents for each 8-hour shift and three registered nurses for every 30 residents for each 8-hour shift. All staff would have the same residents assigned. Staff will work four 8-hour shifts and rotate. Weekdays shift

(continues)

(Monday, Tuesday, Wednesday, and Thursday), Weekend Shift (Friday, Saturday, and Sunday). Rotating weekends.

All state and federal guidelines of care and standards are strictly enforced.

Poetry readings.

Recreation would be staffed to personalize what residents enjoy.

Weekly trips to museums, parks, theatres, and movies.

Art classes and artwork.

Music and memory programs.

Elementary school choirs visit to sing to the residents.

A robust volunteer program where every resident's room has a buddy assigned that they can rely upon to always visit regularly and consistently.

Keep the environment alive.

Dr. Rose: That seems it would be a very viable and comforting environment. Is there a shortcoming of funding for nursing homes in the United States? How can this be alleviated?

Dr. Aaron: This is a very complicated reimbursement system. The system has private, for-profit nursing homes and not-for-profit nursing homes. Many for-profit nursing homes have a targeted bottom line and projected profits. Sometimes, care suffers because of profit margins. Many not-for-profit rates are enough to provide the bare minimum but cannot afford to provide the quality-of-life amenities that make life enjoyable. The reimbursement only covers medical care. Therefore, things like theater and the arts are not included. Many facilities don't have enough funding in the rate to upgrade facilities. To alleviate the identified issues, I recommend a commission on nursing homes to evaluate the future of nursing home care and decide, as a country, how we want to support older adults as we all have that road to travel.

Dr. Rose: How are nursing homes for the older adults funded in the United States?

Dr. Aaron: Nursing homes are funded by Medicaid, Medicare, private insurance, and self-pay.

Dr. Rose: Is there a racial disparity/inequity in terms of nursing homes for older adults?

Dr. Aaron: The research would need to be done, but from my experience, the nursing homes with the primary payor as Medicaid have some significant negative outcomes and are filled with those who cannot afford private insurance and don't have Medicare as a secondary.

Dr. Rose: What are the training requirements for staff/clinicians that work in nursing homes for older adults?

Dr. Aaron: Nursing home staff comprise the following:

- Licensed nursing home administrator
- Medical director who must be a licensed MD and have admitting privileges to an accredited hospital
- Director of nurses who must be a licensed registered nurse with an active license in good standing
- Licensed nursing staff, registered nurses, and licensed nurse practitioners
- CNAs (certified nursing assistants)
- Licensed social worker or an MSW (Master of Social Work)
- Licensed dietician
- Dietary department director

- Certified recreation therapist
- Physical therapist
- Speech therapist
- Occupational therapist
- Plant and maintenance staff
- Housekeeping staff
- Internal and external laundry service
- Oxygen company and oxygen tank room specified by state standards
- Biomedical waste disposal company and process
- Admissions leaders
- Discharges leader
- Business office providing banking service to residents 24/7
- 24/7 security staff and protocol
- Groundskeeper
- Resident council run by the residents with staff support as requested by the residents

Dr. Rose: What are three main problems in nursing homes that older adults face, along with remedies for each problem identified in your opinion?

Dr. Aaron: The three main problems are loneliness/boredom, disrespect, and the high risk of abuse and neglect. Loneliness and boredom are the result of leaving your home, after 50 years, for example, and moving to a new environment with no family. This is a gut-wrenching event. Residents become depressed. Some get introverted, while others become verbally abusive. Some experience health deterioration quickly, and they are no more.

The remedies are to train staff to understand the issues and be more supportive along with:

- locating family to visit often;
- identifying a care plan that would include the resident interests;
- enhancing activities, internal and external;
- developing caring teams with staff and volunteers; and
- being consistent in delivering high-quality person-centered care.

Disrespect occurs as we lose full capacity of our senses with aging and others in our environment tend to see no value in our input to our daily lives. The nursing home is set up to deliver quality care. To do so, the staff must follow protocol in delivering medication, food, and daily hygienist care. All of these are done on a schedule, including the fun things, such as artwork and music. This routine life may sometimes lead to neglect in terms of checking with the resident for input, hence the feeling of disrespect. It is important to remember that these individuals have made all their decisions in life and at one time may have been a professional who was part of the decision-making process.

The remedy entails understanding that many nursing homes have acquired funding from the federal government on person-centered care initiatives. If done correctly, this program includes training staff to involve residents in their care and decisions about their life at the nursing home. By listening to the residents and working with them instead of dictating all elements of care, respect is rebuilt over time.

Lastly, in terms of the high risk of abuse and neglect, all nursing homes across the country must offer the highest quality of delivery of care. A major

(continues)

part of the delivery of care is the appropriate staffing levels of the nursing home and the appropriate training of staff members. For example, if a resident is unable to help support his or her daily hygiene care, and a Hoyer lift must be used, there will be risk of injury if the staff has not been trained within proper guidelines of the use of a Hoyer lift. A Hoyer lift helps elevate the resident so care can be delivered. If a resident has urinary incontinence and is unable to call to be changed and the staff has not monitored to change the resident as often as required, this resident will be at risk for skin breakage. If a resident is not eating meals and staff does not monitor their intake, that resident is at risk. If the facility does not properly staff and staff is not observing every resident, then that resident is at risk. Every year, there are hundreds of nursing home patients who are older adults admitted to hospitals for dehydration. This means the resident's fluid intake was not monitored, putting the resident at risk for hospitalization. Also, every year, there are hundreds of residents admitted to hospitals for urinary tract infections. Again, this is closely related to insufficient hydration. There are many other risk factors that have been studied.

   The remedy is based on the fact that the Centers for Medicare and Medicaid have been developing a measurement for payment directly correlating quality of care for hospitals. I hope to see a similar structure for nursing homes. State survey processes for nursing homes should make better efforts to enforce the standards on substandard nursing homes. More effort and dollars should be put into additional state monitors providing hands-on care. The current monitoring process should be studied and evaluated for effectiveness. Closing the nursing homes is not the remedy. Correcting the delivery of safe care is better, especially in underserved neighborhoods. Ongoing training and competency testing for all staff delivering direct and indirect care is a must.

Dr. Rose: Thank you, Dr. Aaron, for this thorough and comprehensive detail. The remedies are especially appreciated.

Ageism

Jackson, et al. (2019) ask a very important question regarding health systems, which is: "Are existing arrangements institutionally ageist?" One item in a survey by Jackson et al. concerned older adults receiving "poorer service or treatment than other people from doctors or hospitals." The ageism question is very interesting, as some have the belief that once an individual lives beyond the life expectancy of their nation or what may be considered a normal lifespan, healthcare entitlement should be reduced. When considering health inequity and older people, it is important to determine whether discrimination is a factor.

   According to Vespa (2018), per U.S. Census data, by 2035 it is expected that there will be 78 million people over 65 in the United States. This is because the baby boomer generation will reach the ages of over 65 and it was the one of the largest generations in the United States. Per the U.S. Census data, 2020, the older population reached 55.8 million or 16.8% of the population of the United States in 2020 (Caplan, 2023). With this swelling number of older adults, the country could see greater demands for health care, in-home caregiving and assisted living facilities. It could also affect Social Security.

In general, there are myriad problems impacting the older adult population in the United States. This problem is exceedingly worse for those who are in lower socioeconomic status, as well as those who are members of certain emerging majority groups. Therefore, remedies are needed to try to resolve some of these issues and ensure a better quality of life for older adults.

REMEDIES

Societal emphasis on filial piety to endear greater respect and appreciation for older adults, among generations in the United States. Some remedies are as follows:

- Remove financial barriers to care by supporting expanded insurance coverage and free clinical services, such as screening programs (Kendall & Ahmadi, 2021).
- Work to strengthen safety nets and supports for caregivers to ensure long-term care, safe housing, and retirement security.
- Increase access to healthcare services and recreation by improving public transportation and promoting safe, livable communities (Lin & Cui, 2021).
- Develop community education programs led by culturally sensitive community health workers that reach targeted populations.
- Support policies that ensure livable minimum wages, equal hiring, and fair firing, especially as it relates to older adults (National Academies of Sciences, 2022).
- Engage with academic researchers and organizations that highlight issues facing aging people who are experiencing poverty, such as the American Society on Aging, Justice in Aging, and the National Association of Social Workers.
- Implement research or utilize existing data sources that measure health disparities, such as the Elder Economic Security Index, to raise awareness and drive action (National Institute on Aging, 2025).
- Educate others and broaden the conversation on health disparities to include healthy aging to influence systems-level change.
- Implement policies or programs that fight income inequality and the effects of poverty.
- Re-evaluate and tailor existing policies and programs according to what barriers may exist for reaching older people.

Efforts must be made to educate older people on the use of technology, including computers, smart phones, and understanding and utilization of the internet and artificial intelligence. Many older people are adept at using conventional approaches involving technology. According to Faverio (2022), ". . . adoption of key technologies by those in the oldest age group has grown markedly since about a decade ago, and the gap between the oldest and youngest adults has narrowed, according to new analysis of a center survey conducted in 2021."

However, shortfalls must be targeted and remedied to ensure that older people are not experiencing the digital divide in terms of health information and beyond.

WRAP-UP

It is quite a challenging experience to be an older person in the United States. Health-wise, there are significant issues, and although quantity of life exists in terms of longevity, quality of life, in the latter years of one's existence, becomes a problem. Some of the concerns mentioned are chronic illnesses (which older people suffer from disproportionately relative to younger members of the U.S. population), overuse of pharmaceuticals and the ensuing problems associated with these drugs, and nursing homes and the poor treatment received by older people in many of them. This is by no means an exhaustive list, since there is a vast number of problems that older people experience in the United States. But, it is an opportunity to think about their quality of life.

If one does not die prematurely, to be an older person is what every person will experience. It is a frightening prospect for many, particularly for those individuals who are experiencing poverty and who are from certain racial and ethnic groups in the United States who experience lack of health equity throughout in terms of chronic illness. There should be prevention, not only treatment, which in turn would reduce the overuse of pharmaceuticals.

Additionally, as mentioned by Dr. Heather Aaron in this chapter's interview, oversight is the key for nursing homes. It would be best if older people in the United States were taken care of with love and compassion by their family members. However, when this is not possible and nursing homes are needed, care for older people must be done with respect and the preservation of their dignity. Family members must visit their relatives who have reached later stages of age in their lives, on an impromptu basis, with regularity, to ensure that all of their needs are met.

Nursing homes must be monitored to ensure that no older person is harmed during their greatest time of need. Furthermore, mass incarceration of older adults must end. Medical and general parole must be a serious consideration for each older adult in prison along with compassionate release and community service as priority options. If older adults have committed non-violent crimes in their golden years, perhaps it would be best to have them provide lectures at schools to younger people about mistakes/crimes and consequences.

The remedies mentioned here are merely ideas toward solving big problems specifically pertaining to older people in the United States. Health equity must be in place from the cradle to the grave, without exception, for all members of the population in the United States. Older people must be given the utmost respect, with an emphasis on maintaining their dignity, within the context of valuing and appreciating all that they have contributed to society throughout their lives. The latter years of life are the periods of time in which wisdom must be shared and stored by and from older people, so that future generations will have the opportunity to learn from the lives of individuals who preceded them and sit with them, whenever possible, to garner wisdom and insight.

Chapter Problems

1. Define *pharmacokinetics*.
2. According to Healthy People 2030, how many older people are living in the United States?
3. What are the most overly prescribed drugs provided to members of the older adult population?
4. Identify key factors associated with mass incarceration of older adults and list two remedies.
5. There are important steps that can be taken to improve nursing homes. Why is oversight one of the most important?
6. Explain the concept entitled filial piety and how it can be used as an effective approach to care for older adults in the United States?

References

Caplan, Z (2023, May 25). *U.S. older population grew from 2010 to 2020 at fastest rate since 1880 to 1890*. United States Census Bureau. https://www.census.gov/library/stories/2023/05/2020-census-united-states-older-population-grew.html

Chettiar, I. M., Bunting, W., & Schotter, G. (2012). At America's expense: The mass incarceration of the elderly. NYU School of Law, Public Law Research Paper No. 12-38, NYU Law and Economics Research Paper No. 12-19, Available at SSRN: https://ssrn.com/abstract=2120169

Department of Elder Affairs. (2022, June 1). World Elder Abuse Awareness Day. Elder Affairs Florida. https://elderaffairs.org/world-elder-abuse-awareness-day/

Emily, J. & Branham, D. (2018, August 23). Nursing homes that didn't evacuate as Harvey flooding rose now remain closed as state reopens investigation. *Dallas News*. https://perma.cc/W6Z2-W23A

Faverio, M. (2022, January 13). *Share of those 65 and older who are tech users has grown in the past decade* [Report]. Pew Research Center. https://www.pewresearch.org/short-reads/2022/01/13/share-of-those-65-and-older-who-are-tech-users-has-grown-in-the-past-decade/

Gibson, L. (2019). Color and incarceration. *Harvard Magazine, 122*(1), 40–45.

Healthy People 2030. (n.d.-a). *Older Adults*. U.S. Department of Health and Human Services. https://health.gov/healthypeople/objectives-and-data/browse-objectives/older-adults

Healthy People 2030 (n.d.-b). *Increase the proportion of older adults with physical or cognitive health problems who get physical activity — OA-01*. U.S. Department of Health and Human Services. https://health.gov/healthypeople/objectives-and-data/browse-objectives/older-adults/increase-proportion-older-adults-physical-or-cognitive-health-problems-who-get-physical-activity-oa-01

Jackson, S. E., Hackett, R. A., & Steptoe, A. (2019). Associations between age discrimination and health and wellbeing: cross-sectional and prospective analysis of the English Longitudinal Study of Ageing. *The Lancet Public Health, 4*(4), e200–e208. https://doi.org/10.1016/S2468-2667(19)30035-0

Kennedy, M. & Slotkin, J. (2017, September 13). At least 8 dead at Florida nursing home after Irma. *NPR*. https://www.npr.org/sections/thetwo-way/2017/09/13/550695498/at-least-6-dead-at-florida-nursing-home-without-power-after-irma

Lin, D., & Cui, J. (2021). Transport and mobility needs for an ageing society from a policy perspective: Review and implications. *International Journal of Environmental Research and Public Health, 18*(22), 11802. https://doi.org/10.3390/ijerph182211802

Kendall, D., & Ahmadi, L. (2021, September 8) *Capping health costs for Medicare beneficiaries* [Report]. Third Way. https://www.thirdway.org/report/capping-health-costs-for-medicare-beneficiaries

National Academies of Sciences. (2022, May 5). 8 – Public policy. In T. Becker & S. T. Fiske (Eds.), *Understanding the aging workforce: Defining a research agenda*. National Academies Press (US). https://www.ncbi.nlm.nih.gov/books/NBK588540/

National Institute on Aging. (2025, February 5). Health disparities research at NIA. National Institutes of Health. https://www.nia.nih.gov/research/health-disparities

Older Adult Fall Prevention. (2024, October 28). Older adult falls data. Centers for Disease Control and Prevention. https://www.cdc.gov/falls/data-research/index.html

Robnett, R. H., Brossoie, N., & Chop, W. C. (2018). *Gerontology for the health care professional*. Jones & Bartlett Learning.

Span, P. (2019, March 15). Older Americans are awash in antibiotics. *The New York Times*. https://www.nytimes.com/2019/03/15/health/antibiotics-elderly-risks.html

CHAPTER 14

Artificial Intelligence: A Problem or a Remedy for Health Care?

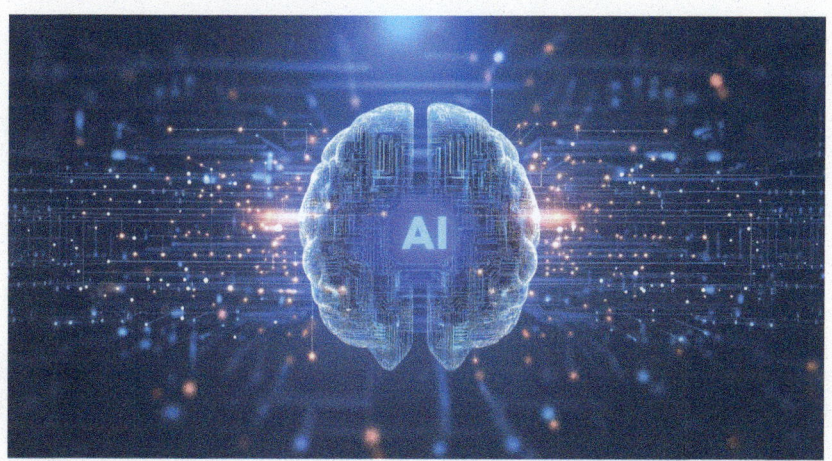

KEY TERMS

algorithms
artificial intelligence (AI)
biometrics

ChatGPT
robots

LEARNING OBJECTIVES

After reading this chapter, you should be able to do the following:

1. Explain the meaning of artificial intelligence (AI)
2. Describe some jobs in the United States that may be replaced by AI both in and out of health care.
3. Identify the difference between AI and robotics
4. Discuss the privacy protection that is needed for customers/patients when AI is utilized in health care.
5. Define algorithm.

Introduction

What is artificial intelligence (AI)? In an effort to determine if AI is a problem or remedy in terms of public health/health care, it is important to understand what AI is. According to McCarthy (2007):

> AI refers to the science and engineering of making intelligent machines, through algorithms or a set of rules, which the machine follows to mimic human cognitive functions, such as learning and problem solving.

The term is also defined by IBM (Stryker, 2024):

> **Artificial intelligence**, or AI, is technology that enables computers and machines to simulate human intelligence and problem-solving capabilities. On its own or combined with other technologies (e.g., sensors, geolocation, robotics) AI can perform tasks that would otherwise require human intelligence or intervention.

On the surface, these definitions seem rather simple, but AI is complicated, in-depth, and applicable to many fields and there are disagreements or different views on the definition. We see it today in terms of robotics, ChatGPT, facial recognition, social media, through our emails with applications such as Grammarly and spellcheck, search engines, SIRI and Alexa, Smart devices, travel apps, banking, streaming apps, and so much more (Marr, 2019).

So what does this have to do with health? There are many challenges in health care that require remedies. As stated by Bajwa et al. (2021), "[a]dvances in AI have the potential to transform many aspects of health care, enabling a future that is more personalized, precise, predictive and portable." But here, we must question, to what end?

AI and Jobs/Livelihoods

The biggest concerns with AI today can be summed up in the question "Will humans lose their jobs/livelihoods if AI plays a significant role in various fields?" To analyze this, it is important to look at where AI has been applied inside and outside of health care and what have been the implications. According to Ellingrud et al. (2023):

> By 2030, activities that account for up to 30 percent of hours currently worked across the US economy could be automated—a trend accelerated by generative AI. He further explains that not all jobs will be impacted but mainly office support, customer service, and food service employment could continue to decline. Many of these jobs involve repetitive actions that could readily be replaced with systems that are automated.

They further state: "These jobs involve a high share of repetitive tasks, data collection, and elementary data processing, all activities that automated systems can handle efficiently." They also mention that fields that should remain intact and perhaps will continue, in terms of growth, are education and training (life-long learning), business, legal professions, management, health care, transportation, construction, and science, technology, engineering, and mathematics, or STEM. Specifically, these authors point out that "[o]verall, we expect more growth in demand for jobs requiring higher levels of education and skills, plus declines in roles that typically do not require college degrees."

The above changes or non-changes pertaining to job loss and job gains are not exclusively attributable to AI. There are other factors, such as a change in the way people are working, post government lockdowns or shutdowns of businesses in recent years, in what were deemed as necessary health measures. Subsequently, new models of work emerged in that many people did not want to return to the office. This led to hybrid models in which people partially or exclusively work from home. This aspect of work environment changes is beyond the scope of this chapter, but suffice it to say that American society is heading toward quite a different work scenario than what is known today, leaving a great deal of opportunity for AI, in all of its various forms, to enter the picture.

As we look at this closely, outside of health care, examples exist to show how automation can truly consume an entity. There is the example of the first fully autonomous restaurant. Per Benedict and Breen (2024), the restaurant is located in Pasadena, California, and is called Cali Express. The restaurant uses a robot, named Flippy, who handles frying, including burgers and fries. The owner of the restaurant laments not being able to get enough workers to handle frying because it is dangerous. This restaurant is just one example, as other restaurant chains also use similar types of **robots**. This type of automation is not AI per se, but the restaurant in Pasadena and others are also using machines for the ordering process. For example, some restaurants take customers' orders through the use of AI facial recognition technology (biometrics) that keeps track of how people pay and what foods they choose. The latter aspect of organizing the process is handled through AI. The initial concerns are where this data is retained and how it is used. Of course, customers are being told that the purpose is not to collect and retain data to surveil customers, but rather about the ordering. The owner of Cali Express indicates that he plans to retain some human employees, but obviously, there will be reduction of humans wherever a robot or automation is in place that can do the work that the humans used to do, for free (**Figure 14-1**).

There must be jobs created to maintain the robots, but it seems quite clear that there will be a differential in terms of numbers. California's new minimum

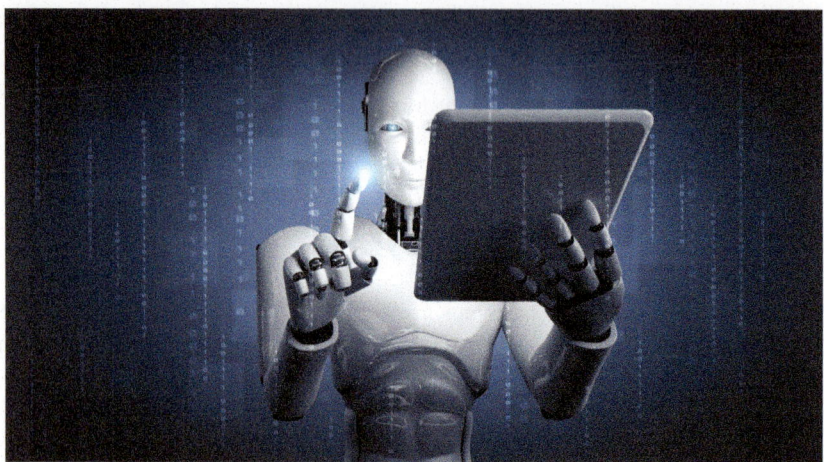

Figure 14-1 An advanced design robot.

wage is $20 per hour for fast food workers, as one example of hourly pay increases. (Sumagaysay and Agrawal, 2023). This is not a position against wage increases, but merely leads to questions about robots. Clearly, no money is paid to a robot. After the initial investment of buying the robot and some maintenance costs, robotic labor is free.

Again, the issue here, in terms of AI, is not the robot that is being used but the facial recognition that remembers what food people are buying and how they are paying. Does this process preclude the customers from being harmed as the data is collected from each person? Where is the data stored and for how long? Will it be shared? Does the customer have a right to privacy around this data collection? These are very relevant questions based on another example of AI facial recognition.

Ethical Concerns and AI

Rite Aid, which is a pharmacy, decided to use AI facial recognition to identify shoplifters. The outcome, per the Federal Trade Commission (FTC, 2023) was as follows:

> Rite Aid will be prohibited from using facial recognition technology for surveillance purposes for five years to settle Federal Trade Commission charges that the retailer failed to implement reasonable procedures and prevent harm to consumers in its use of facial recognition technology in hundreds of stores.

What happened that led to the ban? Per the FTC, Rite Aid's AI facial recognition caused the following problems:

- customer humiliation and other harms;
- consumer's sensitive information was at risk;
- some customers were erroneously accused of shoplifting;
- some customers were falsely flagged as shoplifters or previous trouble-makers;

- customers were not informed that the technology was being used;
- customers were publicly accused;
- people of color were disproportionately accused; and
- the system generated thousands of false-positive matches.

Health Care and AI

AI is rapidly becoming significant in the health care field. According to Price (2019), it is mostly about "automating drudgery and routine tasks in medical practice to managing patients and medical resources." Price further identifies risks and challenges that have to be taken into consideration, "including the risk of injuries to patients from AI system errors, the risk to patient privacy of data acquisition and AI inference and more." It appears that **algorithms** associated with AI can be quite useful. First, it is important to understand what an algorithm is. In the simplest of terms, if you have a specific objective that you want to accomplish, you need steps to do so and they must be clearly defined. Specifically, per Lum and Chowdhury (2021):

> The term implies a set of rules based objectively on empirical evidence or data. It also suggests a system that is highly complex—perhaps so complex that a human would struggle to understand its inner workings or anticipate its behavior when deployed.

The key word here is *complex*. For example, if your objective is to win a chess game, you must know the rules. But, just because you know the rules, will you win every time you play? Of course not. It is because of concepts like anticipation, contemplation, advanced thinking beyond the person you are playing against and vice versa, etc. that impact whether you can apply the rules and out-think the other person. With this being said, using AI in health care will have its advantages, sometimes beyond the human mind, but it is not infallible. There is a significant risk in terms of human lives, privacy regarding data, inferences that may be made, etc., in terms of health care.

Price (2019) points out some of the key roles that AI could play in health care, which include pushing boundaries of human performance, such as medical predictions, democratization of medical knowledge, and excellence. These include sharing the expertise of specialists through images and automating drudgery in medical practice by automating computer tasks and managing medical and patient resources, such as allocating resources, and shaping business. Another area where AI may be helpful is in diagnostics. According to Venkatesh et al. (2023):

> The use of AI for medical diagnosis has found an early home at scale in skin cancer. The complex process of diagnosis can involve integrating data on a patient's symptoms and history, physical exams, lab values, and imaging studies. AI tools, including machine learning and deep learning algorithms, can learn from and efficiently process large volumes of data. Researchers have used AI-based tools to aid in the process of diagnosis in various different contexts, including the detection of diseases of the skin, liver, heart and other organs. Moreover, other tools are made to interface directly with patients and influence their care.

In research by Venkatesh et al. (2023), the benefits and the problems with the use of AI in health care are apparent. In their study, 2.2 million adults were provided with an opportunity (an offer) to use an app for skin cancer detection. The 18,960 participants who used the app were compared with others who did not (controls). The results were interesting. Those who used the app had more claims for pre-malignant (false-positives) and fewer claims for malignant skins legions (true-positives) than individuals who did not use the app. This led to the need for biopsies for those who submitted such claims, and subsequently, higher costs than the non-app users. Essentially, whether for benign or malignant claims, the costs were higher for the app users. There is a clear indication of over-utilization in this study. The authors point out the benefits and the negatives by stating that "[t]hese data fall along similar findings across other areas of digital health, with the benefit of increased access and timeliness balanced by the risk of overutilization." Again, the benefits of AI are indicated but there are inherent risks that must be considered.

Is AI a Problem or Solution for Health Care?

The bottom line, per the examples provided earlier and many others, as AI continues to emerge, it is difficult to determine if AI is a problem or remedy in health care because it is relatively new. Implementation of AI in its various forms, with efficacy studies, would be necessary. However, because AI errors can lead to harm to patients, ethical issues may arise in making these determinations. Data privacy is a major concern. In order for health and medical practitioners to make decisions about patients via some AI initiatives, data would be necessary from electronic medical records, etc. This may cause privacy concerns, subjecting health organizations to lawsuits, as well as invading the privacy of patients. Also, most people do not understand AI, in terms of what it is, why it would be used, and the potential harm that may arise in regard to its use. Hence, it would seem that education is necessary throughout all of the United States to educate people about AI and all of its various forms. In terms of medicine/public/health/health care, this should be deemed as AI health literacy. Without this type of information/insight, informed consent is not possible.

In terms of medical records, use of AI to make determinations about a person's health, use of AI physical technology (such as AI powered clinical robots) and beyond, informed consent would be imperative. Note again that robots are not necessarily AI.

ChatGPT

One of the most commonly discussed uses of AI is **ChatGPT**. What is ChatGPT? To answer that question, one can ask the conversation AI to describe itself. This is the answer it gives:

> ChatGPT is a conversational AI developed by Open AI, based on the GPT Generative Pre-Trained Transformer architecture. It's designed to engage in text-based conversations with users, providing responses that are contextually relevant and coherent.

It is interesting that this form of AI can actually explain to you what it is. Per OpenAI (2022):

> We've trained a model called ChatGPT which interacts in a conversational way. The dialogue format makes it possible for ChatGPT to answer follow-up questions, admit its mistake, challenge incorrect premises and reject inappropriate requests.

Per Hashemi-Pour (n.d.) "Open AI is a private research laboratory that aims to develop and direct AI." Open AI was founded in 2015 by Elon Musk and Sam Altman, and is located in San Francisco, California. Hashemi-Pour (n.d.) also explain the meaning of GPT, which is a "neural network, or a machine learning model, created to function like a human brain and trained on input such as large data sets, to produce outputs—i.e., answers to users' questions." On its surface, it seems like a relatively simple concept. However, it has led to some interesting concerns. As one example, college Professors have experienced the problem of their students using ChatGPT to write their papers. This is clearly leading to concerns of plagiarism and other issues. ChatGPT is more advanced than any other AI platforms of its kind and has gone beyond text to also use voice conversation and images. There have been copyright concerns regarding the data that is used as a basis for ChatGPT, and various copyright holders, including the *New York Times*, have filed lawsuits against Open AI (Brittain, 2024). The *New York Times* lawsuit, among others, raises concerns about the future of this type of AI.

Currently, efforts are underway to utilize ChatGPT AI technology to power robots. As indicated by Kan (2024), the goal is to produce a robot that completes tasks that humans do not want to do. Kan further states:

> [T]he startup Figure, which is developing a general-purpose robot that promises to one day replace what it calls "unsafe and undesirable" human jobs. Last month, the startup announced a partnership with OpenAI to use its AI models to expand the machine's ability to perceive, reason, and interact.

This is an example of a robot (a machine) that can be artificially intelligent, rather than just being created for repetitive tasks. However, robots are another discussion and beyond the scope of this chapter, whether artificially intelligent or not.

REMEDIES

AI in health care must be contained/controlled and regulated to ensure that customers/patients are not harmed. Per the FTC (2023) if biometrics are used:

- Delete collected data within a reasonable time frame.
- Notify customers/patients of the use of AI technology pertaining to them.
- Investigate any complaints posed by customers/patients pertaining to AI usage.
- Provide clear and conspicuous notice to patients/customers that AI is being used.
- Implement a data security program and obtain independent third-party assessments.

WRAP-UP

It seems that it is too soon, at this time, to determine if AI is a remedy for health care. Some would argue that it definitely is. However, given the lack of understanding of AI by most of the population, ethical and efficacy concerns and potential errors that can be harmful/life-threating to people, perhaps more time is necessary to determine if it actually is a remedy in terms of health care. The likely conclusion is that it is a potential remedy for some aspects of health care and as time progresses, there will be a more definitive answer.

The Rite Aid situation, as one example, makes it clear that when AI is used, whether through facial recognition or other means, if consumers/patients are involved, necessary steps must be taken to protect them from harm. Examples of such steps as outlined by the FTC (2023) in this particular example, per their order to Rite Aid, which seems broadly applicable, are to delete collected data within a reasonable time frame, notify customers/patients of the use of AI technology pertaining to them, investigate any complaints posed by customers/patients pertaining to AI usage, provide clear and conspicuous notice to patients/customers that AI is being used, implement a data security program, and obtain independent third-party assessments, particularly if biometric data is being utilized. Although these points are specific to the Rite Aid incident, the need for such guidance, in various forms depending on the circumstances in which AI is used, can be applicable in health care, in general, with some modifications when the matter does not include biometrics.

Per U.S. Department of Homeland Security (n.d.), "**biometrics** are unique physical characteristics, such as fingerprints, that can be used for automated recognition." Healthcare organizations that are using AI involving biometrics and other forms of AI must ensure that customers/patients are protected. This includes all data collected pertaining to them. In order for AI to be a remedy for health care, it must be contained/controlled and regulated to ensure that harm to patients/customers is not the outcome and that is widely understood by the consumer/patient population.

Chapter Problems

1. Why did Rite Aid pharmacy experience problems related to AI and what did the FTC require as remedies?
2. How was utilization a problem for the AI skin cancer screening app?
3. What is the definition of ChatGTP and what are its implications for use in health care?
4. Are robots AI?
5. Is AI a remedy for healthcare problems/concerns?

References

Bajwa, J., Munir, U., Nori, A., & Williams, B. (2021). Artificial intelligence in healthcare: Transforming the practice of medicine. *Future Healthcare Journal*, 8(2), e188–e194. https://doi .org/10.7861/fhj.2021-0095

Benedict, J., & Breen, K. (2024, January 27). California restaurant incorporates kitchen robots and AI. *CBS News*. https://www.cbsnews.com/news/california-restaurant-incorporates-kitchen-robots-and-a-i/

Brittain, B. (2024, February 29). OpenAI hit with new lawsuits from news outlets over AI training. *Reuters*. https://Reuters.com/legal/litigation/openai-hit-with-new-lawsuits-news-outlets-over-ai-training-2024-02-08

Department of Homeland Security. (n.d.). Biometrics. https://www.dhs.gov/biometrics

Ellingrud, K., Sanghvi, S., Dandona, G. S., Madgavkar, A., Chui, M., White, O., & Hasebe, P. (2023, July 26). *Generative AI and the future of work in America* [Report]. McKinsey Global Institute. https://www.mckinsey.com/mgi/our-research/generative-ai-and-the-future-of-work-in-america#/

Federal Trade Commission. (2023, December 19). Rite Aid banned from using AI facial recognition after FTC says retailer deployed technology without reasonable safeguards [Press release]. https://www.ftc.gov/news-events/news/press-releases/2023/12/rite-aid-banned-using-ai-facial-recognition-after-ftc-says-retailer-deployed-technology-without

Hashemi-Pour, C. (n.d). What is OpenAI? TechTarget. https://www.techtarget.com/search enterpriseai/definition/OpenAI

Kan, M. (2024, March 13). Watch this humanoid robot talk and complete tasks thanks to OpenAI tech. *PC Mag*. https://www.pcmag.com/news/watch-this-humanoid-robot-talk-and-complete-tasks-thanks-to-openai-tech

Lum, K., & Chowhudry, R. (2021, February 26). What is an algorithm? It depends whom you ask. *MIT Technology Review*. https://www.technologyreview.com/2021/02/26/1020007/what-is-an-algorithm/

Marr, B. (2019, December 16). The 10 best examples of how AI is already used in our everyday life. *Forbes*. https://www.forbes.com/sites/bernardmarr/2019/12/16/the-10-best-examples-of-how-ai-is-already-used-in-our-everyday-life/?sh=320072df1171

McCarthy, J. (2007, November 12). *What is artificial intelligence?* Computer Science Department, Stanford University. http://jmc.stanford.edu/articles/whatisai/whatisai.pdf

OpenAI. (2022, November 30). *Introducing ChatGPT*. https://openai.com/index/chatgpt/

Price, W. N. II (2019, November 14). Risks and remedies for artificial intelligence in healthcare. *Brookings AI Governance*. https://www.brookings.edu/articles/risks-and-remedies-for-artificial-intelligence-in-health-care/

Stryker, C., & Kavlakoglu, E. (2024, August 9). What Is artificial intelligence (AI)? IBM. https://www.ibm.com/topics/artificial-intelligence

Sumagaysay, L., & Agrawal, S. (2023, December 21). New California laws raise the minimum wage for 2 industries. Others could see pay hikes too. *CalMatters*. https://calmatters.org/economy/2023/12/minimum-wage-2024/

Venkatesh, K. P., Raza, M., & Kvedar, J. (2023). AI-based skin cancer detection: the balance between access and overutilization. *NPJ Digital Medicine, 6*(1), 147. https://doi.org/10.1038/s41746-023-00900-0

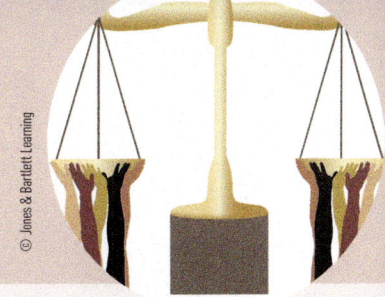

CHAPTER 15

Case Studies: Health Disparities, Diversity, and Remedies

The purpose of this chapter is to review various case studies. The goal for those health professionals who consider ongoing health concerns is not to lament the issues presented, but to generate ideas to remedy the problem(s) that may be applicable in real-world scenarios. This chapter presents various remedies, but the reader should have the aim of adding to those ideas. Readers can agree or disagree with the remedies presented and suggest new case studies based on their experiences in the field of health care. Cases are presented about children, adults, pet owners who encounter veterinary medicine, older people, and people of various races/ethnicities, in healthcare environments and beyond. Remedies, not the problems, are the focus. This book is about achieving health equity and, in order to do so, the emphasis must be on positive change toward ending health disparities and increasing diversity in terms of health care in the United States.

Case 1: Veterinary Medicine

An African American man living in a low socioeconomic community in the city of Baton Rouge, Louisiana, has two mixed-breed dogs and one cat that he acquired from a shelter. He has lost his job, and with it his healthcare insurance. Now living on unemployment and dealing with his ongoing severe rheumatoid arthritis, he is having difficulty caring for his beloved pets. One of his dogs has a problem in which he seems to have to urinate, but when trying to do so, very little urine emerges. The man does not know what to do so he takes his animal to a private Veterinarian near his home.

   As he sits and waits, he notes that all of the magazines primarily show White people and their pets and that there are paintings on the walls with White people in various stages of activity with their pets, including cats, dogs, horses, etc. The Veterinarian, his assistants, and everyone else at the facility are White, except for the receptionist at the front desk. After explaining the dog's symptoms, the

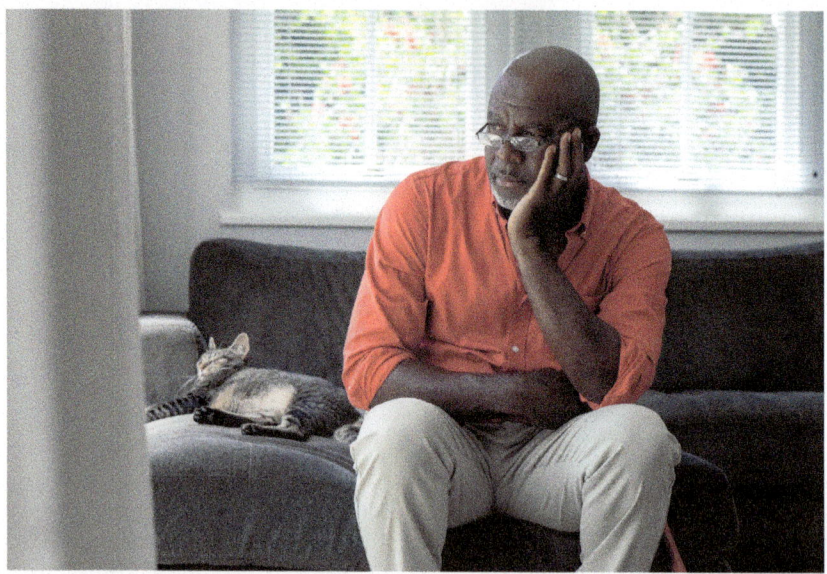

© wavebreakmedia/Shutterstock

Veterinarian advises the man that X-rays and bloodwork will have to be done and, ultimately, medication or beyond will be needed, depending on the outcome of the tests. The man has no money to proceed, so he is advised to go to the veterinary hospital at the nearby university where may be able help him. He does, but with great trepidation, as he is told by the Black woman working at the receptionist desk, "There are no Black people at that veterinary hospital either. I doubt they will help you and yours." He clutches his dog and heads there with worry and concern.

Remedies

A healthcare profession that is rarely included in discussions of health care is veterinary medicine. Veterinarians spend 4 years in professional school, becoming educated in the same subjects as medical doctors as well as public health concerns. Health disparities exist in their field in that there is a correlation between animal health and the socioeconomic status of pet owners. Basically, when people are unable to ensure their own health care due to lack of insurance or accessibility, it can be expected that their pets will have the same experience. In fact, recent research has shown that if humans experience premature deaths in poor neighborhoods, so will their animals. In a study conducted by Dr. Gary Patronek, VMD, PhD, of the Animal Rescue League of Boston and also a Veterinary Epidemiologist, a definite link was established between the socioeconomic status of human pet owners and their health and the health of their pets. Essentially, "[t]he same kinds of things that lead to poor health outcomes in people are leading to poor health outcomes in animals" (Smith & Bonnett, 1998).

Additionally, veterinary medicine is the Whitest profession in the United States (Lee, 2021). The numbers of Black people, and people of color in general, in the profession are dismally low, as is the case with many predominantly White institutions. The man in this case scenario has reason to be concerned. In the first location, there was no visual affirmation of him in the waiting room area. There was nothing to indicate in the images that surrounded him that he was welcome there, hence a seemingly culturally incompetent environment. All healthcare facilities must ensure that visual affirmation in waiting rooms, etc., is in place. People should not feel that they are not welcome because of the images in the room. In a veterinary space, the visuals should merely include a variety of animals without people presented. Otherwise, any depiction of humans with/without pets must be diverse. The receptionist was clearly indicating to him that race matters in terms of the provision of services to his animal. Perhaps the customer should go to the veterinary teaching hospital for care, but his trepidation is due to his concern that he will have the same experience at the next facility. All staff should be trained in cultural competence, which is a skill set. Veterinary schools, and the profession at large, need to diversify so that people will feel comfortable and affirmed in these facilities, eliminating the health disparity of pets of low socioeconomic people of color, as animals need their owners to serve as their healthcare seekers.

Case 2: Tolerance

A Chinese American professor, Dr. Wang, starts a new position as a faculty member at a predominantly White university in a public health program and attends the university orientation for all new employees. Within the context of orientation, a representative of the human resources department announces, with pride, that they have a tolerance program as part of their diversity initiatives. Dr. Wang is concerned about the term, ponders it, and then raises her hand to ask the following questions: How is the term *tolerance* appropriate within the context of this institution? While *tolerance* refers to acceptance, it's usually within the mindset of accepting something that one really disagrees with. Is a parent merely to tolerate his/her children? Should a husband/wife tolerate his/her spouse?

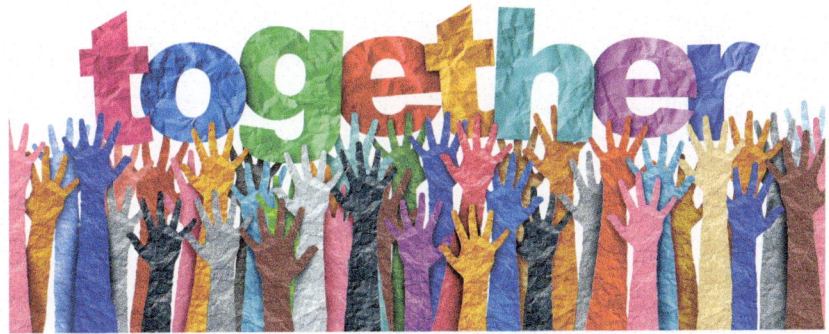

© Lightspring/Shutterstock

What about parents? Should they be tolerated? What about classmates in school? Should they tolerate each other? How about faculty? What if a teacher says to students, at any stage of their education, that in this classroom, "I am going to tolerate your presence?" The answer to some of these questions may be "yes," but is that optimal?

Remedies

In a 2010 article, John Achrazoglou considers the implications of the term *tolerance* (Achrazoglou, 2010):

> Diversity needs to go beyond tolerance. Tolerance is a first step. It is much better than conflict. But tolerance is a somewhat negative word, according to the former lieutenant governor of British Columbia. To "tolerate" and to be "tolerated" involves an unequal relationship. Tolerance implies that the tolerator has the power to not tolerate.

Emerging majorities are members of American society and deserve to be in any place and any space that any other person occupies in the workforce, even if the numbers are low. Often, emerging majority people find themselves as part of a very small group or as the only person from their race/ethnicity in an organization of predominantly White Non-Hispanic people. Emerging majority people do not want to be merely tolerated at such organizations that choose to move forward with diversity initiatives and hiring practices that are inclusive. Diversity is an effort of inclusiveness, to ensure that the workforce is not homogeneous. Homogeneity is not reflective of the American population as a whole; hence, when an organization decides to ensure that diversity happens, it should not be within the context of tolerating people of color, but of valuing and appreciating individuals that will add to a vibrant milieu.

If an organization chooses to have a tolerance program, the term must be clearly defined from a positive vantage point.

But the question is, in reality, are organizations with tolerance programs defining the term this way? Tolerance, if not properly defined, is limiting and demeaning. It is not a step in the right direction. Valuing and appreciating is a better place to begin. Ultimately, all programs using *tolerance* in terms of valuing and appreciating diverse populations should be eliminated.

Case 3: Visual Affirmation

Nurses and staff treated a pediatric hospital volunteer's child, who suffered from cancer and survived, beautifully. This is why she became a volunteer. It was a public hospital, so she decided to give back by decorating a wing of the hospital with art reflective of the varied cultural backgrounds of the patients. Although she is a White person, she realized that the hospital needed to visually affirm the patients and their families, largely emerging majorities, who spent much of their time there as their children were treated. The hospital president supported this endeavor, monetarily and administratively, which led to a wonderful, supportive, diversified atmosphere for the children and their families, allowing the volunteer to feel positive that she was giving back and making a difference.

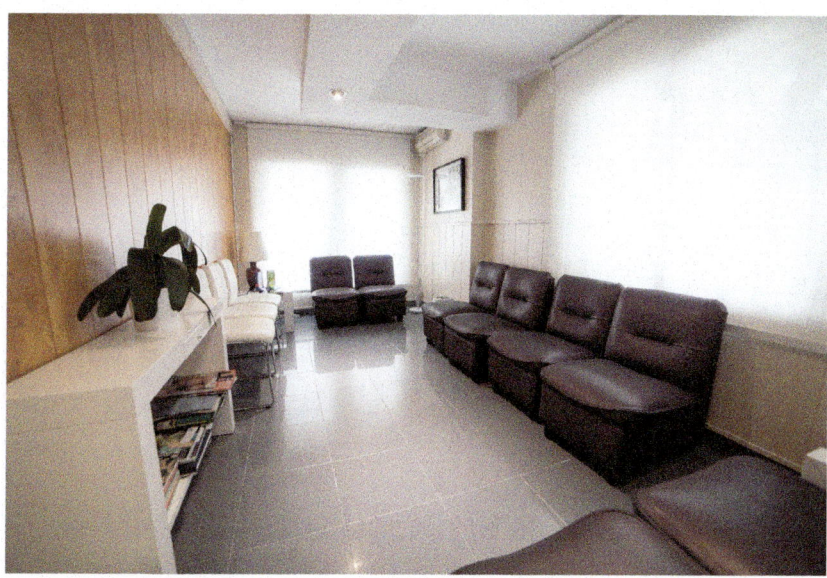

© PabloBenii/Shutterstock

Remedies

Diversity is not merely about the employees at a given organization but also about the environment in which patients/customers are served. Knowing the demographics of patients and creating spaces for them where they feel welcome, comfortable, affirmed, and appreciated enhances the environment of care. In healthcare facilities where the majority of the patients are emerging majorities, the environment should reflect this diversity. Although this is a case where an excellent remedy was applied, generalizing remedies beyond this individual scenario is useful. Hallways and waiting rooms in healthcare facilities should have artwork or images that positively reflect the people being served. There should also be magazines and materials available that are reflective of the people being served. If the majority of the patients/customers being served are Haitian people, for example, then images should be of Haitian people, with magazines and other information in both English and Creole. Visual affirmation is a concept that is easy; it works, and it is the right thing to do.

Case 4: Linguistic Diversity

An older Cuban woman has been in a car accident in Miami, Florida. Subsequently, her doctor recommends that she visit a Physical Therapist so that she can gradually work on her mobility again. Her Physical Therapist is English-speaking and is not a Hispanic person. The family members (her adult son and daughter) request a Spanish-speaking Therapist because their mother is unable to speak any English, having never found the need to learn English while living in Miami. The administrator at the physical therapy facility declines the request, indicating that the simple solution would be to have one of the staff members or one of her children who speaks Spanish present whenever the Physical Therapist is with her. The staff

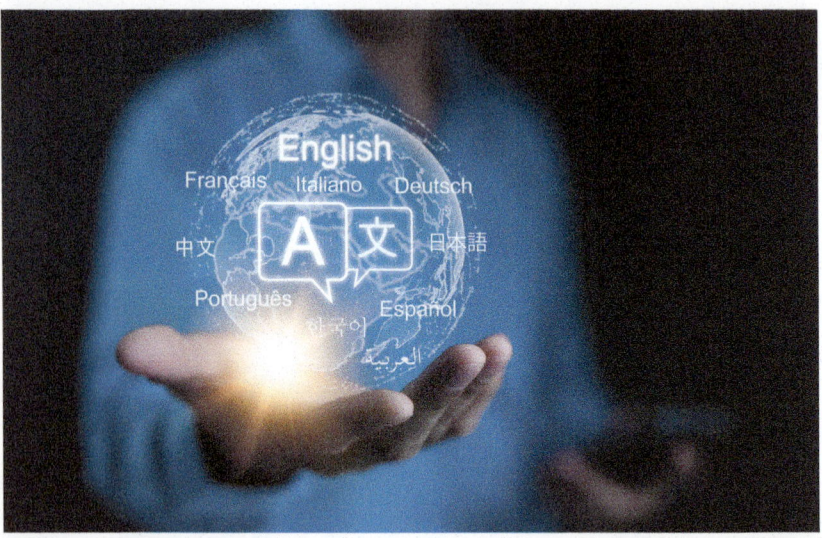

© SuPatMaN/Shutterstock

person selected is not a Physical Therapist, and she is Puerto Rican rather than Cuban. At their first session, the daughter and the staff person get into a conflict in which only Spanish is spoken. The Physical Therapist does not understand their conversation and becomes anxious and frustrated. He is watching the clock because he has another client on his schedule and does not want to be late. Ultimately, the discussion between the staff person and the patient's daughter ends and the staff person interprets the conversation to the Physical Therapist, but by then he is able to work with his patient for only about 10 minutes. The patient is very emotional during the remainder of the session, and very little is accomplished.

Remedies

In this situation, a number of steps could have been taken. First, the administrator should have considered the hiring of a Spanish-speaking Physical Therapist, preferably a Cuban person, given that many individuals seeking care at the facility are Cuban. If a Cuban therapist was not available, a trained, Spanish-speaking interpreter should have been sought, either in person or, if not available, via a language line to ensure understanding of cultural nuances within the communication process, based on nationality. The Health Administrator should have been concerned regarding whether the diversity of the staff met the needs of the clients at the facility. The suggestion of the patient's daughter or a nonclinical staff member being at every one of the client's sessions seemed to be a violation of her privacy and posed a limit to her care.

Linguistic competency must be taken into consideration in facilities that are providing health care. The nationality of the patients/customers is important to consider because the dialects and differences in terms of actual language usage can be quite different from nation to nation even when the same language is spoken. A language line is a good way to go as well as some of the translation/interpretation software that is currently available.

Case 5: The Student Loan Crisis and Its Impact

A young college student who always had an interest in serving low-income communities, given her own rural background, is eager to attend medical school after attending college and completing the medical track. She applies to medical schools and is accepted to several. She needs additional funding, namely a graduate PLUS loan, to complete her financial aid needs. The PLUS loan is a federal student loan that is specifically geared toward graduate students. It requires a credit check. She was not timely with recent credit card payments because she used them to buy books for college and ran out of funds to make her monthly payments. She is denied the PLUS loan and sadly decides she is unable to attend medical school and fulfill her dream to serve in the rural community to help close the health disparity.

Remedies

Given that the current federal debt for student loans is above $1 trillion, with substantial default rates, new ideas besides student loans are needed to assist young people in their endeavors to attend school for medical and healthcare professions and graduate schools. This is especially important in rural communities where lack of access to care is a serious problem. This student should have immediately explored other options, such as scholarships, and approached the universities to find out if they could help her in any way. If a remedy was in place, the financial burden of attending graduate/professional school would not serve as an obstacle. Additionally, high tuition at most graduate schools precludes attendance for potential students. The barrier must be lifted, particularly to assist students in rural communities, as many have great financial need. Programs must be implemented that will allow students from rural communities to attend medical schools and acquire training in other areas of healthcare with low to no tuition, if they commit

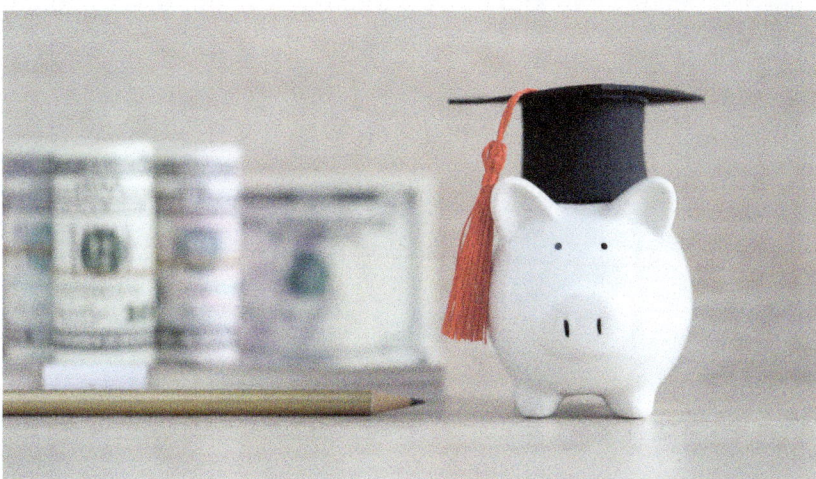

© Monthira/Shutterstock

to serving in rural communities for a significant period of time upon graduation. Payment should be such that these individuals receive salaries at par with those received in urban and suburban communities.

Case 6: Cultural Competence Matters

Melanie is a White Nurse Practitioner at a large community hospital in Los Angeles. She was educated at one of the best nursing programs in a large urban city, and she prides herself on being fair and equal to all of her patients. She turned down many jobs at private hospitals because they did not have a diverse clientele. One day, Melanie is assisting a Hispanic patient who speaks with a heavy accent. As she completes the intake process with him, she becomes a little frustrated and asks the patient to speak more slowly and clearly because she does not understand "Mexican" very well. The patient becomes visibly upset and short with his answers. When the session ends, the patient leaves the room, angrily speaking to himself in Spanish. He was highly offended by her use of the term *Mexican*, as he is from Guatemala, and that she confused nationality with language. Melanie does not understand why the patient was angry and from that point on, she avoids working with Hispanic patients, as she had experienced a similar situation on several occasions previously.

Remedies

The nurse in this case would have benefited greatly from cultural and linguistic competence courses as part of her training or as a requirement at the facility where she is working. Although she is eager to work with a diverse clientele, she is not

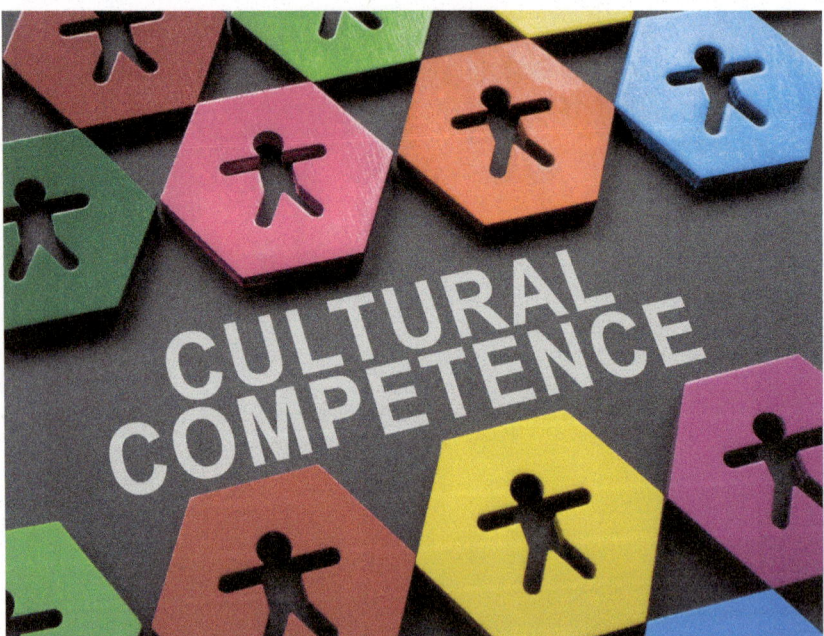

© Vitalii Vodolazskyi/Shutterstock

prepared to do so. She made a tremendous mistake by referring to the Spanish language as "Mexican" and assuming that because the patient is speaking Spanish he is Mexican, which shows a very weak skill set in terms of understanding the nationality aspect of Hispanic people. People who speak Spanish may be from many different Latin American countries, from Spain, or descendants of individuals from those geographic areas. Also, the nurse should have immediately sought out the interpreter at the facility (if available) or used a language line to assist her in communicating with the patient. Cultural competence is a skill set that, unfortunately, many health practitioners are lacking.

Case 7: Cultural Connections

A hospital opens a new walk-in healthcare facility in a community in South Florida where the residents are predominantly Jamaican. The administrator in charge of the facility anticipates that they will be serving a significant number of patients from Jamaica and has openings to recruit several health professionals. He contacts the human resources department and asks them to take this into consideration while hiring. The human resources department decides that because they already hired two African American health professionals, Jamaican health professionals are not necessary.

Remedies

In this case, the human resources department is not recognizing that there are differences between Jamaican and African American people. Although Black Jamaican people are of African descent, as African American people are, the two groups are culturally different. For example, they do not eat the same foods, and so dietary habits would have to be taken into consideration along with health behaviors. Although non-Jamaican people can serve the Jamaican patients optimally, having people who relate to the culture and fully understand it would go a long way. The human resources staff could clearly benefit from cultural competence training, with specific focus on Jamaican culture and beyond.

Case 8: Mental Health

A young Black college student experiences serious health issues, one after another. She complains of lower back pain, pain in her legs, lethargy, and other symptoms. She visits a doctor for various tests, only to be told that there are no identifiable causes for her illnesses. Her mother, with whom she was very close, recently died unexpectedly of a heart attack. She is advised by a doctor to visit a therapist at the mental health center at her school to deal with her grief. Her father advises her that it would be ridiculous to do so. After considerable suffering with no relief, she locates a Black female Psychologist at the center who was recommended by a classmate who meets with her regularly. They work through the grief associated with the sudden loss of her mother. Over time, her physical symptoms gradually dissipate. Her father observes her gradual healing and also decides to see a therapist. He is unable to find a Black male psychologist and refuses to see anyone else,

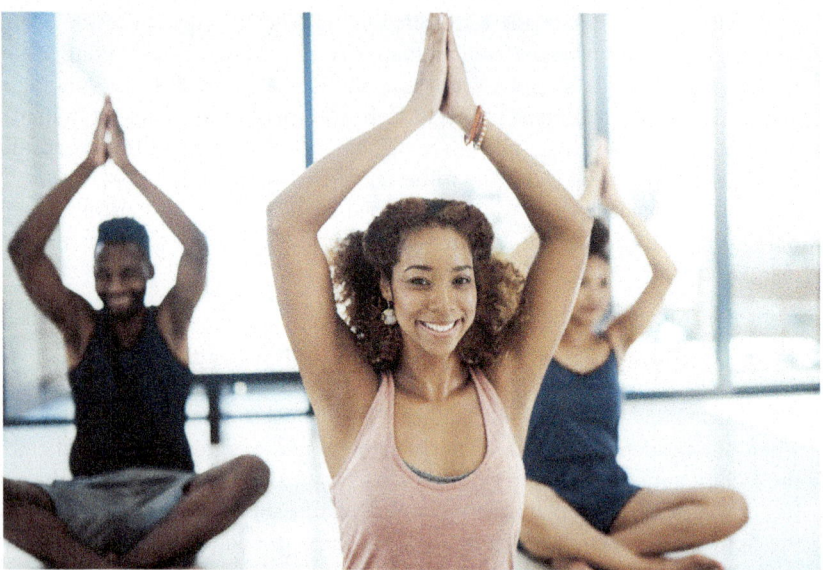

© PeopleImages.com - Yuri A/Shutterstock

deciding that he alone will handle his grief related to the loss of his beloved wife of 35 years. Within 2 years of her death, he also dies of a heart attack. His daughter is saddened but not surprised, as she had heard her father weeping in his room on many nights, grieving for her mother, when she visited him during school breaks. He had refused to discuss his grief with her, or anyone else, and merely endured his pain and sadness.

Remedies

Black men are particularly hesitant to seek mental health care, as pointed out by former U.S. Surgeon General Dr. David Satcher. In a keynote speech for a Black fraternity event titled "Brother, You're On My Mind: Changing the National Dialogue Regarding Mental Health Among African-American Men," he stated the following in regard to the mental health needs of African American men: "We are less likely to seek care because of the stigma associated with mental illness in our community. [But] you shouldn't be embarrassed about having a mental disorder" (Times-Union Editorial, 2015).

Research has supported the idea that race, ethnicity, and culture play an important role in the doctor–patient relationship. Racial and ethnic differences between doctor and patient influence physician communications, but these cross-cultural factors remain relatively unexplored. In fact, those studies that have been done show that communication is enhanced when the patient and physician are of the same race or culture (LaVeist, 2002). Perhaps in this case, if a Black male Psychologist/Psychiatrist had been identified, the father could have worked through his grief under less duress and suffering, possibly extending his life and avoiding his fatal heart attack, as it may have been related to his prolonged, unaddressed grief. Other non-Western approaches, such as yoga and meditation, which can serve to relax the mind and body, offering a calm and soothing effect, may also be very helpful. Such offerings in communities where people are experiencing trauma, grief, poverty, and other serious concerns would provide positive options for those individuals who are not in favor of Western medical approaches, including mental health options, which often involve the use of medication that people are unwilling to ingest.

Case 9: The Spa Effect

A 55-year-old Black woman and a White woman of the same age live in the same city and work at the same office. There is a disparity in their incomes in that the White woman has a very high income and title as compared to the Black woman. The White woman drives a luxury car. The Black woman must take a city bus home after work each day. They both have very stressful jobs, are married, and each has two teenaged children and a toddler. In the community where their job is located, there is a country club that has a very costly membership and no members who are Black. In addition to hosting social events, it has a fitness center, a state-of-the-art gym, including a steam room, sauna, showers, and a spa, to take self-care up to another level. The White woman joins the club and sometimes enjoys time there after work and on weekends, when she experiences pleasant conversations with her peers. She takes fitness classes, such as yoga and cardiovascular exercises, and enjoys the heated swimming pool and other amenities. The Black woman goes to check out the club, hoping somehow she can afford it, but does not feel welcome there. All of the images on the walls, magazines, etc. have images of only White people. All of the workers that she sees cleaning, working in the locker room, etc., during her tour of the facility, are Black and in uniforms, serving others, while all of the people working at reception desks, in the membership office, etc. are White.

She decides not to join based on the latter and because it is too expensive and very difficult to get to by city bus. She has no place for respite to work out in her

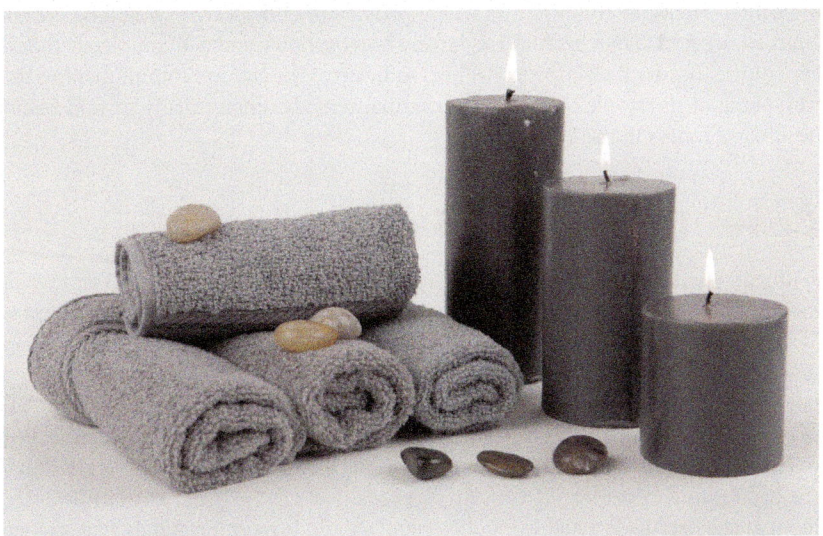

community and enjoy the amenities at the club that her White counterpart experiences and often speaks about at work. Both women are highly stressed, based on their work at the office and managing their home and kids, as their husbands are also very busy. The Black woman finds that she is often very tired, develops hypertension and experiences bouts of depression. Her White counterpart, after joining the club, is refreshed, exuberant and often shares how much she enjoys decompressing at her club, which she says helps to alleviate some of her stress at work. The Black woman reflects on the fact that no place in her community where people are experiencing a lower socioeconomic status has anything of the sort, in terms of recreational clubs, to decompress, in or near her neighborhood. She wonders why.

Remedies

In Iceland, in every neighborhood, regardless of economic status, there is a community pool. These heated pools are not just for swimming but to give community members a chance to relax and recreate. These pool spaces often have a jacuzzi, steam room, sauna, and play and food areas. The entrance fees are minimal and everyone is welcome. Why mention this? In the United States, if these types of recreational facilities were available in every community, it would afford an opportunity for respite from the rigors of daily life. Being able to relax, socialize, and enjoy the comfort of swimming and other forms of exercising at a place where everyone is welcome, at limited costs, would be very helpful. These types of facilities are showing care for the people in communities and providing them with an opportunity for self-care. There are Young Men's Christian Association and Young Women's Christian Association (YMCA and YWCA) in communities in the United States, at lower costs, but there are not many, and they are often not in walking distance of community members and they are not always affordable. There may also be low-cost fitness centers on the outskirts but they are often crowded, have rigorous membership requirements, and are difficult to get to in terms of public transportation. Perhaps ideas toward adding an abundance of these types of facilities described in Iceland in the United States, in communities where people are underserved, would be useful. Granted, Iceland is much smaller, is largely homogenous, and a is completely different culture, but such a simple concept is indicative of a nation's commitment to the well-being of its people. This is one potential remedy among many toward better health and fitness in the United States.

Case 10: The Nail Salon

A Korean woman arrived in Manhattan and found a job working in a nail salon after looking through advertisements in the local Korean newspaper. As she got to know her coworkers on her first day of work, they began to warn her of the hazards of her new job. They explained how one of the manicurist's children was born "slow" and how another manicurist had experienced three miscarriages. They also pointed out that one of their coworkers, who had worked there for many years, had recently died of cancer. Upon the Manicurists' asking her if she was married, she said yes and that she had recently become pregnant. An older Manicurist who heard all of this warned her that she had made a bad work choice and should leave immediately. She advised her that she might lose her baby or have a baby with serious health problems. She

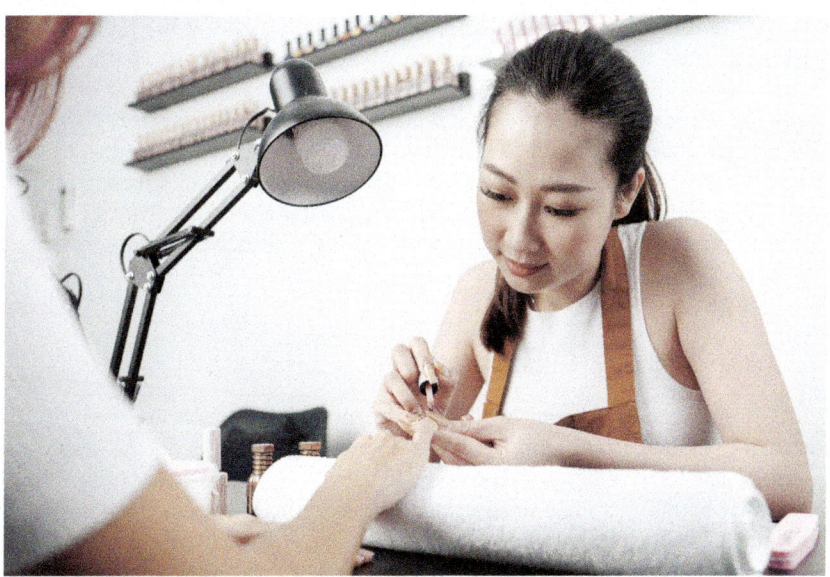

© Dragon Images/Shutterstock

noticed that the older woman had some difficulty breathing as she was speaking. "My breathing problems are from working here," the older woman stated as she noticed that the new, young Manicurist was looking at her curiously every time she spoke.

The young Manicurist, after doing a bit of reading from the material handed to her by the other ladies, in the form of articles and newspaper clippings about the health problems associated with nail salons, the chemicals used there, and the resultant fumes, stood up, took her purse and waved to the other Manicurists as she walked out the door. "I wonder why they didn't tell me this in training," she thought. She never returned to the nail salon to work again.

Remedies

In a *New York Times* article titled "Perfect Nails, Poisoned Workers," which is part 2 of a series on the subject, the author describes an unfortunate situation that primarily affects women who choose to work as Manicurists in nail salons (Nir, 2015). According to Nir, "A growing body of medical research shows a link between the chemicals that make nail and beauty products useful—the ingredients that make them chip-resistant and pliable, quick to dry and brightly colored, for example— and serious health problems." Essentially, this scenario is perhaps a contributing factor to growing health problems that exist primarily among Asian and Hispanic women working as Manicurists. Many nail salons are located in New York City and the wages received by workers are generally low (Nir, 2015). The risks definitely do not seem to outweigh the benefits. So, the young Manicurist in this scenario made the right decision, in the best interest of her and her baby's health.

Regulations must be passed to ensure that individuals are not exposed to toxic products in these environments. In nail salons and similar facilities, information that is linguistically appropriate, must be posted or distributed for all to see, indicating that toxic products are being used. Pregnant women should not be permitted to work in these environments and should be duly warned of the problems and risks associated with doing so. The same advisory should be provided to all customers, especially pregnant women and children. This remedy should be similar to the advisory provided to pregnant women who work in dental offices or utilize the services of dentists, where, when x-rays are taken, they are provided with a lead apron, or the pregnant worker is asked to leave the room. Beyond these remedies, nail salons should be required to use non-toxic, natural products, which currently exist, to preclude harm to their customers and themselves. What additional remedies should be considered?

Case 11: Hair Story

An African American woman, a graduate student in public health, decided that she wanted to launch a research project based on her interest in reducing health disparities. The focus of her project was the impact of the extensive use of hair products used by Black women to straighten and style their hair and the possibilities that the harsh chemicals in these products may cause cancer and other problems. Her research inquiry was based on a literature review that raised speculation about these concerns. She received pushback from her faculty adviser, who indicated that such a study would not constitute a good research project because it was not a real public health issue. The student argued that her research was necessary and proceeded to find a collaborating organization to assist with her project. Her adviser agreed that she should seek out a collaborator, if possible, and proceed accordingly. The student connected with a not-for-profit organization focused on health disparities, which agreed to explore her project with her and to seek funding to do so.

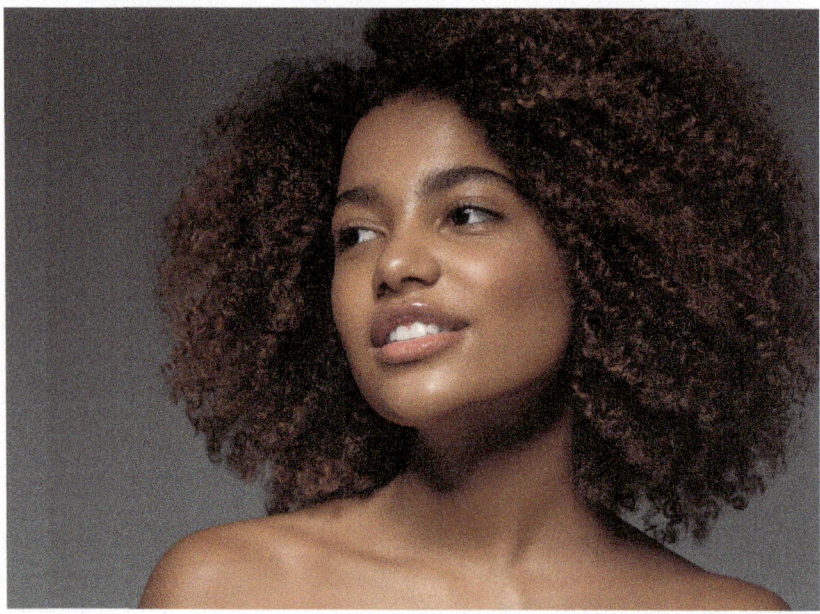

Remedies

Hair is a critical aspect of African American culture, particularly for women, as it has significant cultural and historical implications. During the atrocities of the slave trade, most Black people were brought to the Americas against their will, primarily from the west coast of Africa. This brutal, inhumane process, known as chattel slavery, included removal of the identity of the individuals who were enslaved (cultural genocide). On the ships during the brutal journey to the Americas, enslaved people who spoke the same language or had the same markings of scarification were separated. Africans were no longer able to maintain elaborate hairstyles without their combs and herbal treatments used in Africa. White people looked upon Black people who learned to style their hair like White people as well-adjusted.

Consequently, Black/African American women began to turn to products with harsh chemicals to straighten and style their hair. Currently, there is concern that these straightening products may be contributing to health disparities, as it is suspected that many may be carcinogenic and cause other health issues. The graduate student's project is warranted to investigate whether harsh chemicals found in the hair products used by African American women are a contributing factor to ill health and, consequently, health disparities. Hair products primarily marketed to Black women as straighteners must be pulled from the market. These products must not be sold for use on children, namely little Black girls. Existing lawsuits around these issues must be highly publicized so that Black women and children are made aware of the problem.

All hair straightening products for Black women and children that have toxic chemicals that potentially lead to cancer, or any other health concern, should be removed from the market. Black women should be informed of the potential harmful effects of these products along with advisory information on how to proceed with lawsuits if they have been unknowingly harmed using these products for themselves and their children. Medical practitioners should be advised of the hazards of these products for consideration/discussion with their patients who are using these products. Public health practitioners should conduct extensive research with provision of documented evidence-based publications regarding this issue with potential remedies. This should be a major area of consideration in the above fields and among health educators. Salons should not be permitted to use these toxic hair products. Where usage continues to occur, signage and information must be provided to all customers advising them of the serious risks associated with these products.

Case 12: The Meeting

An Epidemiologist and a Physician meet to discuss the focus of their presentation on health disparities at an upcoming health-related conference. The Epidemiologist believes the focus of their discussion should be on what he believes are the causative factors associated with the health status gap between Black people and White people, with an emphasis on socioeconomic status. The Physician argues that the focus of the presentation should be genetics, as it is his position that Black people are predisposed to those illnesses that are most prevalent among the Black

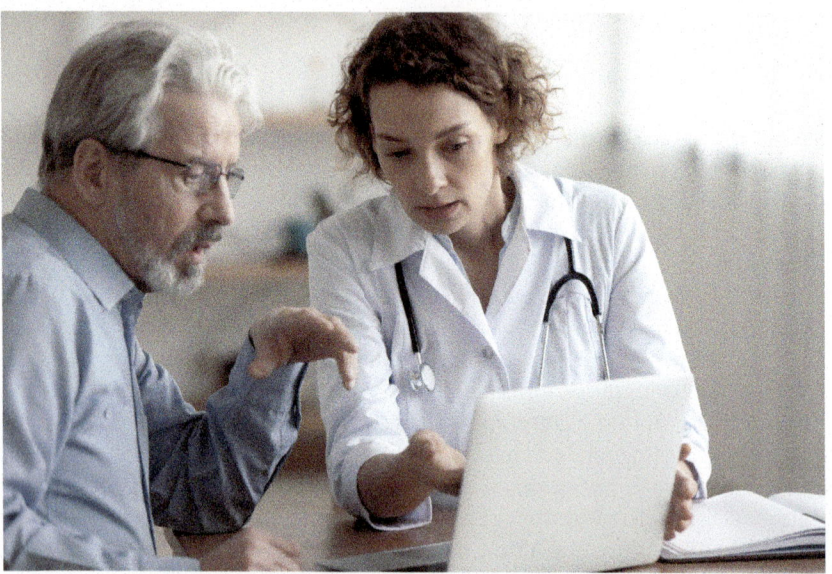

© fizkes/Shutterstock

population. The Epidemiologist asks the Physician if Black people in America suffer from the same illnesses as Black people in West Africa. The Physician is unaware of the answer, so the Epidemiologist informs him that the answer is no, which, he argues, diminishes the genetics perspective. That is, because most African Americans are descendants of West African people, brought over to the Americas as part of the slave trade, it would seem logical, from a genetics perspective, that the two groups would share the same health characteristics, including illness prevalence. However, such similarities are not supported by scientific study, suggesting that an external variable is responsible for the poor health outcomes found in the Black/African American population. The Physician concedes that the point made by the Epidemiologist is an important one, however, unable to agree, they decide to proceed with separate presentations from their respective vantage points.

Remedies

There are varying perspectives on why the African American/Black community experiences poorer health, overall, than the White population. There are many factors, but the overriding issue is seemingly the difference in socioeconomic status between the two groups. A key remedy is to lessen the disparity in terms of income between Black and White people in the United States. This is an oft-discussed topic and for generations this has not been resolved. Until this matter is addressed, the health status of these two groups will remain unresolved. Every effort toward changing this must be pursued beginning with the government of the United States, corporations, banks, and other employers in terms of the provision of loans to Black people to start businesses and buy homes and beyond. What other remedies should be considered?

Case 13: What's in the Water?

An African American woman wakes up in the morning in her Flint, Michigan, home in a low-income community. Like most people, the physical imperative of urinating is first, followed by a toilet flush. She sadly realizes that flushing the toilet is all that the water in Flint is good for. She walks over to brush her teeth and has to use bottled water, now donated to her after her fellow community members, who have been poisoned (based on decisions made by other fellow humans), expressed outrage when city management officials decided to use local water rather than water from Detroit, which had been the case previously. Proper research had not been done to determine if this was a healthy, appropriate choice.

After brushing her teeth, how does she cope with bathing and other uses of water? Warm up bottled water and take a sponge bath every day? What about her two young children, her baby, and her older grandmother who lives with her? She wonders how she will explain this use of only bottled water to her children. She wonders about the homeless people who are already in a dire situation, often relying on water fountains or public bathrooms to take care of their hygiene and hydration needs. What about her dog? What about the stray animals? They drink water, too. Bottled water only? What about the plastic particles in these bottles? Her pipes are ruined from the chemicals placed in the water, which caused them to corrode, resulting in lead poisoning. When will the pipes be replaced? What about the quality of life that water affords all living things? Her questions are endless and she is stressed. All she can do is weep as she goes to her stove and warms bottled water.

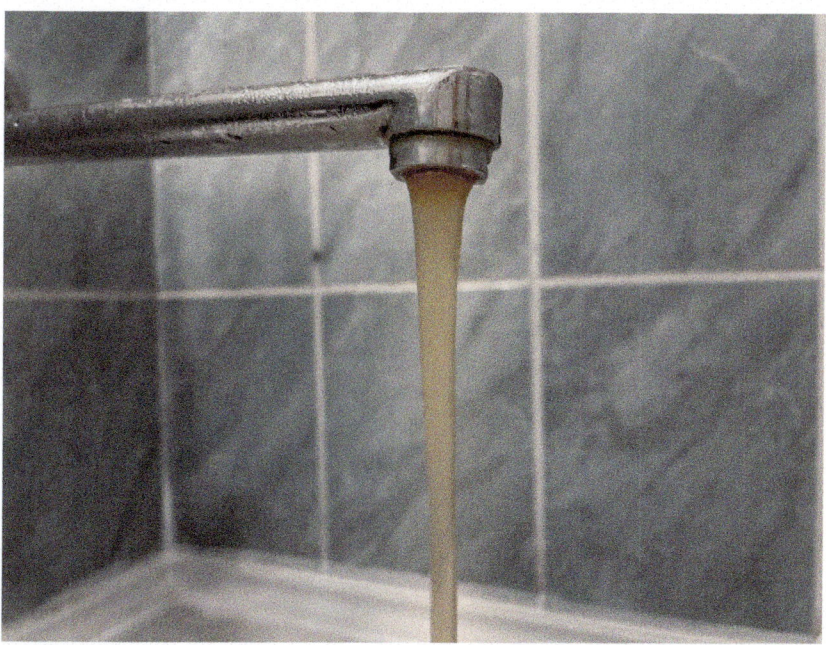

Remedies

Flint, Michigan, is a predominantly Black community with socioeconomic characteristics, namely significant poverty, that have led some to believe that their lives are regarded as insignificant. However, people of all races in Flint are affected. Initially, a state of emergency was declared in Flint, which freed up $5 million in federal aid. A request was submitted for a federal disaster declaration, but that apparently is not available for human-made crises. While this disaster happened in Flint, it is important to understand that there are many more communities that may be at risk for such maltreatment or other types of human-made catastrophes. The what, when, where, and how for these catastrophes should be at the forefront for public health reserachers, given their knowledge, particularly in the area of environmental health.

Epidemiologists and many other experts in public health have the expertise not only to study this matter in Flint but also to ensure that people of all walks of life understand how and why this happened. Water is essential to life and hence to the health of the public. The Federal Emergency Management Agency (FEMA) sent water filter cartridges, bottled water, and water test kits. The actress Cher, in a partnership with Icelandic Glacial, donated 181,440 bottles of water. Other people and organizations also have donated water. This is a step in the right direction but it is not enough. The fact is that this crisis is yet another contributing factor to health disparities. The unfortunate situation continues. There must be a commitment at every level (community, state, and federal) to prevent this from happening and, if it does, there must be a prioritization of the problem, monetarily, time-wise, and resource-wise, to resolve the matter immediately. All community members who are victims of such a crisis should be able to sue and be compensated quickly. The matter should be taken up by the U.S. Department of Justice, with punishments by law for all people who were responsible for this unfortunate scenario. What other remedies should be considered?

Case 14: Criminalization in the Classroom—the School-to-Prison Pipeline

A young Latino high school boy, who lives in a very under-resourced area in the Bronx, New York, has found solace in his life through understanding the music and words of hip-hop artists who have successfully emerged from his community. He spends a significant portion of his time listening to their words and creating his own rhymes to try to express his dismay regarding the rampant poverty and violence in his community. He also uses his words to express his love for his family, his life goals, his desire to learn, and his hope for success through wealth and health in his life. His mother is a drug addict, his father is in jail, and his grandmother is raising him. She cares for him with love and he appreciates her, but she suffers from diabetes and hypertension and he is racked with fear regarding the possibility of her dying. He has no idea how he will function and who will care for him if she becomes seriously ill. None of his teachers at school are Hispanic, and although many are kind to him and recognize his intelligence, they often chide him for not speaking

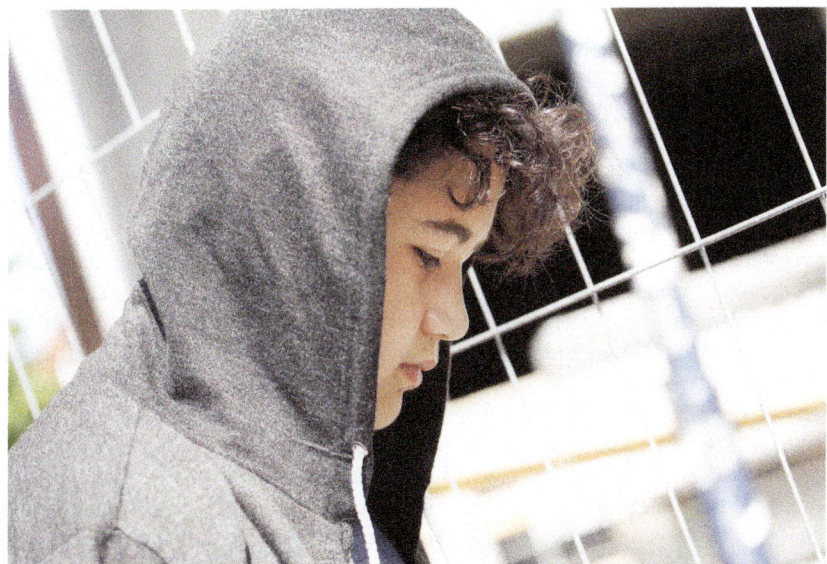

© oleschwander/Shutterstock

up in class and for his many altercations with other students who tease him because his clothes are less than decent. As a result, he is often angry.

He gets into a fight in school and one of his teachers calls the school security officer (who is also a member of the county police force). The boy is taken out of the school in handcuffs, booked, and arrested. This incident ultimately leads to further arrests, as his time in jail enrages him and suppresses his ability to engage with others. He decides that there is no way out for him. His school progress declines and his teachers do not understand his problems, as he never shares them and they do not care to ask. The prospects of high school graduation diminish, and college is possibly not an option that he is able to explore because now he has a record and may not be eligible for financial aid. He feels that all he has left are his words, as he continues to write rhymes, which in his community is known as hip-hop. He shares this ability with no one, but he knows that this is the only medium that resonates with his voice.

Remedies

For minor infractions, children should be reprimanded in school by the Principal's office, Assistant Principals and other Administrators in consultation with parents/guardians rather than arresting the children. Children are the future of the United States. Placing them in prison is not an optimal situation for them or the nation overall. An additional remedy would be to focus on state budgets to ensure that funds are not disproportionately allocated to prisons rather than to public schools. Public schools, particularly in communities where people are experiencing low-incomes, need more funding for schools, which would lead to the improvement of educational facilities. Currently, public schools are funded primarily by local property taxes. This leads to disproportionality because the higher the property taxes, the more resources for schools, hence schools within communities with more expensive homes receive more local funding. Also, higher quality, healthy meals for all students, before and after school programs, fine arts programs, and a variety of exercise programs (besides organized sports) must be in place. These programs should be varied, including yoga, meditation, and other relaxing activities to deal with the stress that children may be experiencing in their lives, in and outside of schools. Furthermore, remedies should include additional structured educational programs for students who need it, offered in a positive way, outside of regular class time. To ensure children are at their grade levels, more resources, such as quality textbooks, computers, school supplies, and the reduction of class sizes are recommended. Students in communities that experience low incomes should have guidance through mental health counselors and social service representatives on site to assist children and their families, especially when arresting students is an option. Before any student is arrested for a minor infraction, there should be a designated review, with assistance where needed, by the campus mental health counselors and social service practitioners. For high schools, the guidance counselors should work with students to ensure that they are on track for graduation and provide assistance in completing college applications or other post-high school plans. These individuals must be trained in working with children and be culturally and linguistically competent. In short, prison is not the remedy to deal with in-school problems with children but rather support on every level is needed. What other remedies should be considered?

Case 15: The Silent Epidemic

A bedridden 61-year-old African American man is in desperate need of a dentist because he has severe pain due to irritation of his gums as a result of ill-fitting dentures and tooth decay. He is unable to sit up after a severe back injury due to a fall.

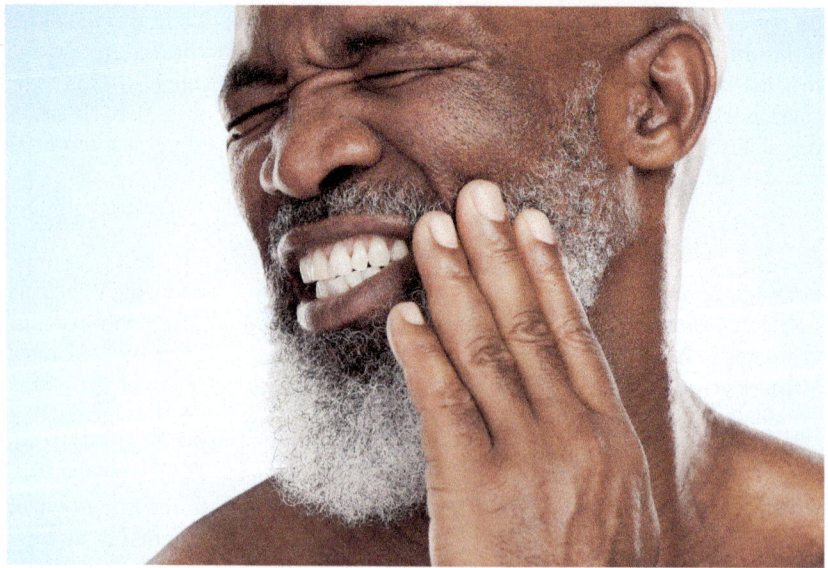

© PeopleImages.com - Yuri A/Shutterstock

His only living relative, his adult son, has contacted several dentist's offices in the community where he resides, only to be told that none of the dentists in his area are able to accept bedridden patients. The man is also uninsured. He cannot afford to be seen in the emergency department, nor can he afford home dentistry beyond his community, which uses mobile dental equipment. He is not eligible for Medicare because he is not yet 65 years old, he has not begun to collect Social Security yet, and he is not considered permanently disabled. His son does not have money to assist his father.

Eventually, his pain becomes unbearable. He is taken via ambulance to the hospital and receives a substantial bill for emergency dental work and for the ambulance transportation cost. In a subsequent follow-up visit to the emergency department by ambulance, the dentist determines that because new dentures are unaffordable for him and his current ill-fitting set have caused substantial tooth decay, removing all of his remaining teeth would be the best option to resolve his problem. The patient and his son agree, as they see no alternative.

Remedies

Oral health has been defined by the World Health Organization (WHO) as a state of being free from chronic mouth and/or facial pain and is an essential component to general health and quality of life (WHO, n.d.). This case highlights the problem associated with dental and oral diseases. Dr. David Satcher, former Surgeon General of the United States, refers to these diseases as the "silent epidemic," a problem impacting Black men at a higher rate than any other group (Satcher, 2000; Centers of Disease Control and Prevention, n.d.). In this scenario, although the quick remedy of pulling all of his teeth was the most expedient way to go, it is definitely not optimal. Extra steps should have been taken to assist him, including having him meet with a social worker to explore other possibilities for accessing care and funding his dental care needs. Transportation possibilities could also have been considered to try to get him to a facility that could have assisted him.

Most people are less than thrilled to visit the dentist and are unaware of the potential ramifications of failing to do so. Oral health can be an indication of overall health quality, as gum disease can lead to, or be an indicator of, other serious health problems. Millions of people in the United States are without dental insurance, and this is especially common among emerging majorities in low-income communities, who are not eligible for Medicaid. Economic barriers significantly impact the likelihood of seeking dental care. For those living in poverty and not eligible for Medicaid, dental care is not typically a priority; needs deemed more pressing, such as housing, food, and medical issues, must be met first. People in lower socioeconomic status scenarios will generally avoid visiting a dentist, particularly if they do not have insurance or have limited Medicaid coverage for dentistry, and opt for tooth extractions if their oral health situation becomes dire, as in this case study. Even with insurance, there are usually additional fees, beyond insurance, which may make the process unaffordable. Thus, the inability to afford appropriate dental care is a major contributor to health disparities. Remedies that would be useful include dental units that visit communities on a regular basis to offer dental care, dental units in schools, the provision of dental care in all health insurance programs, including universal health care, if and when this is implemented in the United States. The teeth should not be considered separately from the rest of the body in terms of health care and insurance, but as a key aspect of health and wellness for every individual. What other remedies should be considered?

Case 16: Testing and Health Disparities

A young Hispanic woman from Honduras, who has lived in the United States for most of her adult life, is proudly working, dating a successful Physician Assistant, and looking forward to a bright future. Her new boyfriend is only the second man with whom she has been intimate, and both relationships, to her knowledge, were/are completely monogamous. She visits the doctor for her annual checkup and is asked if she would like to undergo a full STD (sexually transmitted disease) panel as part of her bloodwork. Since she is sexually active, she agrees. To her shock and dismay, she is told that she is positive for HSV2—genital herpes. She panics and her life is disrupted in a state of hysteria as she wonders how this could have happened to her. Her new boyfriend, whom she has been dating for months, advises her to get a second test at a different lab. Because she is asymptomatic (as is he) and he indicates that he has been completely monogamous, he believes her test is a false positive. He discusses the flawed aspects of the test with her, including lack of specificity, cross-reactions, the various types of tests, and their high rates of false positives. She cries and explains to him that a few of her friends have taken this test and been given positive results and did not consider a second test, and their lives have been deeply impacted, psychologically and beyond, although they were all asymptomatic. She agrees to take another test, finding a different doctor who uses a different lab, as recommended by her boyfriend.

The new lab does not accept her insurance so she has to pay out of pocket for the test, which is costly for her, but she decides to do so anyway. Her second test result is negative, and after thorough review of her history and further exploration by her Physician, a false positive for the first test is the conclusion. She is relieved

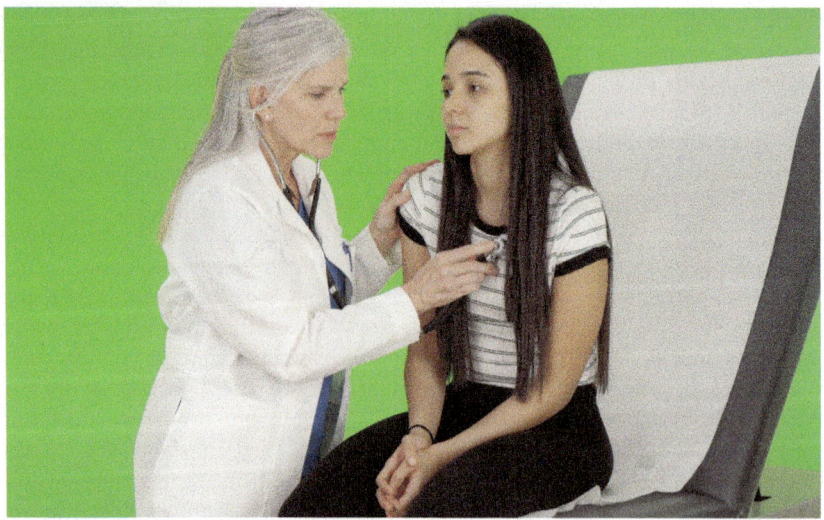

© Rocketclips, Inc./Shutterstock

but then wonders how often this scenario happens and how many people there are walking around, asymptomatic, who tested positive and did not get a second test. She recognizes that many of her friends and family living in the United States are unable to speak English, are experiencing poverty, and have very little understanding of what their doctors explain to them.

Remedies

Health literacy is fundamental to self-advocacy. Often, people are unaware of the fact that Western medicine, like other types of medicine, is not flawless and that various kinds of tests are not standardized or specific and may lead to high rates of false-positive results. Furthermore, they have no idea what questions to ask and may not be able to afford a second opinion/test or consider that they need one. Unfavorable results may lead to psychological dismay, the need for costly medications, and unaffordable retests.

The psychological impact of such tests, without individuals understanding them, magnifies the problem, as explained by Krantz et al. (2004):

> One of the major problems with type-specific testing for genital herpes is false-positive results, particularly since the predictive value of the tests may be low given low prevalence. This may be the case even if the tests have high sensitivity and specificity. For example, in considering STD clinics, diagnosis may occur that is absolutely wrong—10% or potentially 30–40% in lower risk populations. There is an approach to verify these tests, namely Western Blot for HSV2 but unfortunately, this is costly and often not available. When one is diagnosed with genital herpes, there is a psychological impact, particularly because it is an illness that is stigmatized. Therefore, when the diagnosis is not accurate, beyond the trauma caused for the individual there is a serious ethical problem.

Health literacy is also a critical factor in terms of health disparities. Often, data, diagnosis, and ensuing guidance may lead to inaccuracies that further impact the health of communities, psychologically and beyond. In addition to access to care, health education and health literacy are imperative to ensure healthy minds and healthy bodies in emerging majority and low-income communities. Health literacy efforts must be put in place in terms of the provision of information. This can be accomplished by multi-cultural community outreach efforts, mass media and social media efforts to provide health information, apps made available to people, at no cost, which provide health information and the use of colleges/universities to provide health information to students on campus. What other remedies should be considered?

Case 17: Children Need to See

A 6-year-old boy entering the first grade has been diagnosed with a severe vision problem, remedied by glasses. He is on Medicaid, as secured by his mother on his behalf. He lost his first pair of glasses. He is permitted to get a second pair, per Medicaid. Unfortunately, he dropped his second pair in the schoolyard and broke them. Medicaid provides only two pairs of glasses. His mother has no money to get

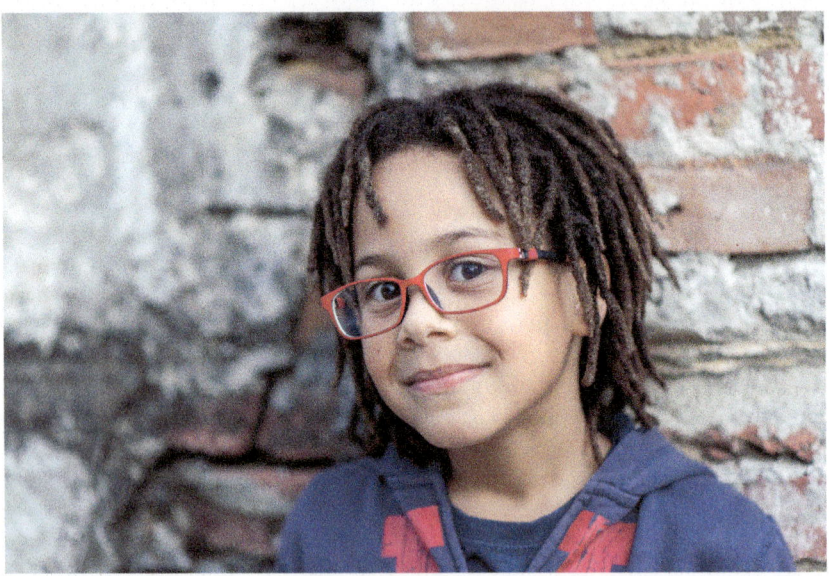

© MaLija/Shutterstock

him new glasses. He is doing very poorly in school because he cannot see without his glasses. His mother seeks help from many venues, but there is no solution. Her young son is now presenting with behavioral problems in the classroom, as he is unable to participate fully in schoolwork with his insufficient eyesight, and it is just halfway through the school year.

Remedies

Eyeglass frames and prescription lenses are often extremely expensive, for both children and adults. A child's inability to see sufficiently, both in the classroom and while doing homework, presents a serious learning problem. Consequently, without glasses for those in need, learning will be limited and the overall outcome is the perpetuation of health illiteracy. Without health literacy, people are unable to resolve the health issues in their lives, which leads to health disparity. The key remedies are that all obstacles leading to children's unsuccessful attempts to learn in the K-12 system must be addressed. Children must be able to see in order to learn, and there must be provisions within the healthcare system to enable children to get or have their glasses replaced if their parents are unable to pay for them. What other remedies should be considered?

Case 18: The Plumber

In 2016, A 63-year old African American unhoused man is sent from a community clinic with a prescription for medication and the advice from a Physician to try to experience better nutrition as he is low body weight and experiencing a severe cough. The Physician also suggests that he visit an Optometrist because his eyesight is weak, to see if he can at least attain glasses, if necessary, or determine if there is a

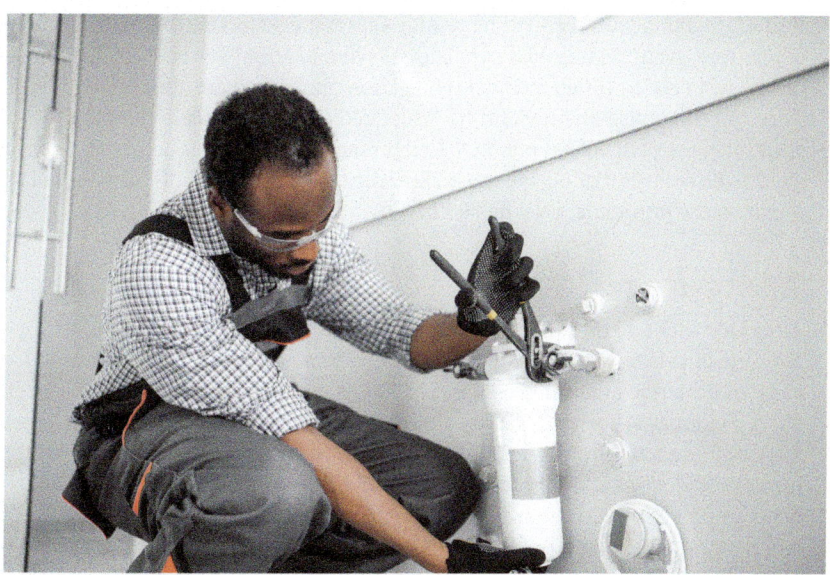

© Hryshchyshen Serhii/Shutterstock

greater problem. He does not have family, and has access to extremely limited funds, which he does not reveal to the Physician. He appeared very clean and neat when he went to the doctor, as he visits local grocery stores and Walmart to wash up daily. He plays his guitar on the street for money and occasionally washes car windows for cars passing by. He doesn't beg as he wants to give some kind of service in order to earn his way. The Physician is unaware that he is unhoused.

The man has a felony conviction and served time, twice, for low-level drug offenses, when he was young, but was never able to sustain a job when he was released due to his felon status. Before prison, he was a plumber, and a good one at that. At that time, he always carried small quantities of marijuana, for personal use, and smoked it with some of his clients after providing plumbing services for them. One of his clients turned him in to the police, unexpectedly, upon his arrival to complete plumbing work at their home. The customer was angry with him because he felt he had charged too much for plumbing services on a prior visit, and he wanted marijuana to settle the matter. When the plumber did not provide the marijuana for him, the customer set him up. The customer had notified the police that he believed that the plumber carried marijuana and the plumber was arrested with marijuana on his person, when he arrived at the customer's house. He had experienced a similar possession conviction in the past, so this arrest was seriously problematic for him. Consequently, because of his felon status, he was not eligible for any of the societal safety nets (public housing, food stamps, etc.) and has lived quietly on the streets, after being released 10 years earlier. No plumbing company will hire him due to his felon status and he is unable to afford or acquire the necessary tools to work as a plumber on his own.

Upon leaving the clinic, he stops at a large pharmacy. He tries on some glasses and finds that with the higher-level readers, he can see better. He slips them into his pocket. He proceeds to the area for cough medicine and puts a bottle in his worn jacket pocket and thinks about using the small amount of money that he has to get fruit to eat along with the food he usually eats at the soup kitchen. As he heads out of the store, security pulls him over and asks him to empty his pockets. He explains that he just needed cough medicine and glasses and begs them not to call the police. They call the police anyway and he is arrested. Due to a three-strikes law, he will spend the rest of his life in prison, based on the mandatory minimum. He is devastated as he realizes that he will most likely die behind prison walls. Although it was tough on the outside, at least he had his freedom.

Remedies

As of December 2018, laws changed. If this man was arrested today, in 2025, perhaps life in prison would not be the outcome because the drug felony would have to be more serious than possession. The law is entitled the First Step Act and this effort continues. This law is better, although it is indeed only a first step, as ideally, the circumstances of this man's experience are such that at the age of 63, with no further convictions after his prior mistakes, perhaps community service would be a better approach to address his crime. Since the First Step Act is not retroactive, he will have no relief based on this new law. It would seem that given his age and his capability as a plumber, he would be in a position to offer plumbing instruction to young people and to be provided with glasses and the necessary medical care that he needs, rather than a sentence to spend his golden years in prison. Although he committed minor crimes of possession involving low-level drugs and had a drug conviction previously, with no indication of committing the latter crime again, long-term sentencing seems unreasonable. His prison sentence for this minor infraction will contribute to the statistics associated with mass incarceration of older people in the United States. Other approaches should be considered in examples like this. Mass incarceration of older people must end.

Remedies for members of the older population who commit non-violent crimes, in lieu of imprisonment, should take into consideration age and the impact that it has on the body and the minds of individuals. Imprisonment of older people is a costly endeavor, as many will need special care to tend to their healthcare needs and daily living activities as they age further. Questions must be considered such as to what extent, based on the nature of the crime, should older people be forgiven, paroled or afforded other options which take into consideration that they are nearing the end of life. Should they, perhaps, be given the opportunity to impart wisdom based on their mistakes, rather than languish in prison cells for extended periods of time, including until death? Compassion for older people must be at the heart of decision-making as to whether to imprison them. In short, remedies for older people, in regard to imprisonment for non-violent crimes, should be based on thoughtful, compassionate consideration, including respect for their wisdom, attempts to understand their mistakes, the provision of mental health and social services, and the reduction of costs. What other remedies should be considered?

Case 19: The Suburban Gap

A 32-year-old Black woman living in a beautiful suburb with her husband and two children was delighted when she learned that she was pregnant with her third child. She and her husband were proud of their accomplishments as she worked

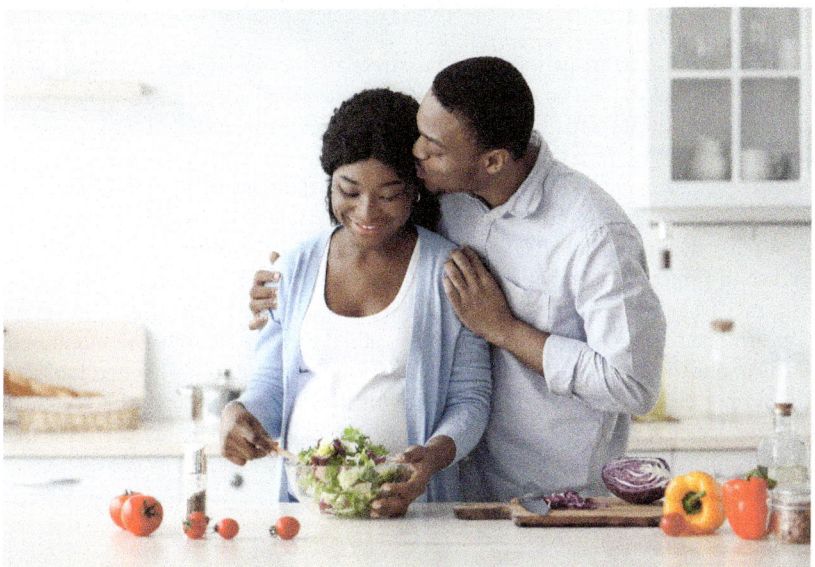

© Prostock-studio/Shutterstock

as an executive at a health insurance company in her community and her husband was a science professor at a local college. As the only Black executive at her firm, she often experienced or heard unfavorable remarks about her hair, Black people in general, and other insults that she brushed off each day, but shared often with her husband. She was also concerned about the number of student loans that she and her husband had acquired while trying to achieve their educational goals and the daily burden of paying them back. When she became pregnant again, she was concerned that perhaps she should discontinue working while pregnant, as it was so difficult to do so with two children, but she decided to press on to continue to help to pay bills for the family, although they lived rather comfortably. She was also concerned because she often worried about matters that were gravely impacting communities of color, namely the Black community, as she reviewed health statistics as part of her daily work. She watched the news because she wanted to be informed but said to her husband, "If I see another shooting of a Black child, I'm not sure if I'll be able to handle it." She tried not to think about what she read and heard too much, but she took many of these matters personally and felt it was her obligation to care. When it was time to deliver her baby, she was quite nervous because she had been experiencing hypertension throughout her pregnancy, which was carefully monitored by her doctor. She never missed a prenatal appointment and her husband was always by her side, for each visit. After she delivered their beautiful baby boy, she suffered a stroke and died suddenly, just a few days after their baby was born. Her husband was shocked. He began to read articles, subsequently, and learned that he was not alone in his grief, as many Black women, even if they are educated and have a higher socioeconomic status, die from maternal mortality. He was absolutely devastated as he thought of his loving wife and realized that he was now the sole parent of two small children and a newborn.

Remedies

Every effort must be made to reduce the stress and burdens that Black women, no matter their socioeconomic status, experience when they are pregnant. This should actually begin during their child-bearing years. Black women should receive mental health care during their pregnancy if it is determined that they are under duress. Alternatives to mental health therapy include meditation, yoga, and other forms of exercise that are appropriate during pregnancy to help assuage stress-induced issues that they may have. Black women often indicate that they are not listened to by health professionals when they share their health problems during pregnancy. This may be helped by having Black women providers care for them. Any and every concern that the pregnant person expresses about their health, must be monitored. Medications that have side effects that may not be appropriate for her and her baby should not be provided, whether they are for hypertension or any other potential or actual health concerns that she may have. The maternal mortality problems that Black women experience must end. What other remedies should be considered?

Case 20: Specialty Care Matters

A 39-year-old man went for his routine optometry appointment. Although he was supposed to go annually to have his prescription reviewed, he had not done so in 6 or 7 years. He had kept his glasses in great shape, so he felt all was fine. What prompted him to go to see an Optometrist was that he was experiencing headaches and dry eyes, the latter now unrelieved by drops.

The Optometrist expressed great concern in examining his eyes and advised that he needed to see a corneal specialist immediately. The Optometrist did not feel comfortable providing a prescription for new glasses. He went to a second Optometrist and did not tell him what the prior doctor indicated so that he could get an

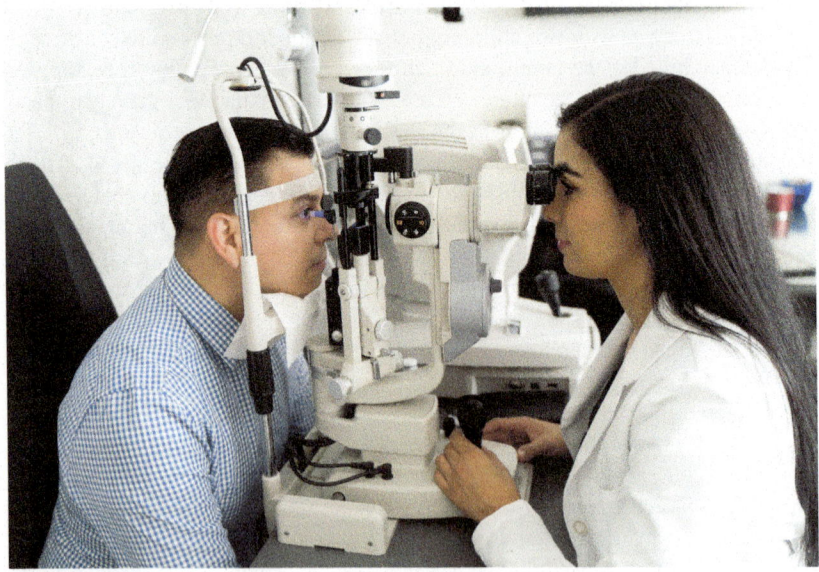

© antoniodiaz/Shutterstock

unbiased second opinion. The second Optometrist expressed similar findings and prescribed glasses with lenses that were deeply uneven in terms of the left vs. right eye because the lack of visual acuity in the right eye was severe. He wrote a referral for him to go to the best eye hospital in the nation, which happened to be in the city where he lived.

The patient had to wait 6 months for an appointment and was promised a significant wait time upon arrival for his appointment. Upon seeing the Ophthalmologist, he was advised that his cornea was cone-shaped and that he had a somewhat rare problem entitled keratoconus, more pronounced in his right eye. He was presented with several options to assist with the problem with the best, from his vantage point, being scleral lenses designed specifically for his eyes. He was told that, with these lenses, 20/20 vision would be a likely outcome. He chose that option, partially covered by his insurance, after his doctor documented that it was a medical necessity. The lenses cost $3,000, not including diagnostics and other appointments necessary to get the lenses. Out-of-pocket expenses added up, causing some distress but what would have happened if he didn't have insurance, as the lenses are not covered by medication, given that he was under 65 and not eligible for Medicare? Upon his visit to get his lenses, the doctor informed him that she had recently resigned and there was no other Ophthalmologist there who specialized in scleral lenses. He became very concerned as now he would have to start from scratch with a new doctor.

Remedies

When a person has a serious eye disease, in this case, keratoconus, given that it is not covered by Medicare and very expensive, there must be a way to provide the person with the specialized scleral lenses necessary for them to see, regardless of their ability to pay. Under no circumstances should a person have to wait 6 months to be seen as this leads to another level of stress. The remedy is to get the patient in quickly to be seen and diagnosed, fitted for, and provided with scleral lenses (contacts) no matter their ability to pay as well as glasses that can be utilized as contacts cannot be worn at all times. The alternative to these remedies is severe visual impairment for people who suffer from this disease. Eye treatment, necessary contacts, glasses, etc. must be included as part of all health insurance including Medicaid, private insurance, Medicare, etc. The eyes are, of course, not separate from the body but part of it. Hence, vision care must not be separate from the rest of health insurance. If a person cannot see, it is very difficult to function. If there is a remedy for an eye disorder, it should be available to everyone, not just those people who can afford to pay. What other remedies should be considered?

References

Achrazoglou, J. (2010, November 8). Perspectives: How diversity goes beyond tolerance. *Diverse: Issues in Higher Education*. http://diverseeducation.com/article/14369

Centers for Disease Control and Prevention. (n.d.). Oral health: Health disparities in oral health. https://www.cdc.gov/oral-health/health-equity/index.html

Krantz, I., Lowhagen, G. B., Ahlberg, B. M., & Nilstun, T. (2004). Ethics of screening for asymptomatic herpes virus type 2 infection. *BMJ (Clinical research ed.), 329*(7466), 618–621. https://doi.org/10.1136/bmj.329.7466.618

LaVeist, T. A. (Ed.). (2002). *Race, ethnicity, and health: A public health reader*. John Wiley and Sons.

Lee, A. (2021, January 22). CVM alums form organizations for cultural change. College Of Veterinary Medicine, University of Georgia. https://vet.uga.edu/cvm-alums-form-organizations -for-cultural-change/

Nir, S. M. (2015, May 8). Perfect nails, poisoned workers. *The New York Times*. https://www .nytimes.com/2015/05/11/nyregion/nail-salon-workers-in-nyc-face-hazardous-chemicals.html

Satcher, D. S. (2000). Surgeon general's report on oral health. *Public Health Reports, 115*. https:// stacks.cdc.gov/view/cdc/64930/cdc_64930_DS1.pdf

Smith, G. D., & Bonnett, B. (1998). Socioeconomic differentials in the mortality of pets: Probably reflect the same differences in material circumstances as in their owners. *British Medical Journal, 317*(7174), 1671–1673.

Times-Union Editorial. (2015, July 16). African-American men must be engaged on mental illness. *The Florida Times-Union*. https://www.jacksonville.com/story/opinion/editorials/2015/07/16 /african-american-men-must-be-engaged-mental-illness/15671890007/

World Health Organization. (n.d.). Oral health: Overview. https://www.who.int/health-topics/oral -health#tab=tab_1

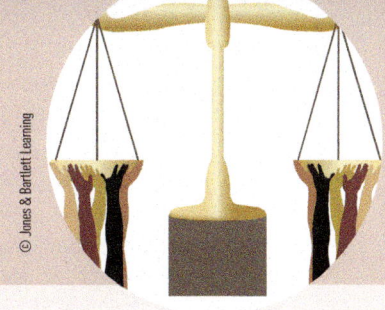

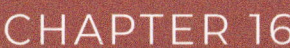

CHAPTER 16

Achieving Health Equity: A Spiritual Approach Toward Remedies

Yolanda Richard, MDiv

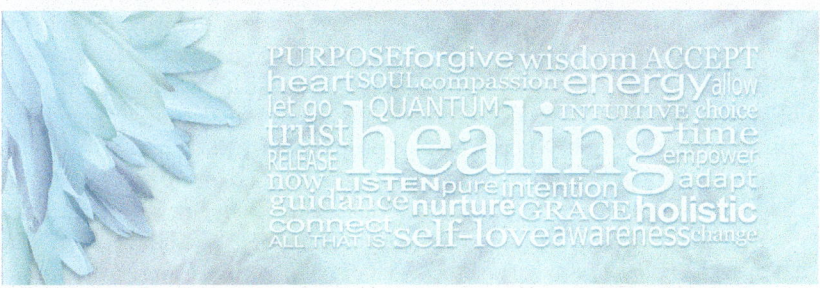

KEY TERMS

Black Sacred Cosmos
Black spirituality
freedom

religion
spirituality

LEARNING OBJECTIVES

After reading this chapter, you should be able to do the following:

1. Understand the importance of religion and spirituality in the lives of racial and ethnic groups, with an emphasis on African American/Black people.
2. Offer alternative definitions and theoretical frameworks for engaging discussion on the role of spirituality in attempts to survey wellness.
3. Consider causes for cultural mistrust of the medical infrastructure.
4. Engage in greater discussion on the need for a broader national identity that includes ethnically and racially marginalized groups.

Introduction

Belief is not simply what one recites at the moment of questioning. Belief is the composition of seemingly insignificant moments that expose the deep thoughts that drive one's engagement with self and others. Belief is the internal matter that accompanies the individual as they both define and navigate the terrain of life. Belief is that undiscovered criterion that lays the foundation for the inconspicuous work of meaning-making. In *Go Tell It on the Mountain*, James Baldwin unveils the unique process of conversion within the African American religious tradition. John, the protagonist, sees God in the ecstatic shouts, songs, and praise of the Black and beaten faces around him. Now their faces, their worship, and their God was in him and it was too late to doubt it. In this revelatory experience, John sees, for the first time, spirituality as a viable resource for the whole of life, the bread of life itself.

Religion and spirituality have always held a central place in the narrative of Black existence in the United States. In the face of severe racism and government-mandated psychological and physical abuse, African American spirituality has operated as a barrier to the external insanity of the nation. It ought to be considerably challenging to discuss Black health without also discussing Black spirituality and its impact on the lives of African American people. In this chapter, the intersection between Black spirituality and the health disparity crisis between Black people and White people will be explored. It is no secret that race, ethnicity, and socioeconomic status are determinant factors in shaping health outcomes.

Health disparity negatively impacts various groups in the United States, including, but not limited to, under-resourced White people, the newly immigrated, Native Americans, non-White Hispanic people, and African American people. Though health disparity impacts various groups in the United States, the gap is widest between Black and White people. This reality is not a new phenomenon; it has held true since the beginnings of the nation. This relationship between White and Black people has also shaped the racial discourse of the United States in such a way that other racial and ethnic emerging majority groups must also confront the consequences of this history. For this reason, this chapter will focus through the lens of the African American religious experience and widen into a discussion about health disparity generally. The goals of this chapter are to highlight the importance of **religion** and spirituality to African American people, offer new definitions and theoretical frameworks for engaging discussion on the role of African American spirituality in attempts to evaluate Black wellness, explore the benefits and challenges of understanding religion and spirituality as a source of resolution for the health disparity crisis, and, finally, explore an expanded national identity as a conceptual response to disparity.

Black Spirituality and the De-Christianization of America

In 2007 and 2014, the Pew Research Center administered virtually identical surveys to a national sample to capture changes in America's religious landscape over the course of 7 years. This comparative study has been quite significant since the U.S. government does not collect statistics on religious composition of the

U.S. public. The 2014 results revealed that there are more Christians in the United States than anywhere else in the world. Seven in 10 Americans identify with some branch of Christianity. The jewel of the study was data showing that overall Christian affiliation in the United States is at a surprising decline. The percentage of American adults who identify with some branch of Christianity had declined by 8%, from 78.4% in 2007 to 70.6% in 2014. Adults who identify as being unaffiliated with any religion had increased by 6%, from 16.1% in 2007 to 22.8% in 2014. Overall, American Christians have declined somewhere between 2.8 and 7.8 million. In spite of the national decline of Christian affiliation, as pointed out by Shelton (2024):

> Baptists comprise the largest Christian tradition in Black America by far at 43%, and they along with Methodists (five percent) help to comprise the "mainline" branch of the Black Church's denominational family tree.

He also indicates that holiness/Pentecostal and those who are nondenominational are at 6% and 12% respectively. These groups are considered the "evangelical" groups.

The significance of Black religious stability is highlighted when juxtaposed to the Pew Research report on the religious portrait of African American people published in 2009. The conclusions of this report were derived from data presented in the 2007 U.S. Religious Landscape Survey. According to this survey, African American people are the most Protestant ethnic group in the country. African American people (78%) far exceed Protestant affiliation compared to Whites (53%), Asians (27%), Latinos (23%), and the overall U.S. population (51%). The survey also showed that Black people are the least likely group to be unaffiliated with any religion. White respondents ranked highest at 24%, compared to 20% of Hispanics and 18% of Black people (Sahgal & Smith, 2009).

The results make clear that African American people are the most religiously affiliated group among the U.S. population. Bolstering this claim, the study shows that 87% of African American people belong to a religious group, while 83% report being affiliated with a specific religion. Beyond religious affiliation, the study shows that religion and involvement in religious life constitute a significant aspect of African American life. Eight in 10 African American people say religion is very important to their lives, compared to 56% of the U.S. population. Even among African American people who identify as being unaffiliated with any particular religion, spirituality is a significant aspect of their lives. According to the study, 45% of unaffiliated African American people say that religion is very important in their lives. A higher percentage (72%) of unaffiliated African American people reported that religion plays at least a somewhat important role in their lives (Sahgal & Smith, 2009).

African American involvement in religious life is also telling. When asked about prayer and attendance at religious services, 76% of African American people say they pray daily (**Figure 16-1**) and more than half report attending religious services at least once a week (Sahgal & Smith, 2009). When asked about the existence of God, 88% report being absolutely certain that God exists. Interestingly, unaffiliated African American people's response to these same categories mirrors the percentages of mainline Protestant and Catholic people (Sahgal & Smith, 2009). Among unaffiliated African American people, 48% pray at least daily compared to

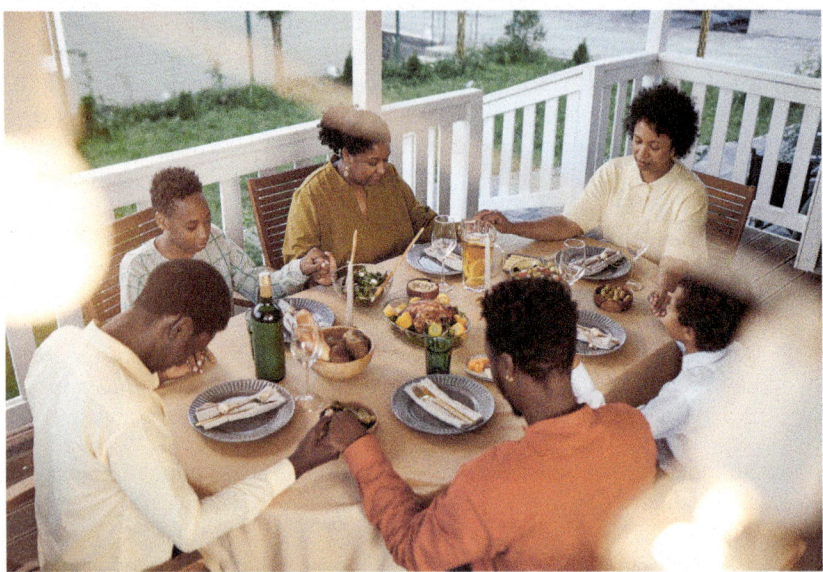

Figure 16-1 Black family praying.
© SeventyFour/Shutterstock

53% of mainline Protestants. Similar to mainline Protestants (73%) and Catholics (72%), 70% of unaffiliated African American people believe God exists with absolute certainty (Sahgal & Smith, 2009). Only 1% of African American people describe themselves as atheists or agnostic (Sahgal & Smith, 2009).

The Role of Spirituality in the Lives of African American people and Wellness

It is essential to acknowledge the critical role of spirituality in the lives of African American people. An assessment of Black wellness without any consideration of spirituality ignores the significant ways in which this group has chosen to lift up religion as central to the Black ethos. The results make clear that religion, particularly Christianity, is not simply important but present in the everyday lives of African American people through engagement with the historically Black church and daily prayer, among other factors.

Furthermore, the results highlight that **Black spirituality** is not only significant but also distinct from the greater population. The stability of religious affiliation is telling of the uniqueness of Black culture and life in the United States. It points to the need for definitions, theoretical frameworks, and models of wellness that do not simply seek to model the normativity of White culture but that generate meaning from a locus point of Black life. (The locus point of Black life and that of the greater populace are not to be seen as mutually exclusive or separate. In this instance, the locus point of Black life refers to a point of cultural saturation along a spectrum of Black embodiment, engagement, and connection with surrounding human expression.) Spirituality has always carried potential for shaping behavior, influencing lifestyle, and defining the parameters for one's understanding of self, others, and the world. Black spirituality deals deeply with the inner workings of Black people and thus plays a major role in influencing the health outcomes of African American people. To be explored later in this chapter is the notion that Black spirituality is not simply professing basic Christian tenets, but is a divinely inspired reframing of Christianity that affirms Black existence in the world. Many scholars have taken on the task of evaluating the role of religion and spirituality in the health outcomes of African American people. In the process, one must determine a definitional framework that will shape how the data are understood in light of the demographic sample. Definitions of religion and spirituality play a major role in framing the discussion of the relationship between Black religious practice and health. Therefore, before delving into a discussion of remedies, a conversation about definitions is at hand.

Religion Versus Spirituality

Religion and *spirituality* are terms that are often used interchangeably, though they describe different aspects of one's relationship to faith. Religion is an infrastructure of belief surrounding a collective understanding of the divine identity. This infrastructure contains a series of theological premises, the conclusions of which determine the boundaries that make the religion distinct from other claims to divine revelation. These theological claims concerning the divine identity manifest into a set of subclaims about the human identity. Understandings of the human identity and the divine identity are not mutually exclusive; in fact, one informs the other knowingly and unknowingly. From an understanding of the divine and self emanates a set of practices and expectations that mediate an individual and collective relationship to the divine being.

In a sense, this religious infrastructure is helpful. Over time, the structure will shortcut centuries of theological developments and debates within the tradition into a series of norms, expectations of membership, catechistic orientations, and periodic chastisement to make one aware of the behavioral boundaries of belonging. Also, devotees will discover language and ritual nuance, the utilization of which further integrates them into the institutional identity. These prepackaged theological bright lines are quite attractive to new converts and members because they ease the process of religious assimilation and create an in-house measurement to gauge religious performance. They are also helpful in providing alternative sources of allegiance. Belonging on the basis of belief subverts the requirements of cultural belonging on the basis of resources the devotee lacks. For marginalized groups, religion provides a sense of belonging to a higher moral order that trumps the social mores of the day. Finally, religion assumes the operationalization of divine engagement and spiritual growth. A common by-product associated with the religious structure is a tendency toward rigidity and the formation of dogma. Such outcomes bolster the pursuit of clearer institutional identity but simultaneously strain one's pursuit of a fluid, organic spirituality.

Spirituality evokes a different relationship to the divine that is not intrinsically associated with the expectations of the religious structure. Spirituality is marked by a comfort with the mysterious quality of the divine and the mysterious quality of the self. This engagement located in the space of mystery operates within a theological assumption of private intimacy with God that generates creative, innovative, and individualized theology. Many turn to spirituality in an attempt to break from the religious institution; however, such a task is quite difficult. Often, this spirituality finds itself bound by the expectations of the religious structure. In other words, how can one completely part from what may be his or her only reference point to divine engagement? The tools one acquires to engage the divine (e.g., prayer, songs of worship, folklore, reading of religious texts, meditation, contemplative practices, retreat to the divine temple) will influence the person's spirituality or at the very least remain as contours to his or her spirituality. In this way, religion and spirituality are bound to overlap. Spirituality makes possible the ability to transcend the religious structure, but the structure will often inform how one understands that transcendence. For example, one can transcend to a higher awareness of the finitude of life via deep reflection on a religious text that acts as a convenient springboard to the place of transcendence. In this sense, some find the contours of the institution as a comforting guide toward their development and connection with the divine. Others find these contours restricting and seek to balance the assumed truths of the structure with suspicion and the development of unique terms for their divine engagement.

Definitions are essential to set a base understanding of key concepts and determine the scope of discussion. Over the years, researchers have gone back and forth concerning definitions and potential distinctions between religion and spirituality. Definitions have been provided earlier in this chapter to weigh in on the matter and to mark the point beyond which we will explore deeper, nuanced, and complex definitions that match the movement of the African American religious experience. Additionally, general definitions are important to provide a context by which alternative definitions are highlighted.

Spirituality, Religion, and Mental Health

In her 1998 dissertation, *The Relationship Among Spirituality, Religion, and Mental Health for African Americans*, Gwendolyn L. Jones provides a slew of definitions of spirituality and religion. Spirituality is described as "a quality deep within all human beings," and "its expression through the individual is one's spiritual perspective" (Jones, 1998, p. 13). Religion is understood as "an integrated set of beliefs, rituals, and institutions through which persons give expression about that which is holy or held in highest esteem in their lives" (Jones, 1998, p. 13). Jones hypothesizes that these two terms are distinct concepts in the lives of African Americans. Ultimately, her study shows that spirituality is a much better predictor for mental health than is religion, suggesting that African Americans understand these two terms as separate and distinct (Jones, 1998). She argues that the lack of definitional autonomy between the terms is due to the difficulty health professionals find in operationalizing these seemingly immeasurable concepts. Also, she finds that mental health practitioners simply lack knowledge about religion and spirituality. Jones argues that research on health outcomes of African Americans should consider not only an individual's relationship to the infrastructure of the church, but also one's perception of self in relation to others (Jones, 1998).

A recent 2010 report on the impact of the two terms showed different results. In the article "Importance of Religion and Spirituality in the Lives of African Americans, Caribbean Blacks and Non-Hispanic Whites," Robert J. Taylor and Linda M. Chatters evaluated the importance of religion and spirituality in the lives of African American people. They cited religion as a three-fold concept: "(1) a multidimensional construct encompassing public and private behaviors, attitudes and beliefs, (2) organizing around a structured system of tenets, practices, and ritual and, (3) characterized as community-focused, formal, and behaviorally oriented" (Taylor & Chatters, 2010, p. 281). Spirituality is defined as "a higher-order endeavor with individual quest that facilitates both greater personal expression and enhanced personal benefits and outcomes, a viewpoint that is particularly ardent among those who are estranged from organized religion" (Taylor & Chatters, 2010, p. 282). The report of Taylor and Chatters is based on the "National Survey of American Life: Coping With Stress in the 21st Century" administered by the Program for Research on Black Americans at the University of Michigan. This survey is one of only a few national probability samples that explore the connection between religion and spirituality (Taylor & Chatters, 2010). The survey sample was composed of 6082 face-to-face interviews from 3570 African Americans, 891 Non-Hispanic Whites, and 1621 Blacks of Caribbean descent. Respondents were asked two questions: "How important is religion in your life?" and "How important is spirituality in your life?" The study found that African Americans are more likely to report that religion and spirituality are very important to their daily lives, at 93%. When the results of African American people and Caribbean Black people are viewed together, results show that both groups were likely to report that spirituality and religion are very important to them (90%). Taylor and Chatters argue that the results are indicative of two things. First, studies that simply concern themselves with institutional engagement with religion (i.e., church attendance and membership) miss the mark at displaying the full range of one's relationship to faith. Second, the results indicate that the larger Black community does not perceive any particular distinction between the two terms—religion and spirituality—to describe the importance of faith in their lives (Taylor & Chatters, 2010).

Both studies confirm that a sole focus on African American involvement to the religious institution does not fully capture what African American people mean when they report that religion and spirituality are important to them. The two studies differ: Jones reports that spirituality is a better indication of African American religious expression, while Taylor and Chatters contend that recent data reveal that African American people do not see these two constructs as mutually exclusive and actually find both valuable for their religious expression. It is clear that African American people engage the terms spirituality and religion when asked to relate them to their religious experience. What is not clear is how effectively these terms capture the religious structure of African American people.

The Black Religious Cosmos and Its Impact on Health

In *The Black Church in the African American Experience*, C. Eric Lincoln and Lawrence H. Mamiya provide a descriptive and historical overview alongside statistical data on the current state of the Black church. Their study is the latest major empirical study of Black churches in the United States since Benjamin E. Mays and Joseph W. Nicholson's study in 1924, published in their book *The Negro's Church*. Lincoln and Mamiya interviewed a national sample of pastors from seven historically Black denominations serving in 2150 urban and rural churches. The study occurred over the span of 8 years, from 1978 to 1986. They provide sociology of the Black church and contribute much-needed theoretical assumptions for engaging the study of the African American religious tradition. They assume a religious dimension spanning over the entirety of Black life they call the "Black Sacred Cosmos."

Like other scholars, Lincoln and Mamiya provide a base definition of religion as a starting point of discussion on the Black religious tradition. They site David Émile Durkheim's 1965 claim in his book *Elementary Forms of Religious Life* that religion is "a social phenomenon, a shared group experience that has shaped and influenced the culture as screens of human communication and interpretation" (Lincoln & Mamiya, 1990, p. 2). Lincoln and Mamiya, however, push beyond this definition and do the work suggested by Taylor and Chatters. They present the concept of the **Black Sacred Cosmos** as a theoretical framework for understanding the religious composition of African American people. For Lincoln and Mamiya, The Black Sacred Cosmos is "the religious worldview of African Americans . . . related to their African Heritage, which envisaged the whole universe as sacred, and to their conversion to Christianity during slavery and its aftermath" (Lincoln & Mamiya, 1990, p. 2). This definition moves beyond base definitions and is tailor-made for a deeper understanding of the African American religious tradition.

The Black Sacred Cosmos provides the framework many researchers lack when trying to evaluate the impact of religious tradition on Black health. Lincoln and Mamiya suggest that scholars have consistently struggled to see African American history, culture, and religion as being distinctly generated from the locus point of Black life. It is only in recent years that scholars have recognized Black cultural creations without assuming Eurocentric origin or the mimicking of mainstream culture. Lincoln and Mamiya make clear that Black culture is a culture valid in itself and generative of itself against external pressures. Assumed lack of innovation on the part of African American people, Lincoln and Mamiya argue, points to the common practice of not granting African American people the same presuppositions as other "hyphenated Americans" (Lincoln & Mamiya, 1990, p. 3), the presupposition that prior to contact with North America they had viable cohesive, and valid cultures through which they developed new creative American identities (Lincoln & Mamiya, 1990). Such an acknowledgement is crucial when one considers the enormity of research on the connection between spirituality and health of African American people that lacks a definitional framework specific to the religious cosmos in which African American people operate. In other words, to simply ask questions of religious involvement or whether religion and spirituality are important not only misses the full picture of the impact of religion on the lives of African American people but also reinforces the idea that the Black religious infrastructure is not unique, independently developed, and distinct from mainstream conceptions of religion and spirituality. It is important for scholars not to dismiss the creative and generative quality of the Black religious infrastructure. To do so is to dismiss a reservoir of unexplored and untapped remedies for Black health that derive from the locus point of Black life. Lincoln and Mamiya teach us how to appropriately match conceptual framework with demographic sample.

Lincoln and Mamiya's theoretical assumption of the Black Sacred Cosmos also allows them to redefine terms typically associated with definitions of religion. For example, they define culture as "the sum of the options for creative survival" (Lincoln & Mamiya, 1990, p. 3). This definition, when situated within the locus of Black life, takes unique shape. When centered on the heritage of African American people, survival is the designated end to the pursuit of cultural production. Lincoln and Mamiya's redefinition of terms through the lens of Black life is indicative of the definitional potential of the use of Black-centered paradigms when surveying African American communities. This is not to say that all Black people will articulate their religious experience specifically as "the Black Sacred Cosmos" or even articulate that survival is at the center of culture. Such theoretical assumptions are meant to posit the unarticulated, lived experience of African American people and frame research in such a way that one's results and discussion of data are appropriately understood in light of the arch of Black religious heritage and history. The Black Sacred Cosmos is marked by the African religious tradition of having a central sacred object. For African American people, the Christian God revealed in Jesus Christ is the central sacred object of the Black Sacred Cosmos (Lincoln & Mamiya, 1990).

Though African American people have operated within the religious structure of White Christian people, African American people are generative in where they choose to place emphasis in the vast tapestry of Christian theology. For example, the imagery of God as a liberating force that avenges on behalf of his children is a powerful emphasis made by African American people. The idea of being children of God directly confronts constitutional definitions (overturned by the 14th Amendment) of Black people as being three-fifths of a person. Even today, several Black churches still place emphasis on this kind of divine imagery. The suffering and humiliation of Jesus is also a point of emphasis that resonates with this community (Lincoln & Mamiya, 1990).

A central concept in the Black Sacred Cosmos is the concept of **freedom**. For Lincoln and Mamiya, freedom is "the absence of any restraint which might compromise one's responsibility to God" (Lincoln & Mamiya, 1990, p. 4). Freedom through the lens of the Black Sacred Cosmos presupposes a call to total allegiance to God alone and free reign over one's life to do as God requires. To not be free would then complicate one's assurance of salvation. If one belongs to an earthly master, how can he or she also belong to God? Freedom through the lens of Eurocentric normativity has always highlighted an American pursuit toward individualism. The pursuit of freedom to follow one's destiny has always been at the center of American identity. For African American people, though, the collective nature of slavery and the pre-eminent identification as Black above all else generated an understanding among African American people that freedom is a communal pursuit (Lincoln & Mamiya, 1990).

Also at the center of the Black Sacred Cosmos is the concept of individual conversion. Though the idea of being "born again" was a theology widely propagated during the first and second religious awakenings in the United States, African American people engaged this theological concept differently than did their White counterparts. Though White Christian people also emphasized personal conversion, African American people encountered conversion with a marked element of ecstatic expression. From its inception, the ecstatic nature of the Black church has remained its most marked distinction and unique quality among other American churches (Lincoln & Mamiya, 1990).

For Lincoln and Mamiya, religion "raises the core values of that culture to ultimate levels and legitimates them.". At the center of the Black Sacred Cosmos are the values of "freedom, justice, equality, an African Heritage, and racial parity at all levels of human intercourse.". Within the cosmos, these values are legitimated and may inform how individuals evaluate their life and determine their level of satisfaction (Lincoln & Mamiya, 1990, p. 7).

Lincoln and Mamiya's work is an optimal example of how one ought to engage definitions and theoretical models for research on the African American religious tradition. It is also significant for its acknowledgement of the role of religion in the formation of Black culture and points to our initial claim that any resolution for health disparity for African American people must be rooted in the locus point of Black life, which naturally assumes a deep engagement with the African American religious tradition and the reclaiming of that tradition as American.

In *Black Spirituality and Black Consciousness*, Carlyle Fielding Stewart describes what spirituality means from the perspective of African American people: "To be spiritual from an African-American perspective, is to live wholly from the divine soul center of human existence. This center is the core of the universe and the quintessential impetus driving the quest for human fulfillment" (Stewart, 1999, p. 2). For Stewart, this definition connotes possession of a "soul force" that allows the individual to transcend the realities of human existence. This soul force "divinely mediates, informs, and transforms a human being's capacity to create, center, adapt, and transcend the realities of human existence" (Stewart, 1999, p. 2). From this soul force derives a "cultural soul" where Black existence resides. This cultural soul force is where African American people discover, analyze, celebrate, valuate, corroborate, and transform the meaning of Black life in society.

Soul force can be understood through a dual praxis: creative soul force and resistant soul force. Creative soul force refers to the elements of spirituality that enable African American people to creatively confront and manage their current reality through the generative construction of Black culture. Resistant soul force is the ability to creatively transcend the barriers and constraints that seek to "enforce the complete domestication to those values, processes, behaviors, and beliefs that reinforce human devaluation and oppression" (Stewart, 1999, p. 2). Simply put, creative soul force is the spirit of creativity to transform and bend reality to support one's existence in the world. Resistant soul force is the part of Black spirituality that resists all attempts to domesticate and annihilate the creative mechanisms of survival of the Black spirit. Culture soul is thus the "archive of values, beliefs, behaviors, practices, and passions that empower and confer value on African-American life" (Stewart, 1999, p. 3).

The concept of creative and resistant soul forces derives from Black people's unique view of themselves as spiritual beings who are yoked with the divine in such a way that freedom, liberation, and positive change are consistently birthed from the connection. African American spirituality is particularly essential to acknowledge because it is the "ultimate reference point for black existence" (Stewart, 1999, p. 3). Since Christianity's introduction to North American Black captives, God and the spirit of the divine became the guarantee that survival was inevitable and freedom imminent.

This definition of spirituality marries well with the concept of the Black religious cosmos, as it is rooted in the belief that freedom is at the center of the Black religious tradition. These two definitions will carry through the rest of this chapter as we consider additional ways of understanding Black spirituality and its impact on the health disparity crisis.

A Spiritual Approach Toward Resolution of Health Disparities: A Personal Case Study

I had a dream that God gave me medicine.

—**Seul Dieu Richard** (father of this chapter's author)

When my father spoke these words, I paused in wonder and in terror. As a person of faith, I didn't disregard the idea entirely. I myself have had dreams, so vivid and mysterious that it could be, for me, nothing less than the presence of the divine revealing itself to me. But this religious declaration seemed to be lodged in a different category entirely. Did he believe that his connection with God somehow made him immune to sickness and death? Was the medicine of God better than the medicine of science? Was he simply avoiding yet another doctor's visit? Was this a classic example of how religion gets in the way of health care?

My father's perspective is quite unsettling for many of us. Immediately, the mind travels to the many consequences of a lack of preventive care. A desire to somehow show him the power of modern medicine and draw him to an enlightened modern socio-perspective subsequently follows. Often, this enlightened modern socio-perspective requires a deconstruction of the divine identity, a psycho-emotional detachment from the divine presence, and a tempering of one's level of dependence on the amorphous acts of the divine. It is believed then that the image of the divine, assumedly crowding the rational judgment of the devotee, will be displaced to make room for the clear choice of modern medicine.

We must move away from cheap evaluations that overestimate religiosity as the Achilles' heel of African American people and other affected communities as it relates to health disparity. To do so is not simply to appease affected groups to make them feel "welcomed"; rather, to highlight an assumed mutual exclusivity between religion and science is to avoid the real issues of health disparity altogether. There are mountains of sociopolitical, socioeconomic, racial, gender, and sexuality-based factors that keep affected groups sick, tired, and poor. Plainly, at the center of health disparity is not a question of one's ability to believe in the efficacy of modern medicine (the long-held biased focus of Western European concern), but one's ability to trust institutions of health that seem to work in tandem with the socioeconomic and sociopolitical forces that have historically pursued, in overt and latent fashions, the domestication and annihilation of non-normative life in the United States. Sadly, the health system has proven over and over again, particularly in the lives of African American people, to be antithetical to the existence of non-normative life.

In her essay "The Underutilization of Health Services in the Black Community: An Examination of Causes and Effects," Daphne Chandler discusses the roots of the Black community's cultural mistrust toward the generally White medical infrastructure. She sees cultural mistrust as being "characterized by a lack of trust in Whites, suspicion of their motives, uncertainty about the sequence of events, a sense of individual powerlessness, and a belief that caution is necessary to avoid trouble" (Chandler, 2010, p. 926). Another source of mistrust is connected to the fear of being misdiagnosed and over-diagnosed. Chandler states, "Blacks are disproportionately misdiagnosed and over-diagnosed for such mental disorders as schizophrenia, due to such factors as counselor incompetence, an outcome of little or no knowledge of the Black culture, and racial or cultural bias" (Chandler, 2010, p. 926). Mistrust is deepened when one considers the history of surgical and disease experimentation on Black bodies and access to these bodies through the medical and prison infrastructure. Unsurprisingly, when interacting with the medical infrastructure, Black people generally have low expectations for the quality of care they will experience, even while being treated by a Black doctor. Ultimately, Chandler posits that this mistrust is rooted in the institutional legacy of racism in the United States (Chandler, 2010, p. 926).

When the conversation centers on trust, the weight of responsibility bears heavily on normative locations of power to restore, retain, and maintain healthy relationships with affected communities. It is imperative that these relationships are mutually committed to fostering a kind of trust that conveys the utmost commitment to affirming the flourishing and survival of people affected by health disparity. Furthermore, centering the conversation on trust reveals that religion and science are not at odds with one another. When imagined comparative evaluations on the efficacy of God versus the efficacy of modern medicine are marginalized, suddenly centuries of historical anecdotes that progressively fostered general mistrust of wellness efforts for marginalized groups materialize. Under such circumstances, normative efforts to engage wellness of non-normative people simply do not carry the same credence as institutions centered on the survival and flourishing of that group (i.e., religion and spirituality). Perhaps there is a reality where religiosity and science will not contend or reach for intellectual authority, but will collaborate in assuring the survival and flourishing of non-normative life. As we have seen, to disregard the role of spirituality is to disregard the cultural psychology of several groups to whom spirituality defines culture and identity. These groups include, but are not limited to, African American people and Native Americans. These groups have historically suffered greatly as a result of health disparity. Thus, it is essential to defend the role of spirituality from swift attempts to supplant it entirely with Eurocentric demands to maintain a mutually exclusive dependence on the efficacy of modern medicine.

How is spirituality a viable lens, though, for envisioning the resolution to health disparity? I begin this exploration by returning to my father's words: "I had a dream that God gave me medicine." What was he saying? And why is it important? In true theological fashion, I have interpreted his statement while considering what I know about the historical context of his life and faith. His beliefs may be expressed in these words:

> I believe in the benevolence of God so deeply that this God can heal me in my sleep of any unknown and known diseases. My connection to the divine does not make me immune to sickness and death, but it says to me every day that I, like anyone else, deserve to live. I believe this so deeply that I do not fear life or death, but am comforted to know that I will be comforted in my departure. If sickness were to take me, I would prefer it be the will of God and not the wielding of strange and unknown men. In this, I am utterly satisfied.

After much coaxing and theological gymnastics, I have still not been able to get my father to the doctor's office. The last time I asked, he said, "They might give me medicine that could end up killing me if it doesn't work with my body." In this comment, I sensed not only a fear of being mishandled or misdiagnosed, but a deeper awareness that his body would not be seen as valuable enough for extraordinarily excellent and accurate care. He was challenging the competence of the medical system in engaging his Black body. He is not a famous Black man, nor does he have many riches. In the walls of a big hospital and local clinic, he is not the beloved Pastor Richard of the local storefront church. He is not immediately known, as I know him, as father, counselor, and friend. He is another patient whose death could be easily explained by medical jargon, without any fear of national press or criticism among colleagues. The fear of being inconsequential in the hands of strange men is real and should not be taken lightly. But God—God, for him, is the only assurance of his survival and existence in this world. Who am I to say that in this day and age he has no right to depend on the divine? One cannot expect those who suffer from health disparity to trust a system that defines them as inconsequential. It is imperative that health frame itself within the various cultural loci of affected groups, which often implies a locus of spirituality. Looking through the lens of Black life reveals spirituality as an integral mode of survival in light of micro-aggression and the external hostility of the nation. In this sense, while we wait for the nation to appropriately respond to health disparity, to create an atmosphere of trust, we will let faith do its work.

The Connection Between Spirituality and Religiosity, Health Outcomes, and Remedies

Several years of research have concluded that there is, in fact, a connection between religiosity and health outcomes. Generally, those who are deeply religious often avoid high-risk behavior, exhibit higher levels of life satisfaction, possess social networks and tools useful to cope with stress and recover from depression from stressful life events, and heal at a much faster rate than do their non-religious counterparts. They also exhibit stronger immune systems, have better cardiovascular health, and fare well as they age and encounter end of life (Koenig, 1999).

Generally, religion and spirituality aid in building resilience, a high level of life satisfaction, and much-needed peace in moments of severe stress and life difficulty that often circumvent risk of disease and sickness. In the face of the effects of health disparity, religion and spirituality provide an internal shield to protect one's internal system of approval and sense of happiness. The more negative the external environment, the deeper the dependence on the internal shield.

Chandler (2010) proposes, "Spirituality can act as a positive or a negative coping strategy depending on one's degree of reliance." She provides an example cited by Fowler and Hill (2004), who found that deeply religious Black women in abusive relationships tend to stay with their partners to uphold religious values of marriage, forgiveness, and steadfast waiting on God to restore the marriage. Chandler concludes that spirituality is not the answer to disparity, but a way of dealing with the stress caused by disparity. She argues that resolution would require a dismantling of the repressive and oppressive forces that are at the root of disparity (Chandler, 2010). It is for this reason that this chapter is subtitled "A Spiritual Approach *Toward* Resolution."

Chandler is right. There can be theological assumptions that emanate out of one's understanding of the divine identity that keep the individual in high-risk unhealthy situations. One's spirituality may be an effective solution to the stress of the situation but is not a solution to the root cause of disparity. The potential of pseudo-harmony does not mean that religion ought to be discarded, but that it is part of a whole approach to address the main issue of disparity. Chandler's critique draws us back to a need to understand spirituality from a perspective of cultural singularity. Spirituality is not a stagnant affair. It is ever evolving as we encounter new and old ideas within our culture. Through the lens of the Black Sacred Cosmos, for example, the value of freedom is viewed in highest esteem, and survival as the end of any attempt of cultural production. One's spirituality, when confronted with moments of oppression, can take the shape of the oppression itself, while simultaneously presenting abundant theological resources for liberation. Such resources will go unnoticed if the religious infrastructure has not been liberated. Chandler's critique is not a wholesale dismissal of spirituality but truly a critique on the impact of dogmatic religious infrastructure that would rather maintain theological claims over the liberation of its people from oppressive forces. Clearly this thinking is not descriptive of all religious encounters, but it is essential to note as a call to religious clergy and spiritual sojourners to actively evaluate the impact of theological claims, affirming claims that liberate, rejecting claims that bind, and creating claims needed to affirm the lives of those we have utterly overlooked.

Furthermore, health disparity points to a greater issue of national identity. Spirituality is not simply understating who God is but also who we are. Definitional frameworks that consider religion and spirituality across racial/ethnic groups are, as we've seen, quite necessary. Taylor and Chatters's request for such definitions ought not be considered as a type of ritualistic checks and balances for academic study. In fact, their request speaks to a greater need for a type of emphasis on cultural singularity that ushers an integration and expansion of the national American identity. In other words, a spiritual approach provokes discourse on identity in such a way that a conversation about national inclusion is inevitable. The hyphen sometimes sandwiched between the terms *African* and *American* is pregnant with the unfinished work of claiming American identity. In the *Souls of Black Folks*, first published in 1903, W. E. B. DuBois (2005) wrote the following:

> Freedom, too, the long-sought, we still seek,—the freedom of life and limb, the freedom to work and think, the freedom to love and aspire. Work, culture, liberty,—all these we need, not singly but together, not successively but together, each growing and aiding each, and all striving toward that vaster ideal that swims before the Negro people, the ideal of human brotherhood, gained through the unifying ideal of Race; the ideal of fostering and developing the traits and talents of the Negro, not in opposition to or contempt for other races, but rather in large conformity to the greater ideals of the American Republic, in order that some day on American soil two world-races may give each to each those characteristics both so sadly lack.

A conceptual emphasis on an integrated national identity speaks directly to the concept of disparity. It short-circuits attempts at making culture the distinctive factor that determines and simplifies methods of care. Establishing cultural singularity is important, but it runs the risk of conceptual reinforcement of racialized binaries that either propagates disengagement by the dominant culture or reaches for parentalist control and judgment of non-normative ways of existing. In other words, when an emphasis on cultural difference is taken too far, cultural difference becomes the scapegoat through which the dominant culture evades responsibility for health disparity. Under such circumstances, narrowing the health disparity gap becomes the task of the non-normative communities and White sympathizers instead of, more appropriately, the responsibility of the national community. Conceptual frameworks for the study of the impact of religion and spirituality on the health outcomes of African American people, for example, must claim the uniqueness of the African American religious tradition, while maintaining a rightful understanding of the broader history of the American religious tradition.

WRAP-UP

This chapter enabled the discovery of the significant role and importance of religion and spirituality in the lives of African American people. It provided the potential for alternative considerations for framing discussions on the impact of religion and spirituality to health outcomes of marginalized groups, through engaging the Black Sacred Cosmos and Black spirituality as definitions that move beyond general and imprecise attempts at matching conceptual frameworks to a demographic sample. Finally, the chapter explored a spiritual approach toward resolving the health disparity crisis. Though research shows that there are major health benefits to religiosity, religion and spirituality are not, per se, the resolution to health disparity but are factors that must be present in any attempt at a resolution, particularly for non-normative ethnic and racial groups who identify deeply with a spirituality as unique to their identity. Approaches to the healthcare disparity crisis must call upon the concepts of religion and spirituality to (1) provoke a deeper definitional framework for discussion that appropriately matches the demographic sample, (2) engage the importance of a psycho-emotional safety net to skillfully manage sickness-inducing stresses caused by disparity, (3) identify misguided attempts at obscuring the central causes of health disparity by a disregard of the importance of spirituality, and (4) engage a discussion on the need for an expanded national identity that embraces the cultural singularity of non-normative groups, particularly those impacted by disparity. A call for an expanded national identity speaks directly to the concept of disparity without reinforcing cultural binaries that re-legitimate segregation-based treatment.

One's unique understanding of the divine, the self, and others is at the center of spirituality. It resides at the core of one's being. To know this core, to see this core, and to affirm its existence is the co-effort of the nation and its Gods. Hand in hand, both must incite belonging and affirm life and wellness.

Chapter Problems

1. Explain the notion of a Black Sacred Cosmos as a conceptual framework and its relevance to health disparities.
2. Is spirituality a concept that should be considered in terms of reducing/resolving health disparities? Explain why or why not.
3. Explain how spirituality may be unique to some individuals.
4. What is the difference between religiosity and spirituality?
5. What racial and ethnic groups are negatively impacted by health disparity in the United States?

References

Chandler, D. (2010, May). The underutilization of health services in the Black community: An examination of causes and effects. *Journal of Black Studies, 40*(5), 915–931. http://www.jstor.org/stable/40648613

Dubois, W. E. B. (2005). *The souls of black folks: Essays and sketches.* Simon & Schuster. (Original work published in 1903.)

Fowler, D. N., & Hill, H. M. (2004). Social support and spirituality as culturally relevant factors in coping among African American women survivors of partner abuse. *Violence Against Women, 10*(11), 1267–1282. https://doi.org/10.1177/1077801204269001

Jones, G. L. (1998, May). *The relationship among spirituality, religion, and mental health for African Americans* [Doctoral dissertation, University of New Orleans].

Koenig, H. G. (1999). *The healing power of faith: Science explores medicine's last frontier.* Simon & Schuster.

Lincoln, C. E., & Mamiya, L. H. (1990). *The Black church in the African American experience.* Duke University Press.

Sahgal, N., & Smith, G. (2009, January 30). *A religious portrait of African Americans* [Report]. Pew Research Center. http://www.pewforum.org/2009/01/30/a-religious-portrait-of-african-americans/

Shelton, J. E. (2024, May 15). *The Black church and the 2024 presidential election.* Brookings Institution. https://www.brookings.edu/articles/the-black-church-and-the-2024-presidential-election/

Stewart, C. F. (1999). *Black spirituality and Black consciousness: Soul force, culture, and freedom in the African-American experience.* Africa World Press.

Taylor, R. J., & Chatters, L. M. (2010). Importance of religion and spirituality in the lives of African Americans, Caribbean Blacks and non-Hispanic Whites. *The Journal of Negro Education, 79*(3), 280–294.

Appendix I

The National CLAS Standards

The National Standards for Culturally and Linguistically Appropriate Services in Health and Health Care (National CLAS Standards) were derived from an analysis of current practices and policies on cultural competence and shaped by the experiences and expertise of healthcare organizations, policy makers, and consumers. Sponsored by the U.S. Department of Health and Human Services, Office of Minority Health, they were developed over a three-year period based on inputs from a number of sources (Rose, 2013).

In *Essentials of Health, Culture, and Diversity*, Edberg (2012) describes the National CLAS Standards:

> These standards . . . have become the key document used to guide cultural competence efforts in the United States. . . . They are organized by theme: standards 1–3 address culturally competent care; 4–7 refer to language access services; and 8–14 refer to organizational supports for cultural competence. (p. 160)

Edberg (2012) describes the first seven clinical/service-oriented standards as follows:

- **Standard 1:** Healthcare organizations should ensure that patients/consumers receive from all staff members effective, understandable, and respectful care that is provided in a manner compatible with their cultural health beliefs and practices and preferred language.
- **Standard 2:** Healthcare organizations should implement strategies to recruit, retain, and promote, at all levels of the organization, a diverse staff and leadership that are representative of the demographic characteristics of the service area.
- **Standard 3:** Healthcare organizations should ensure that staff at all levels and across all disciplines receive ongoing education and training in culturally and linguistically appropriate service delivery.
- **Standard 4:** Healthcare organizations must offer and provide language assistance services, including bilingual staff and interpreter services, at no cost to each patient/consumer with limited English proficiency at all points of contact, in a timely manner, during all hours of operation.

- **Standard 5:** Healthcare organizations must provide to patients/consumers, in their preferred language, both verbal offers and written notices informing them of their right to receive language assistance services.
- **Standard 6:** Healthcare organizations must assure the competence of language assistance provided to limited English proficient patients/consumers by interpreters and bilingual staff. Family and friends should not be used to provide interpretation services (except on request by the patient/consumer).
- **Standard 7:** Healthcare organizations must make available easily understood patient-related materials and post signage in the languages of the commonly encountered groups and/or groups represented in the service area.

Edberg (2012) goes on to describe the organization-oriented standards as follows:

- **Standard 8:** Healthcare organizations should develop, implement, and promote a written strategic plan that outlines clear goals, policies, operational plans, and management accountability/oversight mechanisms to provide culturally and linguistically appropriate services.
- **Standard 9:** Healthcare organizations should conduct initial and ongoing organizational self-assessments of CLAS-related activities and are encouraged to integrate cultural and linguistic competence-related measures into their internal audits, performance improvement programs, patient satisfaction assessments, and outcomes-based evaluations.
- **Standard 10:** Healthcare organizations should ensure that data on the individual patient's/consumer's race, ethnicity, and spoken and written language are collected in health records, integrated into the organization's management information systems, and periodically updated.
- **Standard 11:** Healthcare organizations should maintain a current demographic, cultural, and epidemiological profile of the community as well as a needs assessment to accurately plan for, and implement, services that respond to the cultural and linguistic characteristics of the service area.
- **Standard 12:** Healthcare organizations should develop participatory, collaborative partnerships with communities and utilize a variety of formal and informal mechanisms to facilitate community and patient/consumer involvement in designing and implementing CLAS-related activities.
- **Standard 13:** Healthcare organizations should ensure that conflict and grievance resolution processes are culturally and linguistically sensitive and capable of identifying, preventing, and resolving cross-cultural conflicts or complaints by patients/consumers.
- **Standard 14:** Healthcare organizations are encouraged to regularly make available to the public information about their progress and successful innovations in implementing the CLAS standards and to provide public notice in their communities about the availability of this information.

References

Edberg, M. (2012). *Essentials of health, culture, and diversity* (1st ed.). Jones & Bartlett Learning.

Rose, P. R. (2013). *Cultural competency for the health professional* (1st ed.). Jones & Bartlett Learning.

Appendix II

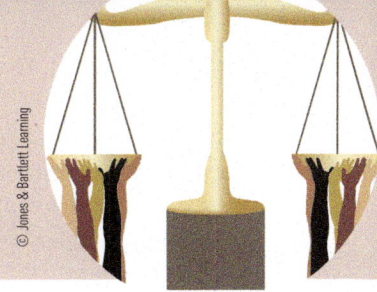

Cultural Competence Assessment Survey: Executive Team and Management

Executive Team and Management

Site: _____

Date: _____

Please place a check mark [✓] next to the selection that best represents your thoughts.

1. I display pictures, posters, and other materials that reflect the cultures and ethnic backgrounds of patients/clients/customers served by my site.

   ☐ Strongly agree   ☐ Agree
   ☐ Disagree   ☐ Strongly disagree
   ☐ Not applicable

2. I speak up when someone is humiliating another person or acting inappropriately.

   ☐ Strongly agree   ☐ Agree
   ☐ Disagree   ☐ Strongly disagree
   ☐ Not applicable

3. I avoid using language that reinforces negative stereotypes.

   ☐ Strongly agree   ☐ Agree
   ☐ Disagree   ☐ Strongly disagree
   ☐ Not applicable

4. I ensure that magazines, brochures, and other printed materials in reception areas reflect the different cultures of patients/clients/customers served by my site.

   ☐ Strongly agree   ☐ Agree
   ☐ Disagree   ☐ Strongly disagree
   ☐ Not applicable

5. When using videos, films, or other media resources for health education, treatment, or other interventions, I ensure that they reflect the culture of the patients/clients/customers served by my site.

☐ **Strongly agree**   ☐ **Agree**
☐ **Disagree**   ☐ **Strongly disagree**
☐ **Not applicable**

6. I assist my new staff members, including people of various cultures, ages, and sizes, to feel welcome and accepted.

☐ **Strongly agree**   ☐ **Agree**
☐ **Disagree**   ☐ **Strongly disagree**
☐ **Not applicable**

7. I disregard physical characteristics when interacting with others and when making decisions about competence and ability.

☐ **Strongly agree**   ☐ **Agree**
☐ **Disagree**   ☐ **Strongly disagree**
☐ **Not applicable**

8. I am culturally competent.

☐ **Strongly agree**   ☐ **Agree**
☐ **Disagree**   ☐ **Strongly disagree**
☐ **Not applicable**

9. I know the definition of cultural competence.

☐ **Strongly agree**   ☐ **Agree**
☐ **Disagree**   ☐ **Strongly disagree**
☐ **Not applicable**

10. I know the definition of cultural proficiency.

☐ **Strongly agree**   ☐ **Agree**
☐ **Disagree**   ☐ **Strongly disagree**
☐ **Not applicable**

11. I am culturally proficient.

☐ **Strongly agree**   ☐ **Agree**
☐ **Disagree**   ☐ **Strongly disagree**
☐ **Not applicable**

12. I intervene in an appropriate manner when I observe my staff or clients/patients/customers engaging in behaviors that exhibit cultural insensitivity or prejudice.

☐ **Strongly agree**   ☐ **Agree**
☐ **Disagree**   ☐ **Strongly disagree**
☐ **Not applicable**

13. Cultural proficiency training sessions/workshops will be helpful to my staff in their overall work performance.

☐ **Strongly agree**   ☐ **Agree**
☐ **Disagree**   ☐ **Strongly disagree**
☐ **Not applicable**

14. My work responsibilities include direct patient/client/customer contact.
    - ☐ **Strongly agree**
    - ☐ **Agree**
    - ☐ **Disagree**
    - ☐ **Strongly disagree**
    - ☐ **Not applicable**

15. I have difficulty communicating with patients/clients/customers who cannot speak English.
    - ☐ **Strongly agree**
    - ☐ **Agree**
    - ☐ **Disagree**
    - ☐ **Strongly disagree**
    - ☐ **Not applicable**

16. All patients/clients/customers who visit my work site for service should know how to speak English if they want help.
    - ☐ **Strongly agree**
    - ☐ **Agree**
    - ☐ **Disagree**
    - ☐ **Strongly disagree**
    - ☐ **Not applicable**

17. Translation and signage should be available for patients/clients/customers with limited English proficiency (LEP).
    - ☐ **Strongly agree**
    - ☐ **Agree**
    - ☐ **Disagree**
    - ☐ **Strongly disagree**
    - ☐ **Not applicable**

18. Ongoing training and education for executives, management, and staff is necessary to promote culturally and linguistically competent/proficient service delivery.
    - ☐ **Strongly agree**
    - ☐ **Agree**
    - ☐ **Disagree**
    - ☐ **Strongly disagree**
    - ☐ **Not applicable**

19. I am interested in attending cultural competency/proficiency workshops/training sessions.
    - ☐ **Strongly agree**
    - ☐ **Agree**
    - ☐ **Disagree**
    - ☐ **Strongly disagree**
    - ☐ **Not applicable**

20. I use bilingual staff or trained volunteers to serve as interpreters during assessment, meetings, or events for clients/patients/customers who would require this level of assistance.
    - ☐ **Strongly agree**
    - ☐ **Agree**
    - ☐ **Disagree**
    - ☐ **Strongly disagree**
    - ☐ **Not applicable**

Thank You

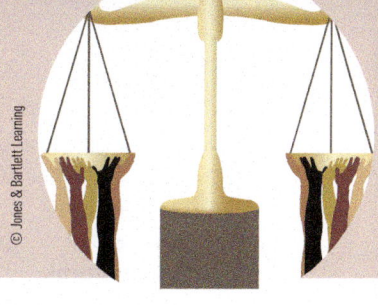

Cultural Competence Assessment Survey: Staff

Staff

Site: _____

Date: _____

Please place a check mark [✓] next to the selection that best represents your thoughts.

1. I avoid imposing values that may conflict, or be inconsistent, with those of cultures or ethnic groups other than my own.

   ☐ **Strongly agree**　　　　☐ **Agree**
   ☐ **Disagree**　　　　　　　☐ **Strongly disagree**
   ☐ **Not applicable**

2. I speak up when someone is humiliating another person or acting inappropriately.

   ☐ **Strongly agree**　　　　☐ **Agree**
   ☐ **Disagree**　　　　　　　☐ **Strongly disagree**
   ☐ **Not applicable**

3. I avoid using language that reinforces negative stereotypes.

   ☐ **Strongly agree**　　　　☐ **Agree**
   ☐ **Disagree**　　　　　　　☐ **Strongly disagree**
   ☐ **Not applicable**

4. I get to know people from different groups and cultures as individuals.

   ☐ **Strongly agree**　　　　☐ **Agree**
   ☐ **Disagree**　　　　　　　☐ **Strongly disagree**
   ☐ **Not applicable**

5. I accept and reinforce the fact that not everyone has to act or look a certain way to be successful or valuable.

   ☐ **Strongly agree**　　　　☐ **Agree**
   ☐ **Disagree**　　　　　　　☐ **Strongly disagree**
   ☐ **Not applicable**

6. I assist new people at the site where I work, including people of various cultures, ages, and sizes, to feel welcome and accepted.

☐ **Strongly agree**   ☐ **Agree**
☐ **Disagree**   ☐ **Strongly disagree**
☐ **Not applicable**

7. I disregard physical characteristics when interacting with others and when making decisions about competence and ability.

☐ **Strongly agree**   ☐ **Agree**
☐ **Disagree**   ☐ **Strongly disagree**
☐ **Not applicable**

8. I am culturally competent.

☐ **Strongly agree**   ☐ **Agree**
☐ **Disagree**   ☐ **Strongly disagree**
☐ **Not applicable**

9. I know the definition of cultural competence.

☐ **Strongly agree**   ☐ **Agree**
☐ **Disagree**   ☐ **Strongly disagree**
☐ **Not applicable**

10. I know the definition of cultural proficiency.

☐ **Strongly agree**   ☐ **Agree**
☐ **Disagree**   ☐ **Strongly disagree**
☐ **Not applicable**

11. I am culturally proficient.

☐ **Strongly agree**   ☐ **Agree**
☐ **Disagree**   ☐ **Strongly disagree**
☐ **Not applicable**

12. I intervene, in an appropriate manner, when I observe other staff or clients/patients/customers within my worksite engaging in behaviors that exhibit cultural insensitivity or prejudice.

☐ **Strongly agree**   ☐ **Agree**
☐ **Disagree**   ☐ **Strongly disagree**
☐ **Not applicable**

13. Cultural proficiency training sessions/workshops will be helpful to me in my overall work performance.

☐ **Strongly agree**   ☐ **Agree**
☐ **Disagree**   ☐ **Strongly disagree**
☐ **Not applicable**

14. My work responsibilities include direct patient/client/customer contact.

☐ **Strongly agree**   ☐ **Agree**
☐ **Disagree**   ☐ **Strongly disagree**
☐ **Not applicable**

15. I have difficulty communicating with patients/clients/customers who cannot speak English.

  ☐ **Strongly agree**   ☐ **Agree**
  ☐ **Disagree**   ☐ **Strongly disagree**
  ☐ **Not applicable**

16. All patients/clients/customers who visit my worksite for service should know how to speak English if they want help.

  ☐ **Strongly agree**   ☐ **Agree**
  ☐ **Disagree**   ☐ **Strongly disagree**
  ☐ **Not applicable**

17. Translation and signage should be available for patients/clients/customers with limited English proficiency (LEP).

  ☐ **Strongly agree**   ☐ **Agree**
  ☐ **Disagree**   ☐ **Strongly disagree**
  ☐ **Not applicable**

18. Ongoing training and education for staff to promote cultural and linguistically competent/proficient service delivery is important.

  ☐ **Strongly agree**   ☐ **Agree**
  ☐ **Disagree**   ☐ **Strongly disagree**
  ☐ **Not applicable**

19. I am interested in attending cultural competency/proficiency workshops/training sessions.

  ☐ **Strongly agree**   ☐ **Agree**
  ☐ **Disagree**   ☐ **Strongly disagree**
  ☐ **Not applicable**

20. I recognize and challenge the biases that support my own thinking.

  ☐ **Strongly agree**   ☐ **Agree**
  ☐ **Disagree**   ☐ **Strongly disagree**
  ☐ **Not applicable**

Thank You

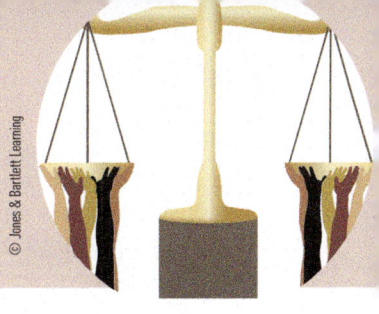
© Jones & Bartlett Learning

Appendix IV

Cultural Competence Assessment Survey: Health Professionals

Health Professionals

Site: _____

Date: _____

Please place a check mark ✓ next to the selection that best represents your thoughts.

1. I display pictures, posters, and other materials that reflect the cultures and ethnic backgrounds of patients served by my site.

   ☐ **Strongly agree**   ☐ **Agree**
   ☐ **Disagree**   ☐ **Strongly disagree**
   ☐ **Not applicable**

2. I make extra efforts to educate myself about the various cultures of my patients.

   ☐ **Strongly agree**   ☐ **Agree**
   ☐ **Disagree**   ☐ **Strongly disagree**
   ☐ **Not applicable**

3. I avoid using language that reinforces negative stereotypes.

   ☐ **Strongly agree**   ☐ **Agree**
   ☐ **Disagree**   ☐ **Strongly disagree**
   ☐ **Not applicable**

4. I ensure that magazines, brochures, and other printed materials in reception areas reflect the different cultures of patients served by my site.

   ☐ **Strongly agree**   ☐ **Agree**
   ☐ **Disagree**   ☐ **Strongly disagree**
   ☐ **Not applicable**

5. When using videos, films, or other media resources for health education, treatment, or other interventions, I ensure that they reflect the cultures of the patients served by my site.

☐ **Strongly agree**   ☐ **Agree**
☐ **Disagree**   ☐ **Strongly disagree**
☐ **Not applicable**

6. I attempt to determine any family colloquialisms used by patients that may impact an assessment, treatment, or other intervention.

☐ **Strongly agree**   ☐ **Agree**
☐ **Disagree**   ☐ **Strongly disagree**
☐ **Not applicable**

7. I accept that religion, and other beliefs, may influence how families respond to illness, disease, and death.

☐ **Strongly agree**   ☐ **Agree**
☐ **Disagree**   ☐ **Strongly disagree**
☐ **Not applicable**

8. I am culturally competent.

☐ **Strongly agree**   ☐ **Agree**
☐ **Disagree**   ☐ **Strongly disagree**
☐ **Not applicable**

9. I know the definition of cultural competence.

☐ **Strongly agree**   ☐ **Agree**
☐ **Disagree**   ☐ **Strongly disagree**
☐ **Not applicable**

10. I know the definition of cultural proficiency.

☐ **Strongly agree**   ☐ **Agree**
☐ **Disagree**   ☐ **Strongly disagree**
☐ **Not applicable**

11. I am culturally proficient.

☐ **Strongly agree**   ☐ **Agree**
☐ **Disagree**   ☐ **Strongly disagree**
☐ **Not applicable**

12. I use bilingual staff or trained volunteers to serve as interpreters during assessment of patients who require this level of assistance.

☐ **Strongly agree**   ☐ **Agree**
☐ **Disagree**   ☐ **Strongly disagree**
☐ **Not applicable**

13. Cultural proficiency training sessions/workshops will be helpful to me in the provision of health care.

☐ **Strongly agree**   ☐ **Agree**
☐ **Disagree**   ☐ **Strongly disagree**
☐ **Not applicable**

14. When possible, I ensure that all communiqués to patients are written in their language of origin.
    - ☐ **Strongly agree**
    - ☐ **Agree**
    - ☐ **Disagree**
    - ☐ **Strongly disagree**
    - ☐ **Not applicable**

15. I have difficulty communicating with patients who cannot speak English.
    - ☐ **Strongly agree**
    - ☐ **Agree**
    - ☐ **Disagree**
    - ☐ **Strongly disagree**
    - ☐ **Not applicable**

16. All patients who need care should know how to speak English if they want help.
    - ☐ **Strongly agree**
    - ☐ **Agree**
    - ☐ **Disagree**
    - ☐ **Strongly disagree**
    - ☐ **Not applicable**

17. Translation and signage should be available for patients with limited English proficiency (LEP).
    - ☐ **Strongly agree**
    - ☐ **Agree**
    - ☐ **Disagree**
    - ☐ **Strongly disagree**
    - ☐ **Not applicable**

18. Ongoing training and education for health providers is necessary to promote culturally and linguistically competent/proficient service delivery, which is important.
    - ☐ **Strongly agree**
    - ☐ **Agree**
    - ☐ **Disagree**
    - ☐ **Strongly disagree**
    - ☐ **Not applicable**

19. I am interested in attending cultural competency/proficiency workshops/training sessions.
    - ☐ **Strongly agree**
    - ☐ **Agree**
    - ☐ **Disagree**
    - ☐ **Strongly disagree**
    - ☐ **Not applicable**

20. I recognize that the meaning or value of medical treatment and health education may vary greatly among cultures.
    - ☐ **Strongly agree**
    - ☐ **Agree**
    - ☐ **Disagree**
    - ☐ **Strongly disagree**
    - ☐ **Not applicable**

Thank You

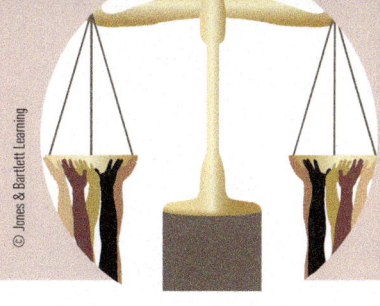

Appendix V

Sample Components of a Diversity Plan

Although *diversity* is a broad term, inclusive of many types of individuals and groups that warrant emphasis, the focus of this brief sample plan is racial and ethnic diversity, as is the case for this text throughout, with the understanding that the information provided may be applicable and revised to suit the needs of groups beyond the scope of this text.

The goal of this sample plan is to provide guidelines and key insight into potentially useful objectives, methods, and action steps relating to the process, and to identify the leaders who may be involved with implementation. This table is intended only to serve as a guide as to components that should be considered. These cursory suggestions are provided in a simple format, as the process should not be complicated but rather easily doable.

Objective	Methods	Action Steps	Leaders
Develop/revise the institutional mission statement to include an emphasis/focus on diversity.	■ Review existing mission statements that have accomplished this. ■ Define the term "diversity" so that it is clear to all members of the organization. ■ The mission and vision statements should be displayed throughout the organization and on the security badges worn by all members of the organization, the organization's web page, and all ingoing and outgoing communications per letterhead or below email signatures.	■ Have a strategic mission statement development/revision meeting with the president and CEO and their cabinet and key staff. ■ Get approval of the board of directors/trustees for the new/revised mission statement.	■ President and CEO ■ Cabinet of the president and CEO ■ Key staff (administrative and nonadministrative) ■ Faculty, administrators, and staff at academic institutions
Create a fully staffed (racially and ethnically diversified) Diversity and Cultural and Linguistic Competence Office with the sole responsibility of racially and ethnically diversifying the organization and handling multicultural affairs.	■ Ensure cultural and linguistic competence training for the board of directors, administrators, faculty, and staff. ■ Maintain and manage a comprehensive budget for all diversity, cultural, and linguistic competence efforts (exclusive of fundraising). ■ Seek ongoing continuing education and developmental training for all diversity and cultural and linguistic staff. ■ Offer educational conferences at the institution to ensure that all members of the organization are provided with timely information about racially, ethnically diverse, cultural and linguistic competence issues.	■ Hire staff for the office that are reflective of the diversity goals of the organization, in terms of administration and staff. ■ Develop a full calendar of events for diversity and cultural competence initiatives (conferences, guest speakers, training sessions workshops, etc.) to be distributed to all members of the organization encouraging and requiring (where appropriate) attendance.	■ Diversity and Cultural and Linguistic Competence Office's vice president and all office staff ■ Chief financial officer ■ President and CEO ■ Board of Directors ■ Human Resources

Objective	Methods	Action Steps	Leaders
	▪ Collect data specific to the definition of diversity for the organization so that efforts are true to the mission of the organization in terms of diversity.	▪ Provide ongoing assessment, evaluation, and review of the efficacy of the office to ensure that all efforts are being met while simultaneously developing and implementing solutions where gaps may exist.	
Create marketing materials that are reflective of a commitment to serve diverse populations and (visual affirmation).	▪ Analyze the sociodemographic characteristics and data of clients/ customers/patients/students served. ▪ Determine the predominant racial/ethnic groups served by the organization.	▪ Budget for, and develop, marketing materials (paper and technological) that are reflective of the populations served based on culturally relevant images and linguistic requirements.	▪ President and CEO ▪ Marketing and relevant administrative staff ▪ Chief financial officer and staff ▪ Practitioners, faculty, and other staff who have direct interactions with clients/ customers/students ▪ Technological staff ▪ Human resources ▪ Diversity and Cultural and Linguistic Competence Office

(continues)

Objective	Methods	Action Steps	Leaders
Recruit a workforce (of clinical and nonclinical staff, administrators, faculty, and beyond) whose demographic makeup is reflective of the population served.	■ Train and advise all staff who will be involved with diversity recruitment on how and where to do so.	■ Develop long-term and short-term recruitment efforts. ■ Develop a multicultural recruitment advisory committee (consisting of members of the recruitment target population). ■ Ensure that all job descriptions include the organization's diversity recruitment aims.	■ Diversity and Cultural and Linguistic Competence Office ■ Human resources ■ Supervisors, managers, directors, and department chairs ■ Marketing department
Organize diversity-related activities that enable cross-cultural learning at all levels of the organization in an atmosphere of positive lighthearted activities.	■ Example: Encourage staff to submit recipes for the development of a company- or institutional-wide cookbook. ■ Have select staff, clinicians, students, faculty present a lecture, in an ongoing seminar series about their culture, language, and family lineage to ensure cross-cultural understanding of diverse cultures.	■ Develop and publish the company- or institution-wide cookbook for all staff to enjoy and experience and for the opportunity to learn about diversity. ■ Prioritize the lecture series as an important and significant aspect of the organization, offering time release and some type of accolades for participation and attendance.	■ Diversity and Cultural and Linguistic Competence Office ■ Human Resources ■ All members of the organization/staff

© Jones & Bartlett Learning

Cultural Competence Plan

Company Analysis

Brief organizational history with cultural competence emphasis.

Community Analysis

- Local demographics
- Patient/client/customer demographics
- Executive and management demographics
- Board of directors demographics
- Provider/health professional demographics
- Staff demographics

Cultural Competence Assessment

- Board and executive team
- Health professionals/providers
- Staff

Facility Assessment (Visual Affirmation and Bi-/Multilingual Signage)

- Waiting areas
- High-traffic areas
- Treatment protocols
- Staff-accessible areas
- Reading materials and written information
- Website review
- Review of procedures and protocols, mission and vision statements

Strategic Cultural Competence Marketing Plan and Development

Strategic Approach

- Expected cultural competence goals and outcomes
- Achieving diversity
- Cultural competence champions (committee)
- Internet cultural marketing and training

Community Partnering

- Community leaders
- Key organizations
- Supporting affiliates/stakeholders

Cultural Competence Project Timeline

- Key elements
- Key points and dates
- Checkpoints

Post-Project Assessment/Evaluation

- Goal measurement
- Continued cultural competence assessment (ongoing)

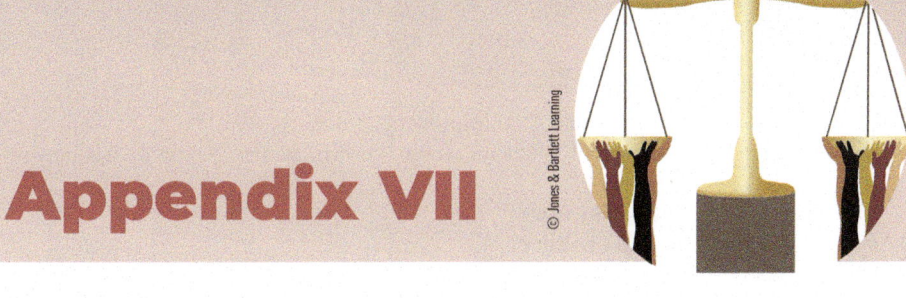

Abbreviations

The following are some abbreviations that are frequently used in this text.

AACTE	American Association of College Teachers
AAMC	Association of American Medical Colleges
ACA	Affordable Care Act (short for Patient Protection and Affordable Care Act)
ACLU	American Civil Liberties Union
AFDC	Aid to Families with Dependent Children
ADL	activities of daily living
AFDC	Aid to Families with Dependent Children
AHRQ	Agency for Healthcare Research and Quality
AIAN	American Indian and Alaska Native
AGS	American Geriatrics Society
AI	artificial intelligence
AVMA	American Veterinary Medical Association
CASSP	Child and Adolescent Service System Program
CBO	Congressional Budget Office
CDC	Centers for Disease Control and Prevention
CEO	Chief Executive Officer
CFO	Chief Financial Officer
CDMP	chronic disease management program
CDOH	commercial determinants of health
CHC	community health center
CIA	Central Intelligence Agency
CLAS	Culturally and Linguistically Appropriate Services
DHHS	Department of Health and Human Services
ELLs	English language learners
EPA	Environmental Protection Agency
FDA	Food and Drug Administration
FPL	Federal poverty level
FQHC	Federally Qualified Health Center
HBCUs	Historically Black Colleges and Universities
HCOP	Health Careers Opportunity Program
HRSA	Health Resources and Services Administration
IHS	Indian Health Service
IMR	infant mortality rate

IHCIA	Indian Health Care Improvement Act
IOM	Institute of Medicine (now known as the National Academy of Medicine)
LBW	low birth weight
LEP	limited English proficiency
MHN	Men's Health Network
MMR	maternal mortality rate
MSAW	migrant and seasonal agricultural worker
MSFW	migrant seasonal farmworker
NAAL	National Assessment of Adult Literacy
NAACP	National Association for the Advancement of Colored People
NAION	non-arteritic anterior ischemic optic neuropathy
NAWS	National Agricultural Workers Survey
NCFES	National Association for Education Statistics
NCACTE	National Council for the Accreditation of Teacher Education
NCES	National Center for Education Statistics
NCHS	National Center for Health Statistics
NEA	National Education Association
NHDR	National Healthcare Disparities Report
NHQR	National Healthcare Quality Report
NIH	National Institutes of Health
NIMHD	National Institute on Minority Health and Health Disparities
OMB	Office of Management and Budget
OMH	Office of Minority Health
PPACA	Patient Protection and Affordable Care Act
PIAAC	Program for the International Assessment of Adult Competencies
PSSA	Pennsylvania System of School Assessment
RCT	Randomized Control Trial
RCM	Reserve Capacity Model
SCF	Survey of Consumer Finances
SDOH	social determinants of health
SIDS	sudden infant death syndrome
SES	socioeconomic status
STEM	science, technology, engineering, and math
TANF	Temporary Assistance for Needy Families
URM	underrepresented in medicine
USDA	U.S. Department of Agriculture
USDOE	U.S. Department of Education
USPHS	U.S. Public Health Service
VPLN	Virtual Professional Learning Networks
WHO	World Health Organization

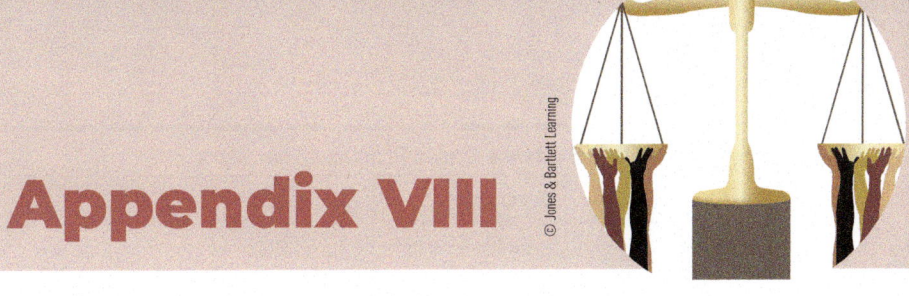

Durant's Model for Diversity and Inclusion

Appendix VIII-1 Evidence-Based Practices That Work

Practice	Description
1. Scholarships	Develop a financial assistance package that includes sources of financial aid.
	Offer competitive funding for reducing cost of degree program, including full and partial scholarships.
2. Mentorship	Develop a mentoring program by providing Black faculty with names and email addresses of Black students each semester.
3. Summer bridge	Identify promising sophomores and juniors for summer enrichment programs.
4. Minority faculty/ administrative representative	Develop an Office of Diversity Affairs to serve the needs of Black students.
	Create paid positions for persons with the responsibility of recruitment.
	Continue to keep open lines of communication between faculty in reference to recruitment and retention of Black students.
5. Recruitment	Hire a recruiter, plan an annual Minority Career Day, and provide rewards to Black faculty who are engaged in recruitment and retention efforts (e.g., reduce teaching load). Provide faculty with recruitment packages to take to local, state, and national meetings, which they attend.
6. Support groups	Develop an administrative unit for planning, programming, and counseling Black students.
7. Institutional linkages	Institute a "buddy" program for new students from the current student body. Form an alumni network of interested Black graduates of your institution to assist with recruitment.

Appendix VIII-1 Evidence-Based Practices That Work

Practice	Description
8. Multimedia advertising	Promote your program and Black students and faculty on social media, with brochures, and in ads.
9. Direct visits	Encourage faculty members to participate in recruiting by visiting Black colleges and universities.
10. Direct visits to the institution	Identify promising sophomores and juniors for summer enrichment programs. Sponsor a reception for Black students.
11. Referrals from alumni	Identify Black alumni faculty at predominantly Black institutions and predominantly White institutions who would be interested in receiving information about the healthcare program at your institution and referring students.
12. Diversity environment	Improve the university's environment so that Black students feel more comfortable. Develop the capacity to monitor the progress disposition and status of Black graduate students. A factual database must be developed from which to establish policy.

Reproduced from Durant, T. J. (2015). *A view from the inside: Thirty-six years of desegregation.* Baton Rouge, LA: Durant Publishing Company.

Appendix IX

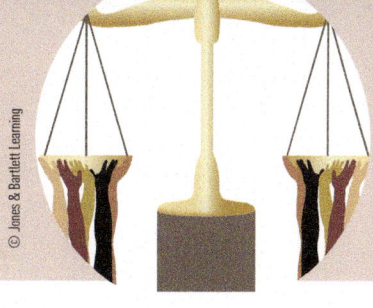

AAMC Diversity Portfolios

Introduction

The Association of American Medical Colleges (AAMC) has created diversity portfolios as part of its commitment to diversity, which includes embracing a broader definition of diversity. The AAMC website describes its Human Capital, Organizational Capacity Building, and Public Health Initiatives portfolios as follows.

Human Capital

The Human Capital portfolio involves impact-driven initiatives, research, and professional development aimed at cultivating and enhancing the knowledge, skills, abilities, and behaviors of individuals. It focuses on cultivating the skills of individuals along the medical continuum from aspiring physicians at the premedical stage to practicing physicians, faculty, researchers, and administrators, through initiatives, programs, and research. Topics include the following:

Premedical

- Enrichment programs on the web
- Medical career fairs
- Medical Minority Applicant Registry (Med-MAR)
- Summer Medical and Dental Education Program (SMDEP)

Medical Students and Faculty

- Herbert W. Nickens Awards
- Grant Writers Coaching Group for NIH Awards
- Minority Faculty Career Development Seminar
- Mid-career Minority Faculty Seminar
- Striving Toward Excellence: Faculty Diversity in Medical Education
- The *Diversity and Faculty Development Digest (DiFac)*

Organizational Capacity Building

The Organizational Capacity Building portfolio is aimed at improving an organization's ability to use diversity as a driver of institutional excellence. It focuses on cultivating organizational capacity building through services, reports, and training that strengthen leadership recruitment, retention, and professional development, cultural competence, and climate and culture assessment, and it addresses diversity issues at the institutional level. Topics include the following:

- Group on Diversity and Inclusion (GDI)
- Tool for Assessing Cultural Competence Training (TACCT)
- Healthcare Executive Diversity and Inclusion Certificate Program
- Learning Lab on Unconscious Bias in the Health Professions
- Diversity Engagement Survey
- Diversity in the Physician Workforce: Facts and Figures 2010
- Diversity Research Forum Publications

Public Health Initiatives

The Public Health Initiatives portfolio is intended to improve the integration of public health concepts into medical education and to enhance and expand a diverse and culturally prepared health workforce. Topics include the following:

- AAMC-CDC Cooperative Agreement
- Urban Universities for HEALTH
- AAMC AHEAD
- LGBT initiatives
- Directory of MD/MPH educational opportunities

© Jones & Bartlett Learning

Resources: Healthcare Academic Program Accreditation Organizations

Accreditation Review Commission on Education for the Physician Assistant (ARC-PA)
3225 Paddocks Parkway, Suite 345, Suwanee, GA 30024. Phone: 770-476-1224
Accreditation: https://www.arc-pa.org/wp-content/uploads/2024/07/Standards-5th-Ed-July-2024.pdf

American Veterinary Medicine Association Council on Education
1931 North Meacham Road, Suite 100, Schaumburg, IL 60173-4360, Phone: 800-248-2862
Accreditation: https://www.avma.org/education/center-for-veterinary-accreditation/accreditation-policies-and-procedures-avma-council-education-coe/coe-accreditation-policies-and-procedures-principles

Commission on Accreditation for Respiratory Care (CoARC)
264 Precision Blvd Telford, TN 37690. Phone: 817-283-2835
Accreditation: https://coarc.com/accreditation/

Commission on Accreditation in Physical Therapy Education (CAPTE)
3030 Potomac Ave., Suite 100, Alexandria, VA 22305-3085. Phone: 703-706-3245
Accreditation: https://www.capteonline.org/faculty-and-program-resources/resource_documents/accreditation-handbook

Commission on Accreditation of Allied Health Education Programs (CAAHEP)
9355 - 113th St. N, #7709 Seminole, FL 33775. Phone: 727-210-2350
Accreditation: https://www.caahep.org/accreditation/accreditation

Commission on Collegiate Nursing Education (CCNE)
655 K Street NW, Suite 750, Washington D.C. 20001. Phone: 202-887-6791
Accreditation: https://www.aacnnursing.org/ccne-accreditation

Council on Education for Public Health (CEPH)
800 I Street NW, Suite 4008, Washington, D.C. 20001. Phone: 202-789-1050
Accreditation: https://ceph.org/about/org-info/criteria-procedures-documents
/criteria-procedures/

Joint Review Committee on Education in Radiologic Technology (JRCERT)
20 North Wacker Drive, Suite 2850, Chicago, IL 60606-3182. Phone: 312-704-5300
Accreditation: https://www.jrcert.org/jrcert-standards/

Liaison Committee on Medical Education (LCME)
330 North Wabash Avenue, Suite 39300, Chicago, IL 60611-5885. Phone: 312-464-4933
Accreditation: https://lcme.org/publications/

National Accrediting Agency for Clinical Laboratory Sciences (NAACLS)
5600 North River Road, Suite 720, Rosemont, IL 60018. Phone: 773-714-8880
Accreditation: https://naacls.org/documents/

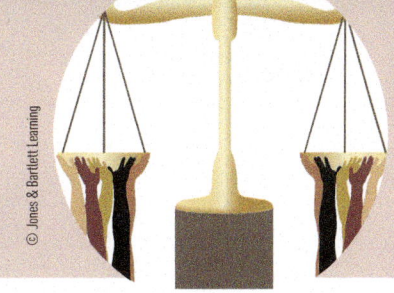

Appendix XI

University of Mississippi Medical Center (UMCC) Pipeline Into Medical School

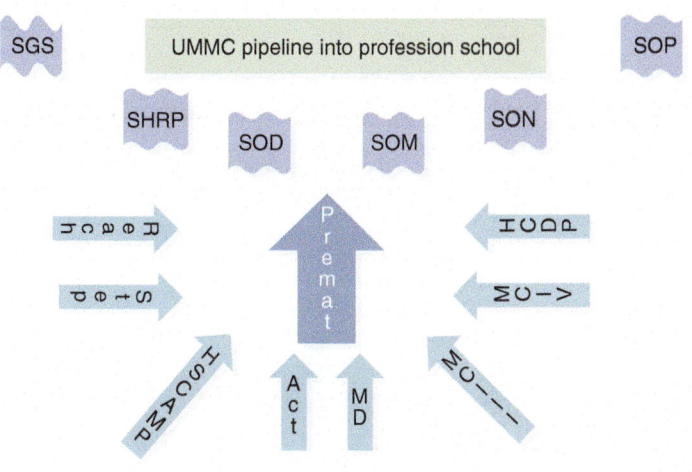

REACH

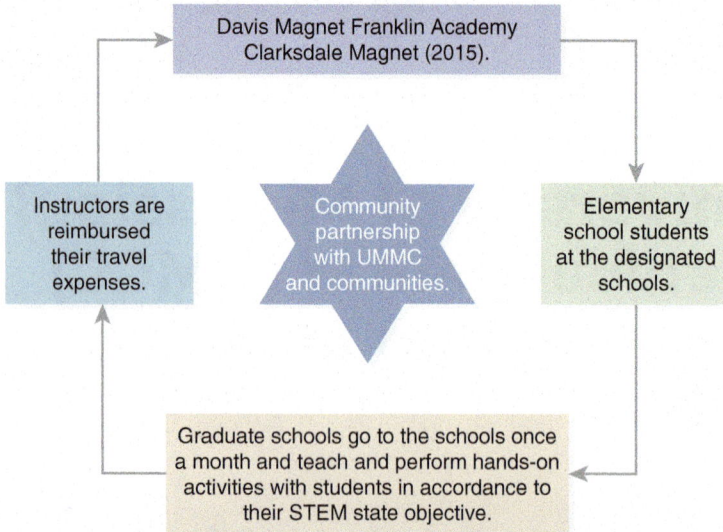

Davis Magnet Franklin Academy Clarksdale Magnet (2015).

Instructors are reimbursed their travel expenses.

Community partnership with UMMC and communities.

Elementary school students at the designated schools.

Graduate schools go to the schools once a month and teach and perform hands-on activities with students in accordance to their STEM state objective.

Science Training Enrichment Program (STEP)

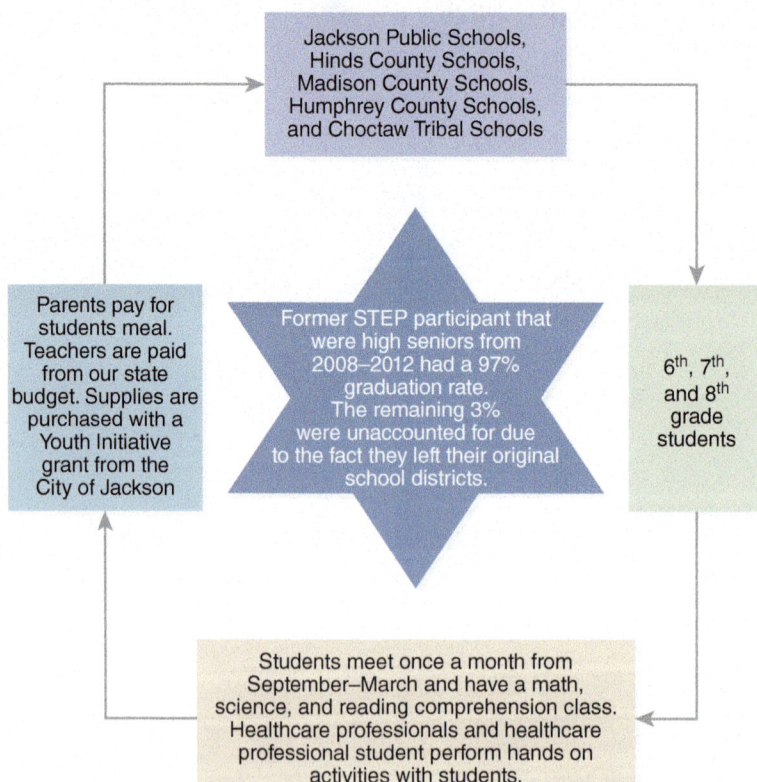

Jackson Public Schools, Hinds County Schools, Madison County Schools, Humphrey County Schools, and Choctaw Tribal Schools

Parents pay for students meal. Teachers are paid from our state budget. Supplies are purchased with a Youth Initiative grant from the City of Jackson

Former STEP participant that were high seniors from 2008–2012 had a 97% graduation rate. The remaining 3% were unaccounted for due to the fact they left their original school districts.

6th, 7th, and 8th grade students

Students meet once a month from September–March and have a math, science, and reading comprehension class. Healthcare professionals and healthcare professional student perform hands on activities with students.

High School Health Care Camp

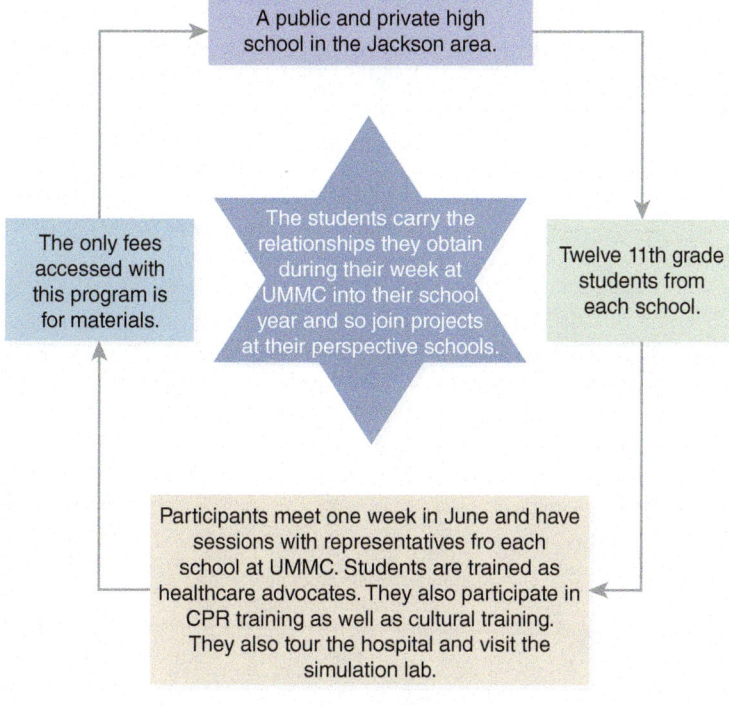

A public and private high school in the Jackson area.

The only fees accessed with this program is for materials.

The students carry the relationships they obtain during their week at UMMC into their school year and so join projects at their perspective schools.

Twelve 11th grade students from each school.

Participants meet one week in June and have sessions with representatives fro each school at UMMC. Students are trained as healthcare advocates. They also participate in CPR training as well as cultural training. They also tour the hospital and visit the simulation lab.

ACT Workshop

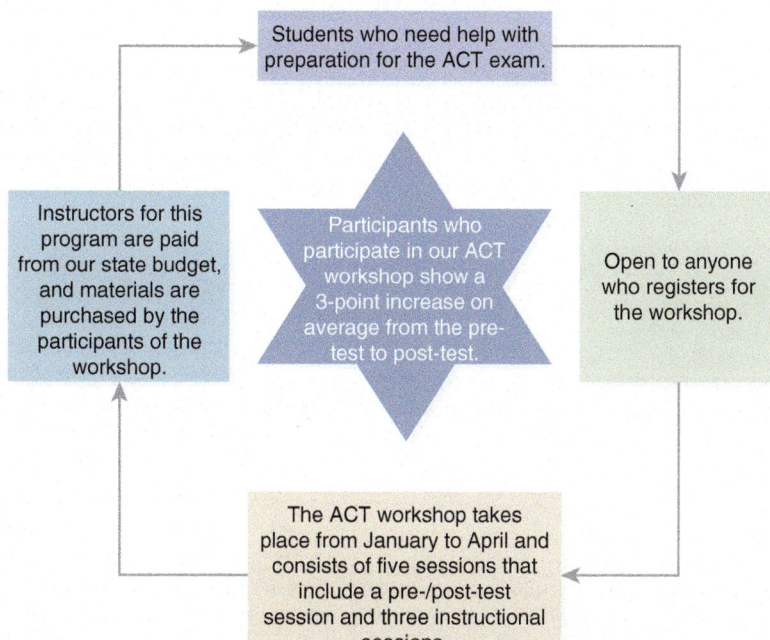

Students who need help with preparation for the ACT exam.

Instructors for this program are paid from our state budget, and materials are purchased by the participants of the workshop.

Participants who participate in our ACT workshop show a 3-point increase on average from the pre-test to post-test.

Open to anyone who registers for the workshop.

The ACT workshop takes place from January to April and consists of five sessions that include a pre-/post-test session and three instructional sessions.

MCAT Workshop

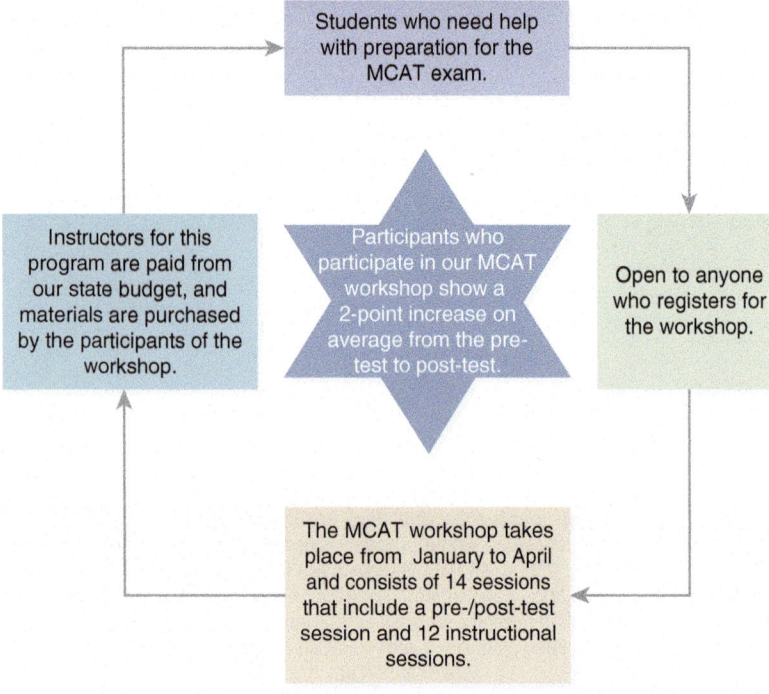

Students who need help with preparation for the MCAT exam.

Instructors for this program are paid from our state budget, and materials are purchased by the participants of the workshop.

Participants who participate in our MCAT workshop show a 2-point increase on average from the pre-test to post-test.

Open to anyone who registers for the workshop.

The MCAT workshop takes place from January to April and consists of 14 sessions that include a pre-/post-test session and 12 instructional sessions.

MedCorp Direct

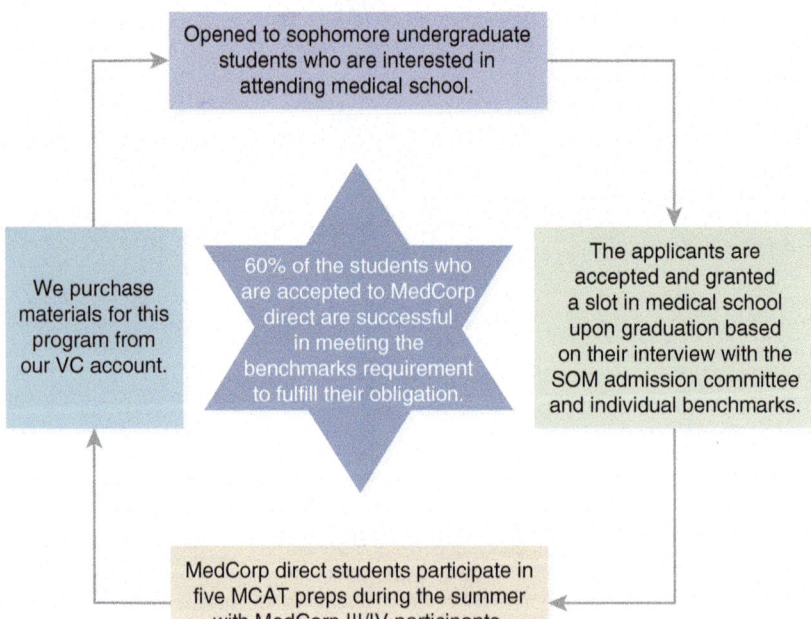

Opened to sophomore undergraduate students who are interested in attending medical school.

We purchase materials for this program from our VC account.

60% of the students who are accepted to MedCorp direct are successful in meeting the benchmarks requirement to fulfill their obligation.

The applicants are accepted and granted a slot in medical school upon graduation based on their interview with the SOM admission committee and individual benchmarks.

MedCorp direct students participate in five MCAT preps during the summer with MedCorp III/IV participants.

MedCorp III (MC-III)

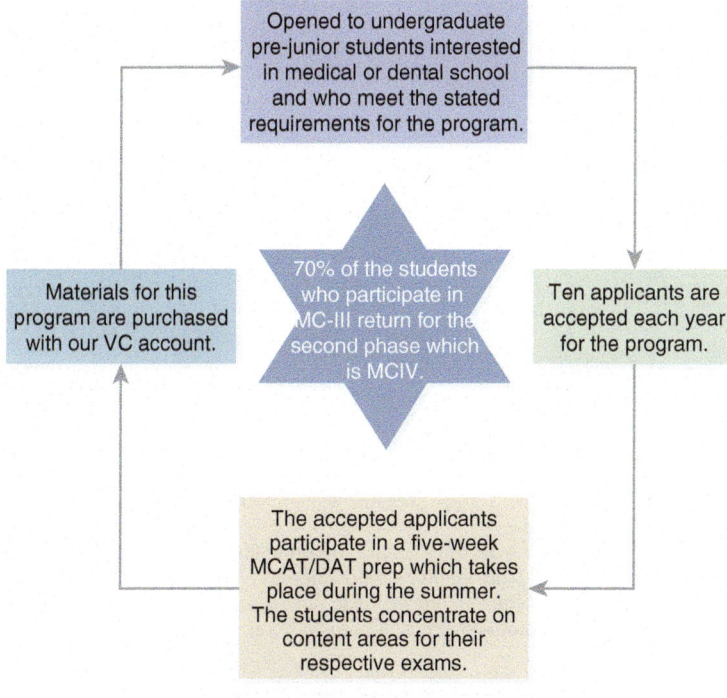

Opened to undergraduate pre-junior students interested in medical or dental school and who meet the stated requirements for the program.

70% of the students who participate in MC-III return for the second phase which is MCIV.

Ten applicants are accepted each year for the program.

Materials for this program are purchased with our VC account.

The accepted applicants participate in a five-week MCAT/DAT prep which takes place during the summer. The students concentrate on content areas for their respective exams.

MedCorp IV (MC-IV)

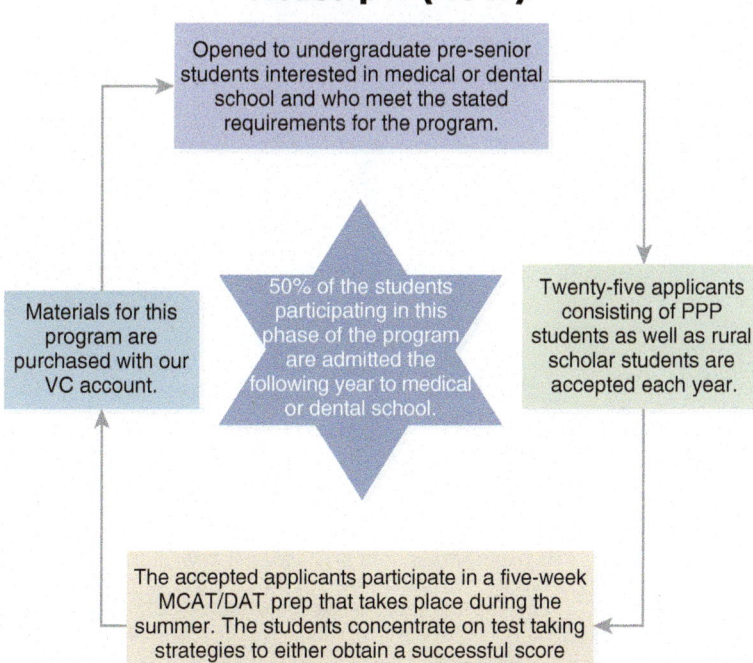

Opened to undergraduate pre-senior students interested in medical or dental school and who meet the stated requirements for the program.

50% of the students participating in this phase of the program are admitted the following year to medical or dental school.

Twenty-five applicants consisting of PPP students as well as rural scholar students are accepted each year.

Materials for this program are purchased with our VC account.

The accepted applicants participate in a five-week MCAT/DAT prep that takes place during the summer. The students concentrate on test taking strategies to either obtain a successful score or improve their current test score.

Health Careers Development Program (HCDP)

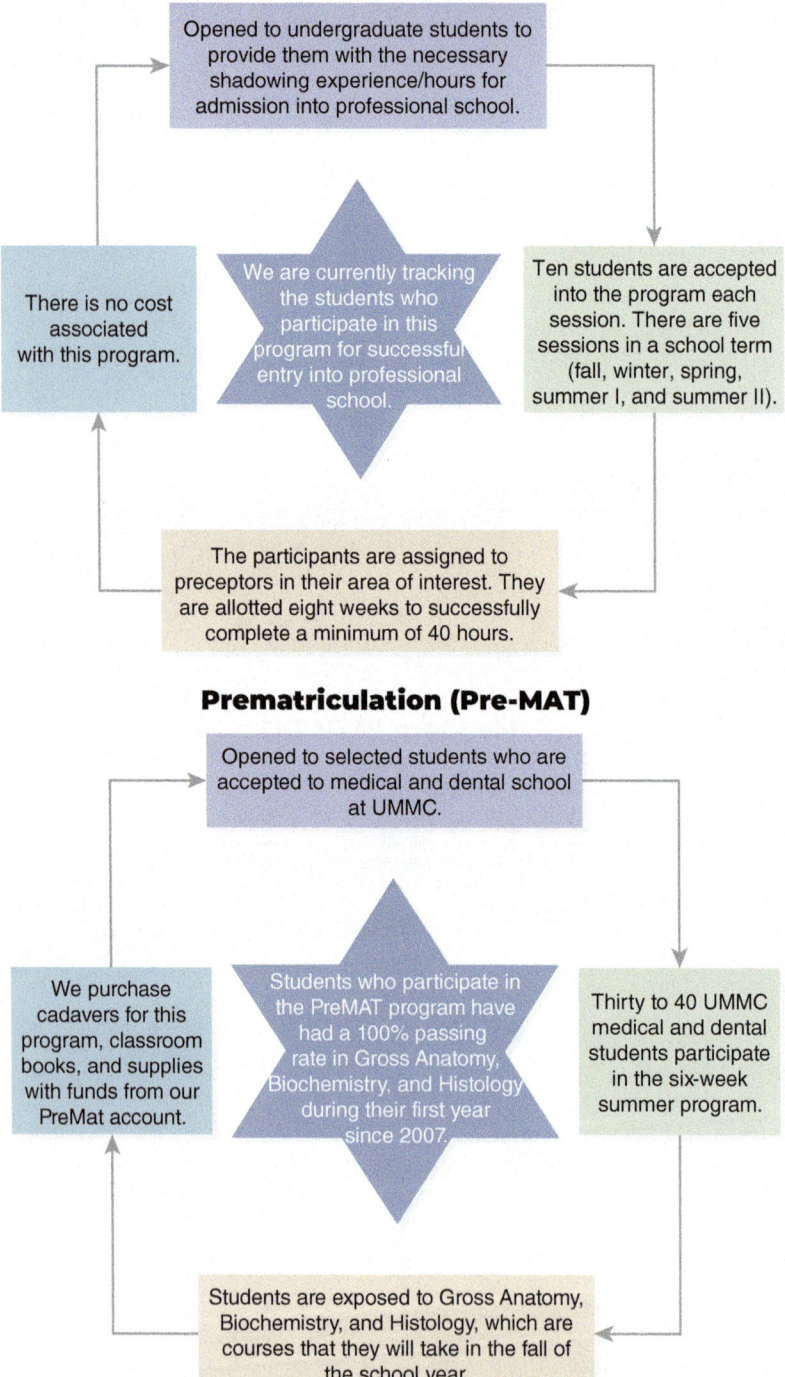

Opened to undergraduate students to provide them with the necessary shadowing experience/hours for admission into professional school.

We are currently tracking the students who participate in this program for successful entry into professional school.

There is no cost associated with this program.

Ten students are accepted into the program each session. There are five sessions in a school term (fall, winter, spring, summer I, and summer II).

The participants are assigned to preceptors in their area of interest. They are allotted eight weeks to successfully complete a minimum of 40 hours.

Prematriculation (Pre-MAT)

Opened to selected students who are accepted to medical and dental school at UMMC.

Students who participate in the PreMAT program have had a 100% passing rate in Gross Anatomy, Biochemistry, and Histology during their first year since 2007.

We purchase cadavers for this program, classroom books, and supplies with funds from our PreMat account.

Thirty to 40 UMMC medical and dental students participate in the six-week summer program.

Students are exposed to Gross Anatomy, Biochemistry, and Histology, which are courses that they will take in the fall of the school year.

Reproduced from Office of health careers opportunity. Dr. Gaarmel Funches, Director of Programs, Ms. LaFreda Sias, Program Administrator, Mr. Jonathan Simmons, Administrative Assistant.

Snapshot of UMMC African American Male Students

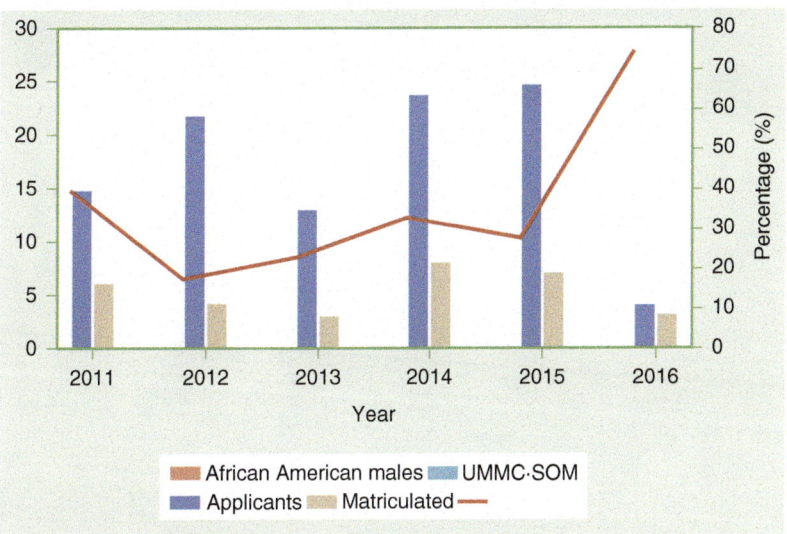

Suggested Readings

Bibliography

Anderson, L. M., Scrimshaw, S. C., Fullilove, M. T., Fielding, J. E., Normand, J., & Task Force on Community Preventive Services. (2003). Culturally competent health care systems: A systematic review. *American Journal of Preventive Medicine, 24*(3S), 68–79. https://doi.org/10.1016/s0749-3797(02)00657-8

Attention-deficit/hyperactivity disorder (ADHD). (n.d.). National Institute of Mental Health. https://www.nimh.nih.gov/health/statistics/attention-deficit-hyperactivity-disorder-adhd#part_2549

Baxter, C. (2001). *Managing diversity and inequality in healthcare*. Bialliere Tindall.

Brach, C., & Fraser, I. (2000). Can cultural competency reduce racial and ethnic health disparities? A review and conceptual model. *Medical Care Research and Review, 57*(S1), 181–217. https://doi.org/10.1177/1077558700057001s09

Broderick, J., Devine, T, Langhans, E, Lemerise, A. J., Lier, S., & Harris, L. (2014, June 5). *Understanding the Relationship between Education and Health* [Discussion paper]. National Academy of Medicine. https://nam.edu/perspectives/understanding-the-relationship-between-education-and-health/

Brondolo, E., Gallo, L. C., & Myers, H. F. (2008). Race, racism and health: Disparities, mechanisms, and interventions. *Journal of Behavioral Medicine, 32*(1), 1–8. https://doi.org/10.1007/s10865-008-9190-3

Brown, C. M., Barner, J. C., & Shepard, M. D. (2003). Issues and barriers related to the provision of pharmaceutical care in community health centers and migrant health centers. *Journal of the American Pharmacists Association (Washington D. C.: 1996), 43*(1), 75–77. https://doi.org/10.1331/10865800360467088

Burgess, D., van Ryn, M., Dovidio, J., & Saha, S. (2007). Reducing racial bias among health care providers: Lessons from social-cognitive psychology. *Journal of General Internal Medicine, 22*(6), 882–887. https://doi.org/10.1007/s11606-007-0160-1

Byrd, M., & Clayton, L. (2000). *An American health dilemma: A medical history of African Americans and the problems of race: Beginnings to 1900*. Routledge.

Chen, F. M., Fryer, G. E., Phillips, R. L., Wilson, E., & Pathman, D. E. (2005). Patients' beliefs about racism, preferences for physician race, and satisfaction with care. *Annals of Family Medicine, 3*(2), 138–143. https://doi.org/10.1370/afm.282

Centers for Disease Control Archive (2020). Population Health. Retrieved from: https://archive.cdc.gov/www_cdc_gov/pophealthtraining/whatis.html

Chettiar, I. M., Bunting, W. C., & Schotter, G. (2012). *At America's expense: The mass incarceration of the elderly* [Research paper]. New York University School of Law, https://www.ojp.gov/ncjrs/virtual-library/abstracts/americas-expense-mass-incarceration-elderly

Chevannes, M. (2002). Issues in educating health professionals to meet the diverse needs of patients and other service users from ethnic minority groups. *Journal of Advanced Nursing, 39*(3), 290–298. https://doi.org/10.1046/j.1365-2648.2002.02276.x

Clark, R., Anderson, N. B., Clark, V. R., & Williams, D. R. (1999). Racism as a stressor or African Americans: A biopsychosocial model. *American Psychologist, 54*(10), 805–816. https://doi .org/10.1037//0003-066x.54.10.805

Churchwell, K., Elkind, M. S., Benjamin, R. M., Carson, A. P., Chang, E. K., Lawrence, W., Mills, A., Odom, T. M., Rodriguez, C. J., Rodriguez, F., Sanchez, E., Sharrief, A. Z., Sims, M., & Williams, O. (2020). Call to action: Structural racism as a fundamental driver of health disparities: A presidential advisory from the American Heart Association. *Circulation, 142*(24). https://doi.org/10.1161/cir.0000000000000936

Diverse Hispanic population to become largest U.S. minority. (1997). *Popul Today, 25*(11), 1–2.

Do, D. P., Frank, R., Zheng, C., & Iceland, J. (2017). Hispanic Segregation and Poor Health: It's Not Just Black and White. *American Journal of Epidemiology, 186*(8), 990–999. https://doi .org/10.1093/aje/kwx172

Dovidio, J. F., Penner, L. A., Albrecht, T. L., Norton, W. E., Gaertner, S. L., & Shelton, J. N. (2008). Disparities and distrust: the implications of psychological processes for understanding racial disparities in health and health care. *Social Science & Medicine, 67*(3), 478–486. https://doi .org/10.1016/j.socscimed.2008.03.019

Emery, J., Crump, C., & Bors, P. (2003). Reliability and validity of two instruments designed to assess the walking and bicycling suitability of sidewalks and roads. *American Journal of Health Promotion, 18*(1), 28–46. https://doi.org/10.4278/0890-1171-18.1.38

Fortmann, A. L., Soriano, E. C., Gallo, L. C., Clark, T. L., Spierling Bagsic, S. R., Sandoval, H., Jones, J. A., Roesch, S., Gilmer, T., Schultz, J., Bodenheimer, T., & Philis-Tsimikas, A. (2024). Medical Assistant Health Coaching for Type 2 Diabetes in Primary Care: Results From a Pragmatic Cluster Randomized Controlled Trial. *Diabetes Care, 47*(7), 1171–1180. https://doi .org/10.2337/dc23-2487

Fry, R., Kennedy, B., & Funk, C. (2021, April 1). *STEM jobs see uneven progress in increasing gender, racial and ethnic diversity* [Report]. Pew Research Center. https://www.pewresearch.org /science/2021/04/01/stem-jobs-see-uneven-progress-in-increasing-gender-racial-and-ethnic -diversity/

Gee, G. C., & Ford, C. L. (2011). Structural racism and health inequities: old issues, new directions. *Du Bois Review: Social Science Research on Race, 8*(1), 115–132. https://doi.org/10.1017 /S1742058X11000130

Gimenez, M. E. (1989). Latino/"Hispanic"—Who Needs a Name? The Case against a Standardized Terminology. *International Journal of Health Services, 19*(3), 557–571. https://doi.org/10.2190 /HN6N-P1TH-8CHL-KW5X

Obesity: Technology-supported multicomponent coaching or counseling interventions – to reduce weight. (n.d.). The Community Guide. https://www.thecommunityguide.org/findings/obesity -technology-supported-multicomponent-coaching-or-counseling-interventions-reduce.html

Hausmann, L. R. M., Jeong, K., Bost, J. E., & Ibrahim, S. A. (2008). Perceived discrimination in Health care and health status in a racially diverse sample. *Medical Care, 46*(9), 905–914. https:// doi.org/10.1097/mlr.0b013e3181792562

Hedegaard, H., Curtin, S. and Warner M., (2018, November). Suicide mortality in the United States. NCHS Data Brief No. 330. https://www.cdc.gov/nchs/data/databriefs/db330-h.pdf

Huntington, S. P. (2004). The Hispanic challenge. In R. Eddy, & V. Villanueva (Eds.), *A language and power reader: Representations of race in a "post-racist" era*, pp. 335–351. University Press of Colorado.

Institute of Medicine (US) Committee on Health Literacy, Nielsen-Bohlman, L., Panzer, A. M., & Kindig, D. A. (Eds.). (2004). Health literacy: A prescription to end confusion. National Academies Press (US). https://doi.org/10.17226/10883

Jones, D. (2006). The persistence of American Indian health disparities. *American Journal of Public Health, 96*(12), 2122–2134. https://doi.org/10.2105/AJPH.2004.054262

Kirsch, I. S., Jungeblut, A., Jenkins, L., & Kolstad, A. (1993). *Adult literacy in America: A first look at the results of the National Adult Literacy Survey (NALS)*. Washington, DC: National Center for Education Statistics, U.S. Department of Education. https://files.eric.ed.gov/fulltext/ED358375 .pdf

Kopp, W. (2011). The newest silver bullet: Providing every child with an effective teacher. *One Day Alumni Magazine*, Spring, Edition XI, 29.

Kuzma, J. (1998). *Basic statistics for the health sciences.* Mayfield.

Ladson-Billings, G., & Tate, W. (1995). Toward a critical race theory of education. *Teachers College Record, 97*(1), 47–68. https://doi.org/10.1177/016146819509700104

Mak, W. W. S., Poon, C. Y. M., Pun, L. Y. K., & Cheung, S. F. (2007). Meta-analysis of stigma and mental health. *Social Science & Medicine, 65*(2), 245–261. https://doi.org/10.1016/j .socscimed.2007.03.015

Massey, D. S. & Denton, N. A. (1993). *American apartheid: Segregation and the making of the underclass* (Chapters 2 & 3). Harvard University Press.

McKinney, J., & Kurtz-Rossi, S. (2000). *Culture, health, and literacy: A guide to health education materials for adults with limited English skills.* World Education.

Men and mental health. (n.d.). National Institute of Mental Health https://www.nimh.nih.gov/health /topics/men-and-mental-health

Milner, H. R. (2012). Beyond a test score: Explaining opportunity gaps in educational practice. *Journal of Black Studies, 20*(10), 1–26. httpS://doi.org/10.1177/0021934712442539

National Center for Education Statistics. (2006). *The health literacy of America's adults: Results from the 2003 National Assessment of Adult Literacy.* U.S. Department of Education.

Naylor, L. (Ed.). (1997). *Cultural diversity in the United States.* Bergin and Garvey.

National Institute of Health (2024). *Office of Management and Budget (OMB) Standards* https://orwh .od.nih.gov/toolkit/other-relevant-federal-policies/OMB-standards

National Institute on Minority Health and Health Disparities (n.d.). NIMHD research framework details. https://www.nimhd.nih.gov/resources/research-framework/nimhd-research-framework -details

Escarce, J. J., Morales, L. S., & Rumbaut, R. (2006). The health status and health behaviors of Hispanics. In M. Tienda, & F. Mitchell (Eds.), Hispanics and the future of America. National Academies Press. https://www.ncbi.nlm.nih.gov/books/NBK19899/

Noe-Bustamante, L., Mora, L., & Lopez, M. H. (2020). *About one-in-four U.S. Hispanics have heard of Latinx, but just 3% use it* (Report). Pew Research Center. https://www.pewresearch .org/race-and-ethnicity/2020/08/11/about-one-in-four-u-s-hispanics-have-heard-of-latinx -but-just-3-use-it/

Orvis, K. (2024). OMB Publishes Revisions to Statistical Policy Directive No. 15: Standards for Maintaining, Collecting, and Presenting Federal Data on Race and Ethnicity. Retrieved from https://www.whitehouse.gov/omb/briefing-room/2024/03/28/omb-publishes-revisions-to -statistical-policy-directive-no-15-standards-for-maintaining-collecting-and-presenting-federal -data-on-race-and-ethnicity/

Passel, J. S., & Cohn, D. (2008). U.S. population projections : 2005–2050 [Report]. Pew Research Center. https://nccd-crc.issuelab.org/resources/11543/11543.pdf

Pratt, B. M., Hixson, L., & Jones, N. A. (n.d.). Measuring Race and Ethnicity Across the Decades: 1790–2010. U.S. Census Bureau. https://www.census.gov/data-tools/demo/race/MREAD_1790 _2010.html

Purnell, L., & Paulunka, B. (1998). *Transcultural healthcare: A culturally competent approach.* F. A. Davis.

Richard, A. (Ed.). (2007). *Eliminating healthcare disparities in America.* Humana Press.

Rose, P. R. (2014). *Effie's soul food recipes and more...with a healthy twist.* Rose Publishing.

Ross, C. E., & Wu, C. (1995). The links between education and health. *American Sociological Review, 60*(5), 719–745. https://doi.org/10.2307/2096319

Rothstein, R. (2004). *Class and schools: Using social, economic and educational reform to close the Black– White achievement gap.* Teachers College, Columbia University.

Armstrong, K., McMurphy, S., Dean, L. T., Micco, E., Putt, M., Halbert, C. H., Schwartz, J. S., Sankar, P., Pyeritz, R. E., Bernhardt, B., & Shea, J. A. (2008). Differences in the patterns of health care system distrust between blacks and whites. *Journal of General Internal Medicine, 23*(6), 827–833. https://doi.org/10.1007/s11606-008-0561-9

Scott, M. G. (2002). Cultural competency: How is it measured? Does it make a difference? *Generations: Journal of the American Society on Aging, 26*(3), 39–45.

Smedley, B., Stith, A., & Nelson, A. (Eds.). (2003). *Unequal treatment: Confronting racial and ethnic disparities in health care.* National Academies Press.

Srivastava, R. (2006). *The healthcare professional's guide to cultural competence.* Mosby.

Taylor, S., & Lurie, N. (2004). The role of culturally competent communication in reducing ethnic and racial healthcare disparities. *American Journal of Managed Care, 10*, SP1–SP4.

Universal health coverage study series (UNICO). (n.d.). The World Bank. http://www.worldbank.org /en/topic/health/publication/universal-health-coverage-study-series

U.S. Department of Health and Human Services. (2001). *National standards for culturally and linguistically appropriate services in health care.* Washington, DC: Office of Minority Health. https://thinkculturalhealth.hhs.gov/assets/pdfs/EnhancedNationalCLASStandards.pdf

U.S. Department of Health and Human Services. (2008). *America's health literacy: Why we need accessible health information.* Washington, DC: Office of Disease Prevention and Health Promotion. https://www.ahrq.gov/sites/default/files/wysiwyg/health-literacy/dhhs-2008-issue -brief.pdf

Waidmann, T. (2009, September). *Estimating the cost of racial and ethnic health disparities* [Report]. The Urban Institute. https://www.urban.org/sites/default/files/publication/30666/411962 -Estimating-the-Cost-of-Racial-and-Ethnic-Health-Disparities.PDF

West-Olatunji, C. (2008). Language as a form of subtle oppression among linguistically different people in the United States. *Social Perspectives, 10*(1), 11–28.

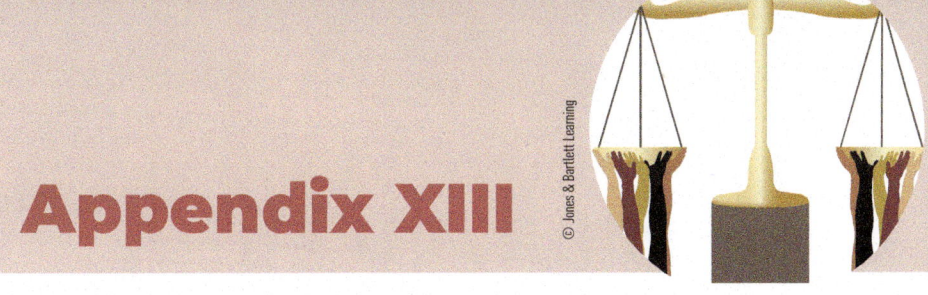

Appendix XIII

First Step Act (H.R. 5682)

Mass Incarceration and Criminal Justice System Reform: First Step Act (H.R. 5682)

ACT SECTIONS

1. Creating Evidenced-based Recidivism Reduction Programs
2. Expansion of Good Behavior and Early Release Programs for Federal Inmates
3. Amend Federal Sentencing Laws
4. Miscellaneous Improvements

Proposed Reform Actions	Responsibility for Reform Actions	Timeline for Reform Actions
Develop a Risk & Needs Assessment System ("system") to be applied to each prisoner upon intake and reassessed periodically	Attorney General (AG) in consult with the Directors of the BOP, Administrative Office of the U.S. Courts, Office of Probation and Pretrial Services, National Institute of Justice, and the National institute of Corrections	Within 180 days of Enactment (after consultation with the Independent Review Committee created by the Act)
Must assess recidivism rate level		
An Independent Review Committee shall assist in developing the system		Independent Review Committee shall terminate 30 days after the release of the risk and needs assessment system
• Two members with published peer-review scholarship	The BOP shall list appropriate recidivism reduction programs for each prisoner	
• Two corrections practitioners who have developed risk and needs assessment tools		
• One person with expertise in assessing risk assessment implementation	The AG shall develop training programs for the BOP officers and employees responsible for administering the system	Phase-in period of 2 years to give BOP time to provide appropriate programming and to develop and validate the system to be used
Assign prisoners to appropriate recidivism rate reduction programs		
Ensure programs are evidenced-based, effective, and efficient		Initial report due to Congress 2 years after enactment. Subsequent reports due each year for the next 5 years
Train Bureau of Prisons (BOP) employees to correctly implement programs		
Conduct annual audits of the BOP to ensure that the system is being used and implemented properly		
Congress must receive regular report of results		

Proposed Reform Actions	Responsibility for Reform Actions	Timeline for Reform Actions
The system shall provide incentives and rewards to prisoners in recidivism reduction programs	AG and Director of BOP	Immediately upon law enactment
■ Telephone and visitation rewards (additional time and video conferencing)	Time credits shall be applied toward time in prerelease custody or supervised release	Immediately upon successful completion of recidivism reduction program
■ Transfer to facility closer to prisoners' home residence upon recommendation of warden and if bed is available	Home confinement: 24-hour electronic monitoring; remain in residence except to participate in work, community service, religious/family activities, medical care, or crime victim restoration activities.	Immediately upon law enactment
■ At least two other incentives as follows: increased commissary spending and offerings, enhanced email access, transfer to preferred housing units, and prisoner-solicited incentives		Immediately upon law enactment
■ Time credits for successfully completing a recidivism reduction program (eligible prisoners only)*	Reentry Center: Used when 24-hour electronic monitoring is not feasible.	Immediately upon law enactment
■ Types of prerelease custody include home confinement and residential reentry centers.	Director of BOP must ensure sufficient capacity for all eligible prisoners exists within the system	
■ Amends the Second Chance Act to make elderly and terminally ill offenders who are eligible for family reunification through home detention instead of being housed in a federal facility	Director of U.S. Pretrial and Probation Services	
■ U.S. Pretrial and Probation Services shall offer assistance to any prisoner not under its supervision during prerelease custody	Director of BOP	
■ All persons released from federal prison must be given their birth certificate and photo identification		

(continues)

Proposed Reform Actions	Responsibility for Reform Actions	Timeline for Reform Actions

Enhanced mandatory minimum sentences for drug felons are reduced
 	
■ The three-strike mandatory penalty is reduced from life imprisonment to 25 years
■ The 20-year mandatory minimum is reduced to 15 years
■ Offenses that trigger these enhanced mandatory minimum sentences are also reformed
    ● Qualifying prior convictions must be serious drug felonies (formerly any drug felonies) or other serious violent felonies**
    ● Prior felonies must have occurred within the past 15 years**
■ Broadens existing safety valve
■ Application of Fair Sentencing Act (2010)
	Eligibility for Safety Valve sentencing expands the number of criminal history "points" for offenders from one to four
	
	Allows offenders sentenced under prior provisions to petition for reductions in sentence consistent with new crack cocaine sentencing law
		Immediately upon law enactment
		
		Immediately upon law enactment

Additional improvements for offenders include, but are not limited to, the following: ■ De-escalation training programs ■ Evidenced-based treatment programs for opioid and heroin abuse ■ Free feminine hygiene products for all female inmates ■ Juvenile solitary confinement adjustment	The Director of BOP must include de-escalation training to teach how to de-escalate encounters between law enforcement, BOP employees, and a civilian or prisoner. BOP must report to Congress it's capacity to treat heroin and opioid abuse through evidenced-based programs. The Director of the Administrative Office of the U.S. Courts must report to Congress a report assessing the availability and capacity for the provision of medication-assisted treatment.	Immediately upon law enactment Not later than 90 days after the date of enactment. Not later than 120 days after the date of enactment. Immediately upon law enactment. Immediately upon law enactment

Proposed Reform Actions	Responsibility for Reform Actions	Timeline for Reform Actions
	Director of BOP	
	The BOP must restrict the use of juvenile solitary confinement for any reason except as a temporary response to a juvenile's behavior that poses a serious and immediate risk of physical harm. Staff must use the least restrictive means, including "talking it out" and attempting care by a qualified mental health professional.	

*Eligibility restricted to prisoners classified as minimum or low risk. Prisoners serving sentence for conviction of certain offenses, including crimes relating to terrorism, murder, sexual exploitation of children, espionage, violent firearms offenses, or those that are organizers, leaders, managers, or supervisors in the fentanyl and heroin drug trade are ineligible to receive these incentives. Deportable prisoners are not eligible for time credits.

**Provision is not retroactive and will not apply to any person sentenced before enactment of this law.

First Step Act Section by Section Summary, December 14, 2018; National Conference of State Legislatures Staff: National Conference of State Legislatures. Retrieved from http://www.ncsl.org/documents/statefed/First_Step_Act _Summary_Dec2018.pdf.
Table prepared by Jeffrey A. Rose, B.A., Economics and Political Science, Yale University, 1984.

Glossary of Important Terms

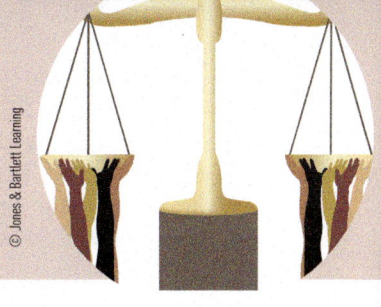

A

Access to care The ability to obtain timely, appropriate, and affordable health services to achieve the best possible health outcomes

Achievement gap The disparity in academic performance and educational outcomes between groups of students, often defined by socioeconomic status, race, ethnicity, or other factors

African American/Black A person having origins in any of the black racial groups of Africa

Agency for Healthcare Research and Quality (AHRQ) A U.S. government agency that develops evidence to improve the quality, safety, efficiency, and effectiveness of healthcare for all Americans

Aid to Families with Dependent Children (AFDC) A federal assistance program in the United States that provided financial support to low-income families with children from 1935 until it was replaced by Temporary Assistance for Needy Families (TANF) in 1996

Algorithms Step-by-step sets of rules or instructions designed to perform a specific task or solve a problem, often used in computing and data processing

Asian Indian American people People having origins in any of the original peoples of the Indian subcontinent, including India, Pakistan, and Bangladesh

American Indian and Alaska Native People having origins in any of the original peoples of North America, and who maintain cultural identifications through tribal affiliations or community recognition

Artificial intelligence The simulation of human intelligence processes by machines, especially computer systems, to perform tasks such as learning, reasoning, and problem-solving

Asian American and Pacific Islander People having origins in any of the original peoples of the Far East, Southeast Asia, the Indian subcontinent, or the Pacific Islands

B

Biometrics Measurable physical or behavioral characteristics—such as fingerprints, facial recognition, or voice patterns—used to identify and verify the identity of individuals

Black/African American People having origins in any of the Black racial groups of Africa

Black Sacred Cosmos A theoretical framework for understanding the religious composition of African Americans

Black Spirituality The notion that black spirituality is not simply the profession of basic Christian tenants, but is a divinely inspired reframing of Christianity that affirms black existence in the world

Brown v. Board of Education A landmark 1954 U.S. Supreme Court case in which the Court unanimously ruled that racial segregation in public schools was unconstitutional, overturning *Plessy v. Ferguson* and declaring that "separate but equal" is inherently unequal

Bureau of Indian Affairs A U.S. government agency within the Department of the Interior responsible for managing and administering federal programs and services for Native American groups and individuals

C

ChatGPT An Artificial Intelligence (AI) language model developed by OpenAI that generates human-like text responses based on user input, enabling natural and interactive conversations

Childhood obesity A medical condition where a child has excess body fat that may negatively affect their health and development, typically measured by a body mass index (BMI) at or above the 95th percentile for children of the same age and sex

Chronic Disease Management Program (CDMP) A coordinated healthcare approach designed to help individuals with long-term conditions effectively manage their symptoms, improve quality of life, and prevent complications through education, monitoring, and support

Colorblindness A vision deficiency that impairs an individual's ability to distinguish certain colors, most commonly red and green

Commercial determinants of health (CDOH) The ways in which corporate practices, products, and policies—such as marketing, production, and distribution—impact population health outcomes and contribute to health risks or benefits

Common school system A publicly funded, locally controlled education system designed to provide free, basic education to all children regardless of background or socioeconomic status

Confucianism A philosophical and ethical system based on the teachings of Confucius, an ancient Chinese philosopher and teacher, that emphasizes moral virtues, social harmony, respect for hierarchy, and the importance of family and community

Cultural capital The non-financial social assets—like education, style, knowledge, and manners—that enable individuals to gain social mobility and influence

Cultural competence A set of congruent behaviors, attitudes, and policies that come together in a system, agency, or among professionals that enables effective work in cross-cultural situations

Cultural incongruence A mismatch or conflict between the cultural values, norms, or behaviors of different groups or settings

Cultural nuances The recognition of subtle differences about a particular culture

Culturally and Linguistically Appropriate Services (CLAS) Standards to address the inequities that exist in the provision of health care and to make services more responsive to the individual needs, on a cultural and linguistic basis, of patients/consumers/clients served

Culturally relevant pedagogy An educational approach that recognizes and incorporates students' cultural backgrounds and experiences to make learning more meaningful and effective

Culture An integrated pattern of learned beliefs and behaviors that can be shared among groups, including thoughts, styles of communicating, ways of interacting, views on roles and relationships, values, practices, and customs

D

Demographic imperative The need to address and adapt to significant shifts in population composition—such as age, race, ethnicity, or immigration patterns—that impact social, political, and economic structures

Diabetes A chronic medical condition in which the body either doesn't produce enough insulin or cannot effectively use the insulin it produces, leading to elevated levels of glucose in the blood

Digital divide The notion that in lower socioeconomic status communities, individuals may not have computers

Discrimination The unjust or prejudicial treatment of individuals or groups based on characteristics such as race, gender, age, religion, or disability, rather than individual merit

Diversity The makeup of the workforce of a given healthcare organization. This includes ethnic and racial backgrounds, age, physical and cognitive abilities, family status, sexual orientation, socioeconomic status, religious and spiritual values, geographic location, and includes all of the dimensions and all of the differences between people

E

Emerging majorities A term used to describe an inevitable change taking place in American society based on the prediction that by the year 2050, in certain geographic areas in the United States, the majority populations will be Hispanic and Black people and other minorities (combined) and White people will be the minority group

Environmental justice The fair treatment and meaningful involvement of all people, regardless of race, income, or background, in the development, implementation, and enforcement of environmental laws and policies

Ethnicity A group or individual's conception of cultural identity that includes a wide variety of learned behaviors that a humans use in their natural and social environment to survive, which may result in cultural demarcation between and within societies

F

Family wage The amount of income for a family to live on, in terms of meeting basic needs

FAST An acronym for recognizing stroke symptoms—Face drooping, Arm weakness, Speech difficulty, and Time to call emergency services—emphasizing the urgency of immediate medical attention

Federally qualified health center (FQHC) Community-based healthcare providers that receive federal funding to offer comprehensive primary care services to underserved populations, regardless of their ability to pay

Filial piety A cultural value, especially prominent in East Asian societies, that emphasizes respect, obedience, and care for one's parents and elders as a fundamental moral duty

Filipino American people Individuals of Filipino descent classified under the broader racial category of "Asian," which includes those with origins in the Philippine Islands

Food desert When supermarkets are built outside of poor communities and individuals cannot get to them and even if they do, they cannot afford what is inside of them

Food injustice Disparity/gap in the offering of quality foods in low-income neighborhoods as compared to higher socioeconomic communities

Food insecurity The lack of consistent access to enough food for an active, healthy life due to financial or other resource limitations

Food mirage When in low-income neighborhoods, there may be actual large grocery stores that include full service, but the individuals, who live in the neighborhood, cannot afford to shop there

Freedom Through the lens of Eurocentric normativity, has always highlighted an American pursuit toward individualism; through the lens of the Black Sacred Cosmos presupposes, a call to total allegiance to God alone and free reign over one's life to do, as God requires

H

Health care disparity Typically refers to differences between groups in health coverage, access to care and quality of care

Health disparity The lack of consistent access to enough food for an active, healthy life due to financial or other resource limitations

Health equity The principle of ensuring everyone has a fair and just opportunity to attain their highest level of health by addressing avoidable inequalities and barriers

Health inequality Healthcare inequality or gaps in the quality of health and

health care across racial, ethnic, and socioeconomic groups and population-specific differences in the presence of disease, health outcomes, or access to health care

Health literacy The ability to obtain, process, and understand basic health information and services needed to make appropriate health decisions

Healthy People A national initiative by the U.S. government that sets science-based objectives to improve the health and well-being of all Americans over a decade

Healthy People 2030 A U.S. federal initiative that provides science-based, 10-year national objectives aimed at improving the health of all Americans by promoting health, preventing disease, and eliminating health disparities

Healthy people initiative A nationwide effort by the U.S. Department of Health and Human Services to set measurable, science-based objectives every decade to improve the health and quality of life for all Americans

Heterogeneity Another way of describing diversity

Hispanic A person of Mexican, Puerto Rican, Cuban, Central or South American or other Spanish culture or origin, regardless of race

Hispanic health paradox The epidemiological finding that Hispanic/Latino populations in the U.S. often have health outcomes that are comparable to or better than those of non-Hispanic Whites, despite having lower average socioeconomic status

Hypertension Also known as high blood pressure, a chronic medical condition in which the force of the blood against artery walls is consistently too high, increasing the risk of heart disease, stroke, and other health problems

I

Indian Health Care Improvement Act (IHCIA) A 1976 legislation that is aimed at improving health care services American Indians and Alaska Natives

Indian Health Service (IHS) A federal agency within the U.S. Department of Health and Human Services that provides comprehensive health care services to American Indians and Alaska Natives

Infant Mortality Rate (IMR) The number of infant deaths per 1000 live births

J

Jim Crow laws State and local laws in the United States, primarily in the South, that enforced racial segregation and disenfranchised Black Americans from the late 19th century through the mid-20th century

L

Latina birth outcomes paradox The phenomenon where Latina women, particularly recent immigrants, tend to have birth outcomes—such as low infant mortality and healthy birth weights— that are as good as or better than those of more socioeconomically advantaged groups, despite facing significant social and economic disadvantages

Linguistic competence The capacity of an organization and its personnel to communicate effectively and convey information in a manner that is easily understood by diverse audiences including persons of limited English proficiency, those who have low literacy skills or are not literate, and individuals with disabilities and the ability to communicate effectively and accurately with individuals whose primary language is other than English

Low birth weight (LBW) Less than 2500 grams at birth

M

Mass incarceration The large-scale imprisonment of people, particularly from marginalized communities, often resulting from strict sentencing laws and systemic inequalities in the criminal justice system

Maternal Mortality Rate (MMR) The annual number of female deaths per 100,000 from any cause aggravated by pregnancy or its management, excluding accidental or incidental causes

Mainstream Term often used to describe the "general market" and usually refers to a broad population that is primarily White and middle class

Medicaid A means tested (income-based) program for low-income individuals including children

Medicare A program that originated for Americans over 65 years of age, individuals with long-term disability or end stage renal disease and was signed into law by President Lyndon Baines Johnson on July 30, 1965

Men's Health Network A national non-profit organization dedicated to improving the health and wellness of men and boys through advocacy, education, and outreach

Migrant and seasonal agricultural worker (MSAW) An individual who moves from place to place to perform agricultural labor on a seasonal basis, often facing temporary employment, low wages, and limited access to healthcare and social services

Mission (of an organization) Generally formulated into a brief statement that attempts to answer the question of why an organization exists and states the purpose of an organization, namely to those in it and to the public

Model Minority A term used to describe groups of people who immigrate to the United States and appear to assimilate easily into the mainstream

Morbidity rates The frequency or proportion of individuals in a population who suffer from a particular disease or health condition over a specified period

N

National Healthcare Disparities Report (NHDR) An annual report by the Agency for Healthcare Research and Quality that assesses and tracks disparities in access, outcomes, and quality of healthcare across different populations in the United States

Nationality An identity that can be defined by a person's place of legal birth or by a person's associational citizenship status governed by where an individual resides and works, which may defy national boundaries and sovereignty

O

Office of Management and Budget (OMB) A U.S. federal agency that assists the President in preparing the federal budget and oversees the administration of executive branch agencies to ensure effective implementation of government policies

Ozempic A prescription medication primarily for type 2 diabetes that is also purported to help with weight loss and reduce the risk of major

cardiovascular events in people with known heart disease

P

Patient Protection and Affordable Care Act (PPACA) A federal statute, pertaining to health insurance, that was signed into United States law by President Barack Obama on March 23, 2010

Patriarchal society A social system in which men hold primary power and dominate roles in leadership, moral authority, social privilege, and control of property

People of color Individuals classified in the emerging majority groups, namely Black or African American, Native American or Alaska Native, Asians and Pacific Islander, and Hispanics or Latino people

Pescatarian A person who primarily follows a vegetarian diet but also includes fish and other seafood as their main source of protein

Pharmacodynamics The study of how a drug affects the body, including the mechanisms of action, the relationship between drug concentration and effect, and the biological responses it produces

Pharmacokinetics The study of how the body absorbs, distributes, metabolizes, and excretes a drug over time

Population health The study and management of the health outcomes of a group of individuals, including the distribution of such outcomes within the group, to improve overall health and reduce health disparities

Poverty The condition in which individuals or communities lack the financial resources and essentials needed to maintain a minimum standard of living, including adequate food, shelter, and healthcare

Prostate cancer A malignant tumor that develops in the prostate gland, a part of the male reproductive system, and is one of the most common types of cancer in men

R

Race Biological variation including phenotypical differences in stature, skin color, hair color, facial shape, and other inherited characteristics that may or may not be mutually exclusive in each individual

Religion An integrated set of beliefs, rituals, and institutions through which persons give expression about that which is holy or held in highest esteem in their lives

Reparation The act of making amends for a wrong or harm done, often through compensation, restitution, or other forms of redress to those who have been wronged

Reserve Capacity Model (RCM) A theoretical framework that explains how individuals with greater social, psychological, and economic resources are better able to cope with stress and maintain health, while those with fewer resources are more vulnerable to its negative effects

Risky behaviors Actions that increase the likelihood of negative health outcomes or harm, such as substance abuse, unsafe sex, reckless driving, or poor dietary choices

Robots Programmable machines capable of carrying out a series of tasks automatically, often used to perform work that is repetitive, dangerous, or requires precision

Rural health The study and practice of improving health outcomes and access to healthcare services in sparsely populated areas, addressing the unique challenges faced by rural communities

Rural Healthy People A companion initiative to the national Healthy People program that adapts and sets 10-year health objectives, specifically, to identify and address the priority health needs of rural communities

Rural Healthy People 2030 The 2030 iteration of the Rural Healthy People initiative, offering evidence-based objectives and measurable targets to improve health outcomes and equity in rural areas by the year 2030

S

School to Prison Pipeline When policies and practices are leading to children being sent into the criminal justice system rather than the pursuit of education in the United States

Semaglutide A GLP-1 receptor agonist medication used to manage type 2 diabetes and support weight loss by mimicking a natural hormone that regulates blood sugar and appetite (see also Ozempic)

Social injustice The unfair treatment or systemic inequality experienced by individuals or groups based on characteristics like race, gender, socioeconomic status, or religion, limiting their rights and opportunities

Social determinants of health (SDOH) The non-medical factors— such as income, education, housing, and access to nutritious food—that influence a person's health outcomes and quality of life

Soul food A typical food preparations style of the American South, which emerged from slavery in the U.S., typically eaten by some African American people

Spirituality A higher-order endeavor with individual quest that facilitates both greater personal expression and enhanced personal benefits and outcomes, a viewpoint that is particularly ardent among those who are estranged from organized religion

Stereotypes Exaggerated beliefs or fixed ideas about a person or group of people

Suburban communities Residential areas located on the outskirts of urban centers, characterized by medium-density housing, commuter-based economies, and distinct social and infrastructure dynamics

Temporary Assistance for Needy Families (TANF) Welfare reform, which emerged in 1995; a state-by-state administered program based on federal grants

Tolerance Respect, acceptance, and appreciation of the rich diversity of our world's cultures, our forms of expression, and ways of being human; it is fostered by knowledge, openness, communication, and freedom of thought, conscience, and belief

Tracking The practice of grouping students into different classes or educational paths based on their perceived ability or achievement levels to provide tailored instruction

Trinidadian people Individuals originating from or descended from Trinidad, the larger of the two main islands of the Republic of Trinidad and Tobago, known for their diverse cultural heritage influenced by African, Indian, European, and Indigenous roots

Tuskegee Syphilis Study An unethical government-sponsored clinical study conducted from 1932 to 1972 that deliberately withheld treatment from African American men with syphilis to observe the disease's natural progression without their informed consent

Urban communities Densely populated areas characterized by developed infrastructure, diverse populations, and a concentration of economic, cultural, and social activities

Virtual professional learning network (VPLN) A technology that extends a local area network (LAN) across multiple geographic locations over the internet, allowing devices to communicate as if they were on the same physical network

Visual affirmation The physical surroundings of healthcare organizations, such as artwork and images, that reflect the customers/patients/clients served

W

Watchful waiting A medical approach that involves closely monitoring a patient's condition without immediate treatment, intervening only if symptoms worsen or change

Wegovy A prescription medication containing semaglutide, used by some adults with obesity or overweight conditions to lose weight by reducing appetite and increasing feelings of fullness

White Person having origins in any of the original peoples of Europe, North Africa, or the Middle East (note that there is great debate regarding North

Africa, as it is located in Egypt, which is in Africa and the people, are largely Arab and African)

White hindrance The ways in which White individuals or systems may actively or passively obstruct progress or equality for others, sometimes through resistance to change or internal conflicts, in contrast with White privilege, which is the societal advantage that White people experience by virtue of their race, with or without conscious awareness, giving them easier access to opportunities and resources

Index

© Jones & Bartlett Learning

Note: Page numbers followed by *f* and *t* refer to figures and tables, respectively.

A

access to care, 107
achievement gap, 116, 122–123
activities of daily living (ADL), 193
Affordable Care Act, 106, 145
African Americans, 119. *See also* Black/African American
ageism, 198–199
Agency for Healthcare Research and Quality (AHRQ), 91, 168
Aid to Families With Dependent Children (AFDC), 142
Alaska Natives, 100
    community-based care providers, 100–101
    cultural nuances, 65–66
    definition, 63
    evidence-based practices, 66–67
    leading causes of death, 65*f*
algorithms, 207
all-cause mortality, 9
American adults
    achievement gap, 122–123
    Brown v. Board of Education, 123–125
    common school system, 120
    culturally relevant/responsive education, 127–128
    demographic landscape, 125–126
    Health Education in Schools, 118–119
    social media and education, 128
    sorting game, 120–121
American Association of Colleges for Teacher Education (AACTE), 127
American Civil Liberties Union (ACLU), 144
American Indians, 100
    community-based care providers, 100–101
    cultural nuances, 65–66
    definition, 63
    evidence-based practices, 66–67
    leading causes of death, 65*f*
American schooling system, 116
America's Public Education System, 125–126
Antibiotics, 191

artificial intelligence (AI)
    ChatGPT, 208–209
    definition, 204
    ethical concerns, 206–207
    health care, 207–208
    jobs/livelihoods, 204–206
    remedies for, 209
    solutions, 208
Asian American and Pacific Islander
    Asian Indian American People, 46–51
    definition, 42
    Filipino American People, 43–46
    health concerns, 42–43
Asian Indian American People
    definition, 46
    health issues, 47
    remedies for, 47–48
    West Indian culture, 49–51

B

biometrics, 210
Black/African American. *See also* Black Sacred Cosmos; Black spirituality
    barrier care, 21
    community-based care providers, 100–101
    definition, 16
    diet-related diseases, 26–27
    emerging majority group, 16
    food deserts and food mirages, 28–33
    health disparities, 23–26
    historical overview, 17–18
    medical exploitation, 18–20
    minimum race, 16–17
    myriad reasons, 21
    role of spirituality, 246–247
    soul food, 26–27
    white privilege *vs.* white hindrance, 21–22
Black, Indigenous, and People of Color (BIPOC), 1
Black Sacred Cosmos, 250, 256
    health impact and, 249–253